OXFORD MEDICAL PUBLICATIONS

Myeloproliferative Neoplasms

Oxford Specialist Handbooks published and forthcoming

General Oxford Specialist Handbooks
Addiction Medicine
Applied Medicine and Surgery in Dentistry
Day Case Surgery
Infection in the Immunocompromised Host
Perioperative Medicine, 2e
Pharmaceutical Medicine
Postoperative Complications, 2e
Renal Transplantation
Retrieval Medicine

Oxford Specialist Handbooks in Anaesthesia
Anaesthesia for Emergency Care
Global Anaesthesia, 2e
Neuroanaesthesia
Obstetric Anaesthesia, 2e
Paediatric Anaesthesia, 2e
Regional Anaesthesia, Stimulation and Ultrasound Techniques
Thoracic Anaesthesia
Vascular Anaesthesia

Oxford Specialist Handbooks in Cardiology
Adult Congenital Heart Disease, 2e
Cardiac Catheterization and Coronary Intervention
Cardiovascular Computed Tomography, 2e
Cardiovascular Imaging
Cardiovascular Magnetic Resonance
Echocardiography, 2e
Fetal Cardiology, 2e
Heart Disease in Pregnancy
Heart Failure, 2e
Hypertension
Inherited Cardiac Disease
Nuclear Cardiology
Pacemakers and ICDs, 2e
Pulmonary Hypertension
Valvular Heart Disease

Oxford Specialist Handbooks in Critical Care
Advanced Respiratory Critical Care
Cardiothoracic Critical Care

Oxford Specialist Handbooks in End of Life Care
Dementia
Heart Failure
Kidney Disease
Respiratory Disease

Oxford Specialist Handbooks in Infectious Disease
Infectious Disease Epidemiology

Oxford Specialist Handbooks in Neurology
Parkinson's Disease and Other Movement Disorders, 2e
Stroke Medicine, 2e

Oxford Specialist Handbooks in Oncology
Practical Management of Complex Cancer Pain
Myeloproliferative Neoplasms

Oxford Specialist Handbooks in Paediatrics
Community Paediatrics
Manual of Childhood Infections, 4e
Paediatric Dermatology 2e
Paediatric Endocrinology and Diabetes
Paediatric Gastroenterology, Hepatology, and Nutrition, 2e
Paediatric Intensive Care
Paediatric Nephrology, 3e
Paediatric Neurology, 3e
Paediatric Palliative Medicine, 2e
Paediatric Radiology
Paediatric Respiratory Medicine
Paediatric Rheumatology

Oxford Specialist Handbooks in Pain Medicine
Spinal Interventions in Pain Management

Oxford Specialist Handbooks in Psychiatry
Addiction Medicine, 2e
Forensic Psychiatry
Medical Psychotherapy

Oxford Specialist Handbooks in Radiology
Head and Neck Imaging
Interventional Radiology
Musculoskeletal Imaging
Thoracic Imaging

Oxford Specialist Handbooks in Surgery
Burns
Cardiothoracic Surgery, 2e
Colorectal Surgery
Current Surgical Guidelines
Gastric and Oesophageal Surgery
Hand Surgery, 2e
Oral and Maxillofacial Surgery, 2e
Otolaryngology and Head and Neck Surgery
Plastic and Reconstructive Surgery
Surgical Oncology
Urological Surgery
Vascular Surgery, 2e

Oxford Specialist Handbooks in Oncology

Myeloproliferative Neoplasms

EDITED BY

Tariq I. Mughal
Clinical Professor of Medicine in Hematology/Oncology
Tufts University Medical Center
Boston, MA, USA

Tiziano Barbui
Professor of Hematology
Scientific Director, Research Foundation
Ospedali Riuniti di Bergamo, Italy

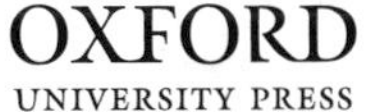

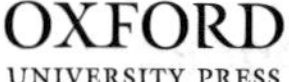

Great Clarendon Street, Oxford, OX2 6DP,
United Kingdom

Oxford University Press is a department of the University of Oxford. It furthers the University's objective of excellence in research, scholarship, and education by publishing worldwide. Oxford is a registered trade mark of Oxford University Press in the UK and in certain other countries

First Edition published in 2020

Impression: 1

Published in the United States of America by Oxford University Press
198 Madison Avenue, New York, NY 10016, United States of America

British Library Cataloguing in Publication Data

Data available

Library of Congress Control Number: 2020937768

ISBN 978–0–19–874421–4

Printed and bound in China by
C&C Offset Printing Co., Ltd.

Preface

The remarkable story of the chronic myeloproliferative neoplasms (MPN), a group of clonal haematological malignancies characterized by excessive accumulation of one or more myeloid cell lineages, continues to evolve. Arguably, despite significant advances in the treatment of some of the subtypes, in particular chronic myeloid leukaemia (CML), polycythaemia vera (PV), and myelofibrosis (MF), many important issues remain unexplored. To mention just a few, the emergence of resistance to treatment, the unexpected clonal heterogeneity, and we still need to clarify how best to treat adult patients, children, and adolescents with MPN. In this inaugural edition of the Oxford Specialist MPN book, we have collated contributions from renowned experts in the field, to provide important preclinical and clinical aspects of all MPN for haematologists, oncologists, and other healthcare professionals interested in the field.

Tariq I. Mughal
Clinical Professor of Medicine in Hematology/Oncology
Tufts University Medical Center
Boston, MA, USA

Tiziano Barbui
Professor of Hematology
Scientific Director, Research Foundation
Ospedali Riuniti di Bergamo, Italy

Foreword

Students of myeloproliferative neoplasms (MPN) have been richly rewarded with the progress made in understanding the molecular biology of these disorders over the past four decades. Even more importantly, the speed at which many of these findings have been translated into survival benefits for MPN patients has been truly remarkable. Today chronic myeloid leukaemia (CML) is undoubtedly one of the great success stories of medicine over the past half-century. The discovery of the Philadelphia chromosome in 1960, the characterization of the (9:22) translocation in the 1970s, and the identification of the *BCR-ABL1* fusion gene in the 1980s paved the way for the introduction of the tyrosine kinase inhibitors (TKIs) in the 1990s. In the other MPN, polycythaemia vera (PV), essential thrombocythaemia (ET), and primary myelofibrosis (PMF), the important landmarks began with identification of the V617F mutation in JAK2 exon 14 in 2005. This was followed by the discovery of other 'phenotypic' mutations in JAK2 exon 12, MPL exon 10, and CALR, all of which are essentially restricted to the MPN, together with mutations in a number of epigenetic regulators, such as TET2, DNMT3A, and ASXL1, which are altered in a wider range of malignancies. Indeed, these and other efforts have allowed us to identify distinct genetic subgroups of MPN and enhanced our understanding of the biology and risk stratification, which in turn enables us to consider personalized therapies for these patients.

In this inaugural edition, Tariq I. Mughal and Tiziano Barbui, with help from several renowned international MPN experts, have compiled a detailed and accessible evidence-based guide to the pathogenesis and management of the MPN. I hope you will enjoy reading it as much as I have.

Anthony R. Green
Professor of Haematology
Director, Academic Department of Haematology
and the Stem Cell Institute
University of Cambridge
Cambridge, UK

Foreword

Acknowledgements

We thank our patients, past, present, and future, who not only inspired us, but made our clinical and academic careers possible. We thank all of the authors who helped collate this book, working patiently to ensure the latest thoughts were included. We thank Nicola and Caroline and their publishing team at Oxford University Press for their professionalism with the preparation of this inaugural edition. TIM thanks his parents and Alpa for their love, patience, and support, and his long-term mentor, friend, and confidante, John Goldman, who is much missed. TB thanks Sylvana for her love.

Contents

Contributors *xiii*

Abbreviations *xvii*

1 History of the myeloproliferative neoplasms 1

2 Genomic landscape of myeloproliferative neoplasms 15

3 Pathogenesis of myeloproliferative neoplasms 32

4 Haematopathology of classic myeloproliferative neoplasms 45

5 Prognostic factors of chronic myeloid leukaemia 63

6 Molecular risk stratification of myeloproliferative neoplasms 79

7 Chronic myeloid leukaemia 93

8 Polycythaemia vera 113

9 Myelofibrosis 126

10 Essential thrombocythaemia 151

11 Systemic mastocytosis 168

12 Myelodysplastic syndromes/myeloproliferative overlap neoplasms 191

13 Eosinophilia-associated myeloproliferative neoplasms 204

14 Transformation of myeloproliferative neoplasms to acute leukaemia 222

15 Monitoring efforts in myeloproliferative neoplasms 234

16 Stem cell transplantation for BCR-ABL1-positive and negative myeloproliferative neoplasms 249

17 Assessment of disease burden in patients with myeloproliferative neoplasms 267

18 Clinical trials in myeloproliferative neoplasms 286

Index *305*

Contents

Contributors

Omar Abdelwahab
Professor, Memorial Sloane Kettering Cancer Center, New York, NY, USA
Chapter 14

Alberto Alvarez-Larrán
Consultant Haematologist, Hematology Department, Hospital Clínic, Barcelona, Spain
Chapter 10

Michele Baccarani
Professor of Haematology, Chair, GIMEMA CML and ELN CML working groups, S. Orsola-Malpighi University Hospital, Bologna, Italy
Chapter 10

Tiziano Barbui
Professor of Hematology, Scientific Director, Research Foundation, Ospedale Papa Giovanni XXIII, Bergamo, Italy
Chapters 1, 8

Giovanni Barosi
Senior Consultant, Department of Anestesia, Rianimazione ed Emergenza Urgenza IRCCS Ca' Granda Foundation, Ospedale Maggiore Policlinico, Milan
Chapter 18

Yan Beauverd
Consultant Haematologist, Department of Haematology Geneva University Hospitals, Geneva, CH
Chapter 9

Beatriz Bellosillo
Professor and Head, Molecular Diagnostic Laboratory, Department of Pathology, Hospital del Mar, Barcelona
Chapter 10

Carlos Besses
Professor and Head, Department of Haematology, Hospital del Mar, Barcelona, Spain
Chapter 10

Fausto Castagnetti
Senior Assistant Professor, Department of Haematology, S. Orsola-Malpighi University Hospital, Bologna, Italy
Chapter 5

Nicholas C.P. Cross
Professor and Chair of Genetics, University of Southampton, Wessex Regional Genetics Laboratory, Salisbury, UK
Chapter 13

Michael W. Deininger
Professor and Head, Division of Hematology-Oncology, Huntsman Cancer Institute, Salt Lake City, UT, USA
Chapter 2

Daniel Egan
Swedish Cancer Center, Seattle, WA, USA
Chapter 15

Richard A. Van Etten
Professor and Director, Chao Comprehensive Cancer Center, Irvine, CA, USA
Chapter 3

Guido Finazzi
Consultant Haematologist, Department of Haematology, Ospedale Papa Giovanni XXIII, Bergamo, Italy
Chapter 8

Angela G. Fleishmann
Hematology Specialist, Department of Hematology/Oncology, Chao Comprehensive Cancer Center, Irvine, CA, USA
Chapter 3

Holly L. Geyer
Hospital Internal Medicine Practitioner, Department of Hematology, Mayo Clinic, Scottsdale, AZ, USA
Chapter 17

Jason Gotlib
Professor, Division of Hematology, Stanford University Cancer Center, Stanford, CA, USA
Chapter 11

Paola Guglielmelli
Associate Professor of Haematology, Dip. Medicina Sperimentale e Clinica, University of Florence, Florence, Italy
Chapter 6

Gabriele Gugliotta
Hematology Specialist, Department of Haematology, S. Orsola-Malpighi University Hospital, Bologna, Italy
Chapter 5

Claire Harrison
Professor and Clinical Director Haematology, Guy's and St Thomas' NHS Foundation Trust, London, UK
Chapter 9

Catriona Jamieson
Professor and Director, Stem Cell Program, University of California La Jolla, La Jolla, CA, USA
Chapter 14

Jamshid S. Khorashad
Professor, Department of Hematology, Huntsman Cancer Institute, Salt Lake City, UT, USA
Chapter 2

Nicholas Kröger
Professor and Medical Director of the Department of Stem Cell Transplantation, University Hospital, Hamburg-Eppendorf, Germany
Chapter 16

Hans Michael Kvasnicka
Professor, Department of Pathology, University of Frankfurt, Frankfurt, Germany
Chapter 4

Alan F. List
Professor of Medicine, Moffitt Cancer Center, University of Florida, Tampa, FL, USA
Chapter 12

Donal McLorran
Guy's and St Thomas' NHS Foundation Trust, London, UK
Chapter 9

Ruben A. Mesa
Director, Mays Cancer Center at UT Health San Antonio MD Anderson Cancer Center, Professor of Medicine, San Antonio, TX, USA
Chapter 17

Tariq I. Mughal
Clinical Professor of Medicine in Hematology/Oncology, Tufts University Medical Center, Boston, MA, USA
Chapters 1, 7, 8, 10, 12, 14

Eric Padron
Lead Investigator, Assistant Professor, MDS/MPN program, Moffitt Cancer Center, University of Tampa, Tampa, FL, USA
Chapter 12

Francesca Palandri
Professor, Department of Haematology, S. Orsola-Malpighi University Hospital, Bologna, Italy
Chapter 5

Deepti Radia
Consultant Haematologist, Guy's and St Thomas's Hospital, London, UK
Chapter 17

Jerald P. Radich
Member, Clinical Research Division, Fredrick Hutchinson Cancer Research Center, Seattle, WA, USA
Chapter 15

Alessandro Rambaldi
Professor, Department of Oncology-Hematology, University of Milan and Ospedale Papa Giovanni XXIII, Bergamo, Italy
Chapters 6, 16

Raajit Rampal
Hematologic Oncologist, Division of Hematology/Oncology, Memorial Sloane Kettering Cancer Center, New York, NY, USA
Chapter 14

Andreas Reiter
Professor, III. Medizinische Klinik, Universitätsmedizin Mannheim, Theodor-Kutzer-Ufer, Mannheim, Germany
Chapter 13

Gianantonio Rosti
Professor and Head, Department of Haematology, B S. Orsola-Malpighi University Hospital, Bologna, Italy
Chapter 5

David Sallmann
Assistant Professor, Department of Hematology, Moffitt Cancer Center, Tampa, FL, USA
Chapter 12

Nicholas Sarlis
Chief Medical Officer, Sellas Life Sciences, New York, NY, USA
Chapter 17

Simona Soverini
Professor and Department of Hematology, S. Orsola-Malpighi University Hospital, Bologna, Italy
Chapter 5

Srinivas K. Tantravahi
Department of Hematology, Huntsman Cancer Institute, University of Utah, Salt Lake City, UT, USA
Chapter 2

Jürgen Thiele
Professor and WHO Myeloid and Acute Leukemia Panel, Institute for Pathology, University of Cologne, Cologne, Germany
Chapter 4

Gianni Tognoni
Professor, Consorzio Mario Negri Sud, Santa Maria Imbaro, Italy
Chapter 18

Alessandro M. Vannucchi
Full Professor of Haematology, Dip. Medicina Sperimentale e Clinica, University of Florence, Florence, Italy
Chapter 6

Abbreviations

ACA	additional cytogenetic abnormalities
aCML	atypical chronic myeloid leukaemia
AE	adverse events
AHN	associated haematologic neoplasm
AHNMD	Associated with clonal haematological non-mast cell lineage disease
ALL	acute lymphoblastic leukaemia
ALT	alanine transaminase
AML	acute myeloid leukaemia
AP	advanced phase
ASCT	autologous stem cell transplant
ASM	aggressive systemic mastocytosis
ASM	airway smooth muscle
AVT	abdominal venous thrombosis
BAT	best available therapy
BC	blast crisis
BCR	breakpoint cluster region
BFI	Brief Fatigue Inventory
BM	bone marrow
BMI	body mass index
BP MPN	blast phase myeloproliferative neoplasm
BPI	Brief Pain Inventory
CBA	chromosome banding analysis
CCA	clonal chromosome abnormalities
CCyR	complete cytogenetic response
CE	clonal evolution
CEL	chronic eosinophilic leukaemia
CGL	chronic granulocytic leukaemia
CHIP	clonal haematopoiesis of indeterminate potential
CHR	clinical and haematological remissions
CI	clinical improvement
CIBMTR	Center for International Blood and Marrow Transplant Research
CM	cutaneous mastocytosis
CML	chronic myeloid leukaemia
CMML	chronic myelomonocytic leukaemia
CMR	complete molecular remission
CNL	chronic neutrophilic leukaemia
CP	chronic phase
CR	complete remission
CT	computed tomography
CV	coefficient of variation
DEXA	dual-energy X-ray absorptiometry
DFS	disease-free survival
DIPSS	Dynamic International Prognostic Scoring System
DLI	donor lymphocyte infusion
DOR	duration of response
EBMT	European Group for Blood and Marrow Transplantation
ECD	extracellular domain
ECNM	European Competence Network on Mastocytosis
EEC	endogenous erythroid colony
EFS	event-free survival
EGF	epidermal growth factor
ELN	European LeukemiaNet
ELTS	EUTOS Long Term Survival Score
EM	extracutaneous mastocytosis
EMA	European Medicines Agency
EMR	early molecular response
EORTC	European Organization for Research and Treatment of Cancer
ESA	erythropoiesis-stimulating agents
ET	essential thrombocythaemia
EUTOS	European Treatment and Outcome Study
FDA	Food and Drug Administration
FGF	fibroblast growth factor
FGFR1	fibroblast growth factor receptor 1
FISH	fluorescence *in situ* hybridization
GEP	gene expression profile

GVHD	graft versus host disease
GVL	graft versus leukaemia
HEUS	hypereosinophilia of unknown significance
HLA	human leukocyte antigen
HMR	high molecular risk
HR	hazard ratios
HRQoL	health-related quality of life
HSC	haematopoietic stem cell
HSCT	haematopoietic stem cell transplantation
HU	hydroxyurea
IPSS	International Prognostic Scoring System
IS	International Scale
ISM	indolent systemic mastocytosis
ITD	internal tandem duplication
JAK	Janus kinase
JMD	juxtamembrane domain
KI	kinase insert
LFS	leukaemia-free survival
LMR	low molecular risk
LMWH	low molecular weight heparin
LOH	loss of heterozygosity
LSC	leukaemic stem cells
MAPSS	mutation-augmented prognostic scoring system
MC	mast cells
MCAS	mast cell activation syndrome
MCD	mast cell disease
MCL	mast cell leukaemia
MDS	myelodysplastic syndrome
MF	myelofibrosis
MIPSS	Mutation-Enhanced International Prognostic Scoring System
MIS	mastocytosis in the skin
MMAS	monoclonal mast cell activation syndrome
MMR	major molecular response
MPD	myeloproliferative disorder
MPN	myeloproliferative neoplasm
MQLQ	Mastocytosis Quality of Life Questionnaire
MR	major response
MRD	measurable residual disease
MSAF	Mastocytosis Symptom Assessment form
MSAS	Memorial Symptom Assessment Scale
NCCN	National Comprehensive Cancer Network
NGS	next generation sequencing
NK	natural killer
NRM	non-relapse mortality
OIS	optimal information size
OS	overall survival
PB	peripheral blood
PCR	polymerase chain reaction
PCV	packed cell volume
PCyR	partial cytogenetic response
PDGF	platelet derived growth factor
PDGFRA	platelet derived growth factor A
PDGFRB	platelet derived growth factor B
PFS	progression-free survival
PGIC	Patient Global Impression of Change
PMF	primary myelofibrosis
PPI	proton pump inhibitors
PR	partial responses
PRO	patient-reported outcome
PS	progression-free survival
PTD	phosphotransferase domain
PV	polycythaemia vera
PVSG	Polycythemia Vera Study Group
QoL	quality of life
RARS	refractory anaemia with ringed sideroblasts
RCM	red cell mass
RIC	reduced intensity conditioning
RNA	ribonucleic acid
ROS	reactive oxygen species
RPSFT	rank-preserving structural failure time
SCF	stem cell factor
SCT	stem cell transplantation
SEER	Surveillance, Epidemiology, and End Results
SM	systemic mastocytosis
SNP	single nucleotide polymorphism
SSM	smouldering systemic mastocytosis
STAT	signal transducer and activator of transcription
TFR	treatment-free remission
TK	tyrosine kinase

TKI	tyrosine kinase inhibitor
TMD	transmembrane domain
TRM	transplant-related mortality
TSS	total symptom score
TTE	time-to-vascular-event
UPD	uniparental disomy
VEGF	vascular endothelial growth factor
VT	variant or atypical translocations
WBC	white blood cell
WHO	World Health Organization

Chapter 1

History of the myeloproliferative neoplasms

Tariq I. Mughal and Tiziano Barbui

Introduction *2*
The seventeenth and eighteenth centuries *2*
The nineteenth century *4*
The twentieth century *6*
The twenty-first century *11*
Conclusion *12*

Introduction

Arguably, the story of what we now know as myeloproliferative neoplasms (MPN) began in the early nineteenth century as a result of astute clinical observations. As illustration, Alfred Velpeau (Paris) is credited with the first description of 'leukaemia' in 1827, when he described a 63-year-old florist and lemonade salesman who presented with gross hepatosplenomegaly and was noted to have 'globules of pus' in his blood. The precise diagnosis, however, remained elusive. The term MPN was introduced in 2008, by a World Health Organization (WHO) appointed panel of experts, to replace the term 'myeloproliferative disorders' (MPDs), which had been coined by William Dameshek in 1951, in alignment with the enhanced molecular biology and clinical knowledge. Dameshek's initial schema of MPDs described several unique haematopoietic stem cell disorders that shared some biological and clinical features, and comprised of chronic myeloid leukaemia (CML), polycythaemia vera (PV), essential thrombocythaemia (ET), and primary myelofibrosis (PMF), previously known as idiopathic myelofibrosis (IMF), and also included megakaryocytic leukaemia and erythroleukemia. The WHO expert panel first published the MPD classification in 2001, and in a revised form in 2008 and 2016. And as a reference to Dameshek's MPD conception, PV, ET, and PMF are often referred to as 'classic' MPN (also known as *BCR-ABL1*-negative MPN), and includes patients who transform to myelofibrosis (MF) from PV (post-PV MF) or ET (post-ET MF). In this chapter we present a brief history of the biological and therapeutic milestones, many of which were seminal, and should interest both the student and scholar of MPN. Moreover, it can often be daunting to obtain detailed historical accounts from most, if not all, of the 'modern' search engines such as PubMed, Google Scholar, and the like. The principal milestones in the study and treatment of CML are depicted in Figure 1.1.

The seventeenth and eighteenth centuries

Microscopy was first introduced by Robert Hooke in England in 1665 and Anton van Leeuwenhoek in the Netherlands in 1674. Many efforts were undertaken thereafter to study blood cells. Initial descriptions of red blood cells appear to have been made by Jan Swammerdam in 1668 and Leeuwenhoek in the Netherlands in 1674, and of white blood cells by Joseph Lieutaud in France in 1749 and William Hewson in England around 1765. The description of platelets, however, did not occur until the nineteenth century, just ahead of the efforts led by Paul Ehrlich in Germany in the use of chemical dyes for better morphological assessment of the various blood cells. It is, of course, likely that one of the first people to publicize the potential role of bone marrow and blood might have been William Shakespeare, who at the end of the sixteenth century wrote '*Thy bones are marrowless, thy blood is cold*'.[1]

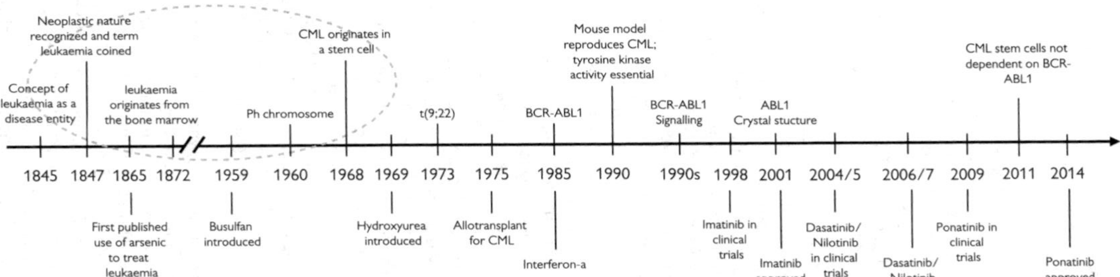

Figure 1.1 Milestones in the study and treatment of chronic myeloid leukemia.

Adapted with permission from Mughal T I and Goldman J M (Eds.) (2008). *Chronic Myeloproliferative Disorders*. London, UK: Informa Healthcare.

The nineteenth century

The first plausible references to the entity now known as CML were probably made in 1845, almost simultaneously, by John Bennett in Edinburgh, who reported a 28-year-old slater, and Rudolf Virchow in Berlin, who reported a 50-year-old cook. They both described autopsy reports in their respective patients who appeared to have been unwell for about 2 years before their deaths and were noted to have very large spleens and an unusual consistency of the blood, which Virchow described as 'weisses blut' and for which Bennett proposed the term 'leucocythaemia'. Such was the interest in these initial clinical descriptions, that by 1846 a further nine cases were documented by Virchow (Figure 1.2). Thereafter cases were described by Craigie, Fuller, and others with increasing frequency. Wood in 1850 is credited with the initial description of CML in the United States, coincidentally as it turns out in the city of Philadelphia. Gustav Heuck in Germany in 1879 recognized what he thought was a variant of leukaemia when he described two cases of young patients presenting with massive splenomegaly, circulating 'nucleated red cells', and 'abnormal leukocytes', and termed this 'splenic-medullary leukaemia', an entity subsequently known by a number of names, including Heuck-Assmann syndrome (1902), agnogenic myeloid metaplasia (1940), chronic idiopathic myelofibrosis (2001), and more recently, in 2006, termed primary myelofibrosis by the International Working Group for Myelofibrosis Research and Treatment.

Though Alfred Donne in France is credited with the initial description of platelets in 1842, both Max Schultze in Germany and Giulio Bizzozero made significant contributions. In 1868 Ernst Neumann in Germany introduced the concept of blood cells being formed in the bone marrow and the notion of 'leucocythemia' arising in the marrow rather than the spleen, as Virchow and others had thought. The 'modern' era of medical microscopy began in the 1880s with the introduction of panoptic staining methods by Paul Ehrlich in Germany. By this time Neumann was already working on a remarkably detailed description of the cellular components of the bone marrow and probably introduced the notion of an 'ancestral cell' that resulted in the production of circulating red cells. In 1891 Ehrlich compiled the first classification of 'leukaemias' with the description of not only 'myeloid' and 'lymphoid' types, but also the various major subtypes of leukaemias, including a better microscopic description of CML. Remarkably he also speculated that the 'ancestral cell' proposed by Neumann might actually represent a cell which gave rise to not only circulating red cells, but also white cells and platelets.

IMF has been recognized since 1879, when Heuck described two cases that differed from classical CML on the finding of extramedullary erythropoiesis and bone marrow fibrosis. Efforts to improve the quality of life by controlling the symptoms attributed to CML probably began with the use of arsenicals by Thomas Fowler in 1865, and (Arthur) Conan Doyle in 1882, who is, of course, rather more famous for his stories of Sherlock Holmes (Figure 1.3). Blood transfusion was performed, but largely without success, and did not become a safe procedure until the discovery of the human blood groups by Landsteiner in 1935. Splenectomy was also used but often resulted in the death of the patient.

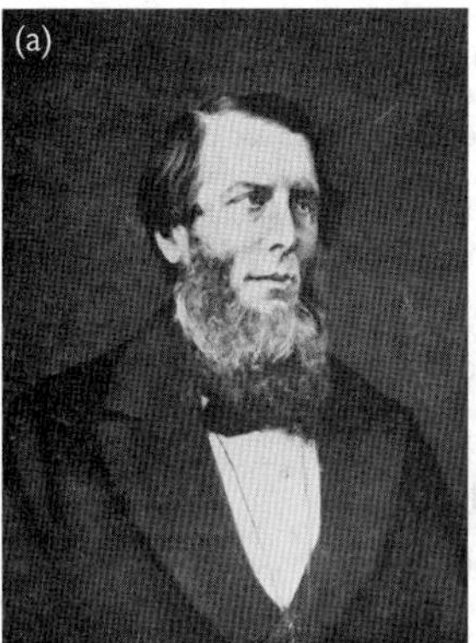

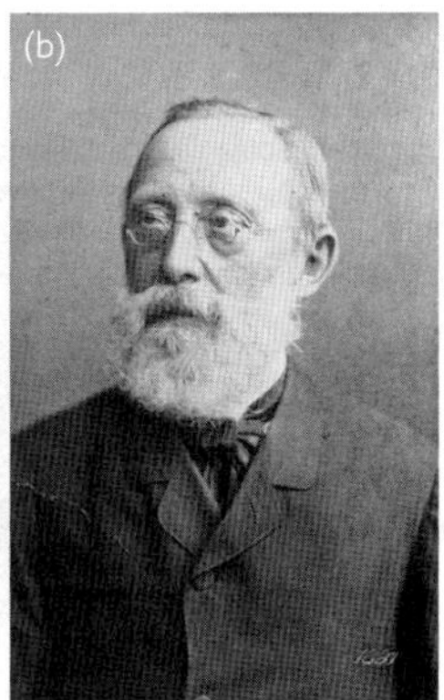

Figure 1.2 Leukaemia pioneers. (a) John Huges Bennett (1812–1875); (b) Rudolf Virchow Rudolf Ludwig Karl Virchow 1981.

(a) 'John Hughes Bennett (1812–1875)'. Wellcome Collection. Reproduced under Creative Commons Attribution 4.0 International (CC BY 4.0); (b) 'Rudolf Ludwig Karl Virchow. Photograph by J. C. Schaarwächter, 1891'. Wellcome Collection. Reproduced under Creative Commons Attribution 4.0 International (CC BY 4.0).

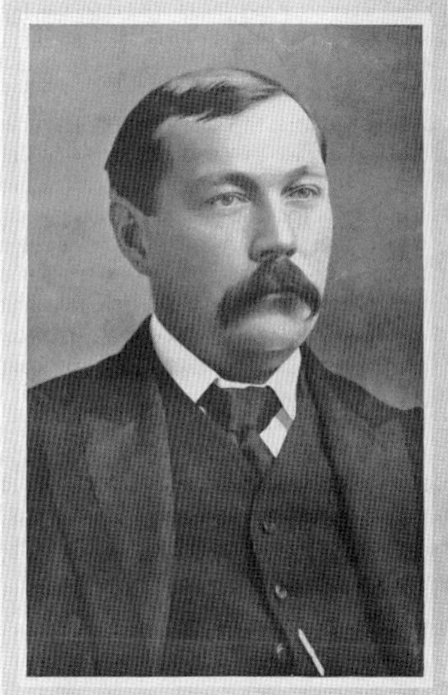

Figure 1.3 Sir Arthur Conan Doyle.

'Portrait of Sir Arthur Conan Doyle, head and shoulders' by Martin and Sallnow. Wellcome Collection. Reproduced under Creative Commons Attribution 4.0 International (CC BY 4.0).

Towards the end of the nineteenth century, an increasing number of cases were described in different parts of the world characterized by an increase in the number of the different blood cells and often accompanied by an enlarged spleen. Louis Vaquez in France in 1892 described the case of a middle-aged man with marked erythrocytosis, hepatosplenomegaly, and a 'ruddy' complexion. Though it was initially thought that the underlying disease was 'congenital heart disease', an autopsy revealed a normal heart; in view of the enormous hepatosplenomegaly, it was speculated that the underlying disease was probably haematological, and it was given the term 'maladie de Vaquez'. In 1899, Richard Cabot in America described additional cases of PV.

The twentieth century

‡At the turn of the twentieth century, Osler, Turk, and Parkes-Weber provided detailed descriptions of PV and its features which overlapped with the leukaemias in general. Osler delineated PV as a 'new' clinical entity characterized by 'cyanosis with polycythaemia and enlarged spleen with symptoms somewhat indefinite and with pathology quite obscure'. These clinicians thought PV was marked only by the increase of red cell count not secondary to congenital heart disease and failed to recognize that the process resulted from a global bone marrow proliferation, as evidenced by concomitant hyperplasia of granulocytic and megakaryocytic cell lines. As a consequence, erythrocytosis was considered the most prominent cause of clinical manifestations and, accordingly, much of the research regarding the pathogenesis of PV focused on erythropoiesis. In 1917, a further entity was added to this list of blood disorders, when Giovanni Di Guglielmo in Italy coined the phrase 'eritroleuco-piastrinaemia' to describe a patient with circulating erythroid progenitors, myeloblasts, and megakaryoblasts.

In 1938, Rosenthal and Bassen described the natural history of PV in some detail. By reviewing the reported cases, they divided the clinical course of PV into the asymptomatic phase, the subsequent polycythaemic and symptomatic phase, and the terminal phase, called by the authors 'anaemic and spent phase'. These investigators pointed out the chronicity of the disease and recognized that acute leukaemia and myelofibrosis were part of its natural evolution. In 1954, Wasserman advanced a hypothetical concept for the course of PV and distinguished subsequent stages of this disorder. The first stage is featured by pure erythrocytosis with increase of haematocrit but with normal platelet and leukocyte counts and no splenomegaly. This description may correspond to an initial phase of PV or to the so called 'idiopathic erythrocytosis', and was the subject of subsequent clinical studies in Europe. The second stage, according to Wasserman, included the overt picture of PV and the subsequent phases represented the evolution to myelofibrosis that can be suspected when an apparent spontaneous remission of PV is occurring. The incidence, type of complications, and causes of death were reported some years later in 1962. European

‡ Section 'The 20th century' adapted with permission from Mughal TI, et al. (2016). Chronic myeloid leukemia: reminiscences and dreams. *Haematologica*. 101(5):541–58. DOI:10.3324/haematol.2015.139337.

investigators followed up a cohort of PV patients left untreated and calculated a median survival varying from 6 to 18 months from diagnosis. With modern therapy, the life expectancy of PV patients in the first decade after diagnosis is not different from that of a matched population whereas a slight difference is seen after 10 years, due to increase of malignancy.

For the CML aficionados, the clinical features were well characterized in a classical paper by Minot and colleagues in 1924. This work also recognized that age was an important prognostic factor. In 1934 Emil Epstein and Alfred Goedel in Austria described a patient with 'extreme' thrombocytosis, absence of 'panmyelosis', and an enlarged spleen, and termed this 'haemorrhagic thrombocythaemia' (later termed 'essential thrombocythaemia'). The notion of trilineage haematopoietic proliferation was introduced by Vaughan and Harrison in 1939. By now efforts were in place to recognize MPD as a separate entity from 'acute leukaemias'.

In 1951, William Dameshek, an American haematologist who started the journal *Blood*, grouped CML with PV, ET, and IMF (myelosclerosis). To elucidate his unifying theory, Dameshek postulated two different pathogenetic mechanisms: the first was that, in response to unrecognized stimulus, the myeloid, erythroid, megakaryocytic, and fibroblastic elements of the bone marrow proliferated *en masse*. The second possibility he advanced, was that the entire process of excessive myeloproliferation could be the result of a lack or diminution of inhibitory factors controlling the haematopoiesis. He also suggested that dormant embryonal haematopoietic cells in extramedullary sites could become activated.

In 1960, in the city of Philadelphia, Peter Nowell and David Hungerford, described the presence of an abnormally small acrocentric chromosome, which resembled a Y chromosome, in two male patients with what was then called chronic granulocytic leukaemia (CGL). Thereafter they described the presence of this chromosomal abnormality in a further seven patients, including two females, with CGL, and speculated that the abnormal chromosomal abnormality was causally associated. Indeed, in 1960, at the First International Conference on Chromosomal Nomenclature in 1960 in Denver (Colorado), it was heralded as the first consistent cytogenetic abnormality in a human cancer., and the abnormal chromosome was named the Philadelphia (Ph^1) chromosome, after the city of its discovery. The superscript '1' was added on the premise that additional abnormalities originating from Nowell and Hungerford's work would be discovered in Philadelphia. This, of course, did not occur and the superscript had been dropped by most haematologists by 1990. The formal recognition that a human cancer might be caused by an acquired chromosomal aberration, of course, vindicated to some degree the hypothesis postulated by Theodore Boveri in Germany in 1914 that cancer may be caused by acquired chromosomal abnormalities.

The next important observations which established that CML was a stem cell-derived clonal disease came from Phillip Fialkow and colleagues in 1967. They applied a genetic technique developed by Susumu Ohno, Ernest Beutler, and Mary Lyon, based on X-chromosome mosaicism in females, and by exploiting the polymorphism in the X-linked glucose-6-phosphatase dehydrogenase locus in female patients, they established the clonal nature of not only CML, but also PV, ET and PMF (albeit in later papers published in 1976, 1978, and 1981, respectively). In 1972, Janet Rowley in Chicago described the morphological aspects of the Ph chromosome in some detail and confirmed that it arose as a consequence of a reciprocal translocation of genetic material between the long arms of chromosomes 9 and 22, t(9;22)(q34;q11). She deserves much credit for making an observation that strongly supported the notion that cytogenetic changes play an important role in leukemogenesis (Figure 1.4). The molecular events underlying the genesis of the Ph chromosome began to unfold in 1982, and established *BCR-ABL1* as the principal pathogenetic event leading to the chronic phase (CP) of CML. The cytogenetic and molecular events are addressed in Chapter 7.

At about the same time efforts were made to distinguish PV from secondary diseases associated with erythrocytosis. True polycythaemia was differentiated from chronic relative polycythaemia occurring in patients with intravascular fluid depletion and without splenomegaly. The concept of secondary polycythaemia was further elucidated by Gaisbock in 1905 who described the association of polycythaemia with hypertension and regarded this picture as a separate entity distinct from PV. Subsequently, many other authors reported cases of polycythaemia associated with obesity, anxiety, and smoking. Noteworthy was the observation by Russell and Conley that, in contrast to patients with PV, individuals with secondary polycythaemia had little improvement in symptoms after phlebotomy, suggesting that in these secondary erythrocytoses there was no cause–effect relationship between the increased haematocrit and vascular disturbances. These early

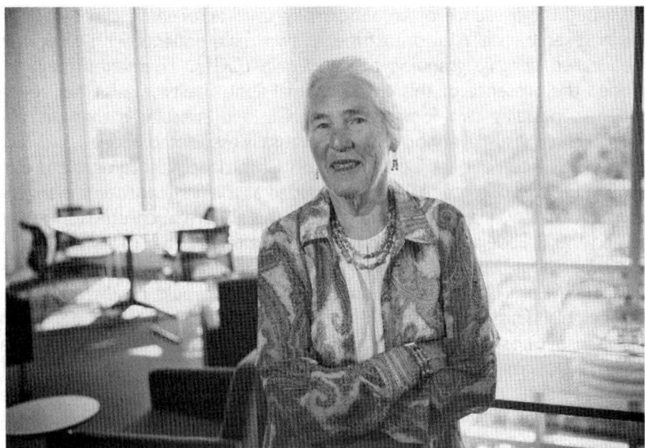

Figure 1.4 Janet Rowley, who described the translocation of chromosomal material in the Philadelphia chromosome.

Reproduced with permission from Mughal TI, et al. (2016) Chronic Myeloid Leukemia: Reminiscences and Dreams. *Haematologica*. 101(5):541–58. DOI:10.3324/haematol.2015.139337. Copyright © 2016 Ferrata Storti Foundation.

publications set the stage for more reliable and accurate classification of the polycythaemic states.

In 1974, haematopoietic stem cells derived from bone marrow or peripheral blood of PV patients were found to proliferate in serum containing cultures in the absence of exogenous erythropoietin. Initially, some concerns on these experiments were raised since these 'endogenous erythroid colonies' or 'EECs' could be driven by minimal traces of erythropoietin (EPO) contamination in the serum but, subsequently, any doubts were dispelled by using an improved serum and EPO-free medium. EECs are one the current WHO criterion for the diagnosis of PV. In the same year, studies based on X-chromosome inactivation in women with PV found that these disorders were derived from a clone of a single multipotent haematopoietic stem cell. Thus, the question whether PV was a benign condition, as interpreted by Osgood, Ward, and Block, or a neoplastic process, as claimed by Wasserman years before was answered.

The measurement of red cell mass (RCM) by the *in vitro* labelling of autologous erythrocytes with ^{51}Cr sodium chromate, as described by the International Committee for Standardization in Hematology in 1973, was considered an essential element in establishing the diagnosis of absolute erythrocytosis. Further advances in the differential diagnosis of polycythaemic states came from the work done in France by Najean and colleagues. These investigators demonstrated that the simultaneous measurement of red cell and plasma volume was more reliable than either the haematocrit evaluation or the measurement of a single volume to differentiate PV from ET, pure erythrocytosis, spurious, and secondary polycythaemia.

In contrast to PV, the history of ET and IMF is less rich. The first description of ET was reported by Epstein and Goedel in 1934, but it should be mentioned that there was a considerable controversy as to whether this condition truly represented a distinct entity. McCabe and colleagues claimed that if patients were followed for a sufficient length of time, some other underlying haematologic diseases would eventually emerge. It was not until the classic papers of Gunz and Ozer in 1960, both of whom critically reviewed their experience and other reported cases of haemorrhagic thrombocythaemia, that ET became widely accepted as a separate myeloproliferative disorder. However, despite its recognition, the lack of uniform diagnostic criteria made ET the least well-defined of the MPDs. That IMF were a unique pathological entity became apparent after the work of Ward and Block in 1971, who presented evidence that this myeloid disorder had to be distinct from the others. In the 1980s, the German pathologist Burkhardt and colleagues described typical histopathological features from bone marrow biopsy material for the diagnosis and classification of PV, ET, and IMF. These pathological findings inspired the WHO to include bone marrow morphology in the diagnostic criteria of MPDs.

The notion of using arsenicals to improve symptoms related to CML continued in the first half of the twentieth century with radiation therapy to the spleen in 1902, antileukocyte sera in 1932, benzene in 1935, urethane in 1950, and leukapheresis in the 1960s. There were a number of other notable treatment attempts, but most, if not all, were unsuccessful. Busulfan, an alkylating agent, was introduced largely by David Galton in London, in

1953. Galton then carried out the first prospective randomized study in CML, comparing busulfan and splenic radiation, and showed improved survival in the busulfan cohort. In the mid-1960s, busulfan was replaced by hydroxycarbamide (previously hydroxyurea, HU), a ribonucleotide reductase inhibitor, following the recognition of busulfan being mutagenic and a randomized study confirming HU's superiority, though neither drug was able to reduce the proportion of Ph positive haematopoiesis or prolong the overall survival (OS). Interferon alpha (IFN-α) was introduced into the clinics in the mid-1980s and proved popular, despite frequent side effects such as flu-like symptoms and fatigue. In the early 1990s several randomized studies comparing IFN-α or interferon-α n1 (wellferon) with HU or busulfan, were undertaken and demonstrated an improvement in OS from by about 2–3 years with IFN-α. In addition, a French study testing the addition of cytarabine to IFN-2b found this to result in an increased proportion of patients achieving a cytogenetic response. Thereafter interferon, either alone or in combination with cytarabine, replaced HU as the preferred treatment for CML in the CP. The precise mode of action of IFN-α remains unelucidated but probably related to its immunomodulatory properties, a principal reason for its resurgence in studies addressing patients who remain in the CP but do not fare well with tyrosine kinase inhibitors (TKIs). IFN-α was replaced by imatinib as the preferred treatment for patients with CML in the CP in summer 2001, following a randomized study comparing imatinib with IFN-α plus cytarabine. The results proved very impressive and established the firm place of imatinib mesylate (imatinib), exclusively with efforts from Brian Druker, and scientists from Ciba-Geigy (now Novartis Pharmaceuticals) in the first-line therapy of patients with CML. The success of imatinib also constituted the final proof of the importance of the BCR-ABL1 oncoprotein to CML. Imatinib was rapidly followed by the development of the next generation-TKIs. This is discussed in detail in Chapter 7.

For patients with PV, venesection as a form of treatment was introduced in the years between 1903 and 1908. In the late 1930s, Lawrence introduced radiophosphorus as treatment for PV and the first recorded case of acute leukaemia associated with the use of radiophosphorus was reported some years later. In a landmark debate in 1955 by led by Dameshek, venesection and radiophosphorus were critically assessed and a consensus was reached to recommend radiophosphorus as the first-line therapy of PV. However, soon thereafter, Dameshek supported the notion of using venesection as the preferable initial treatment. Around the same time, several chemotherapeutic agents, such as thiotepa, busulfan, chlorambucil, cyclophosphamide, and melphalan, entered the clinics and were considered as alternatives to venesection or radiotherapy for the treatment of patients with PV. These drugs were thought to have advantages over phlebotomy since they were able to control not only the excessive erythrocytosis but also the thrombocytosis, leukocytosis, and splenomegaly.

A great impetus to solving the uncertainties in the management of these disorders was given by Wasserman who established in 1967 the Polycythemia Vera Study Group (PVSG), comprising of international haematologists. The group's principal objectives were to define very stringent diagnostic criteria for future clinical trials, to delineate the epidemiology, natural history, and pathophysiology, and to determine the optimal treatment. The group went to conduct several trials and significantly influenced the worldwide clinical practice of PV. From these studies, the recommended treatment for PV was phlebotomy for the low-risk patients and HU for high-risk cases. The group also initiated a series of studies for patients with ET confirming the preference to use HU if and when therapy was indicated. Much controversy with regards to this recommends remains, in particular the risk to develop acute leukaemia and myelodysplasia.

Bone marrow (now stem cell) transplantation began soon after the description of the histocompatibility system in 1958. Much of the pioneering work was carried out by the Nobel laureate Donald Thomas in Seattle. In 1978 John Goldman in London showed that marrow-populating stem cells were present in the peripheral blood of untreated CML patients. This led to the use of an autograft for patients ineligible for an allo-SCT, and though in some patients Ph-negative haematopoiesis was restored, very few patients remained Ph-negative for extended periods. Subsequent efforts in allo-SCT using sibling and volunteer unrelated donors were increasingly successful, as a result of the recognition that the graft-versus-leukaemia effect plays a major role in eradicating CML after allo-SCT and the improvements in the conditioning regimens. The potential to accord long-term survival and probable cure for patients with CML in the CP was firmly established by the early 1990s and an allograft was then considered the first-line treatment for all eligible patients in the CP. The use of donor lymphocyte infusions to treat early relapse after allograft by exploiting the graft-versus-leukaemia effect became popular in the mid-1990 and confirmed the importance of the donor derived immune system to overcome residual leukaemic cells. Allo-SCT was introduced for the treatment of patients with MF in the 1980s and at present remains the only treatment which can accords long-term remission and potential cure. Allo-SCT is discussed in detail in Chapter 16.

The twenty-first century

The genetic landscape of the MPN began to unfold in 2005, with the discovery of the deregulated JAK2 signalling and a recurrent somatic mutation involving *JAK2*^{V617F}, now considered to be a pivotal genetic driver mutation of *BCR-ABL1*-negative MPN. This, and other seminal observations, such as the demonstration of the pathogenetic role of the thrombopoietin receptor (MPL) and the calreticulin (CALR) genes, were made by investigators on both sides of the Atlantic (Kralovics, Skoda, Green, Vainchenker, Gilliland, and others). Thereafter, many efforts led to the introduction of Janus kinase (JAK) inhibitors into the clinics in 2007, and the licensing of the first JAK1 and JAK2 inhibitor, ruxolitinib, in 2011 and 2015, for patients with advanced MF and selected patients with PV, respectively. The drug affords substantial symptomatic benefits, reduction in splenomegaly, and improved survival, but has no significant impact on the malignant clone. These treatments are discussed in detail in Chapters 8 and 9.

Recent efforts examining MPN through genetics, epigenetics, and physiology has revealed several important biological findings which are now being incorporated into tools to help optimize the clinical management, and also helps understand the treatment resilience of some of the subtypes of

MPN. We have also learned how different genetic findings, and the order in which they are acquired, may influence the phenotypes and prognosis.

Conclusion

§It is remarkable to have witnessed how the biology and therapy of patients with MPN has evolved since the earlier historical observations and how profoundly the recent translational research findings have impacted the treatment algorithms. For patients with CML in CP, there are now five TKIs in the clinics: imatinib, nilotinib, dasatinib, bosutinib, and ponatinib. The first three are currently licensed for first-line use, in addition to other drugs such as interferon and omacetaxine. One of the principal clinical challenges now is the efforts to discontinue TKI therapies safely once a durable complete molecular response has been achieved. In sharp contrast with the success in the treatment of CML, which is contingent upon the *BCR-ABL1* being the founder mutation in every CML cell, the impact of JAK2 inhibitors in selected patients with MF and PV, so far, is limited to the control of splenomegaly and symptomatic improvement, with scarce current evidence in support of deeper effects on disease pathophysiology. Furthermore, unlike CML, patients with *BCR-ABL1*-negative MPN demonstrate much genetic diversity and of course complexity. Acquired clinical resistance to JAK2 inhibitor therapy is being observed, possibly due to novel mutations, and might represent a challenge for the future therapies. Combining JAK inhibitors with other targeted drugs, including immunomodulators, epigenetic agents, and telomerase inhibitors, are now being pursued, in tandem with efforts to unravel the underlying molecular complexities. Much work lies ahead.

Reference

1. Shakespeare W. The Tragedy of Macbeth, Act 3, Scene 4, Page 6. 1606.

Further reading

Assman H. Beitrage zur osteosklerotischen anamie. *Beitr Pathol Anat Allgemeinen Pathologie (Jena)*. 1907;41:565–95.

Baxter EJ, Scott LM, Campbell PJ, et al. Acquired mutation of JAK2 in human myeloproliferative disorders. *Lancet*. 2005;365:1779–90.

Bennett JH. Case of hypertrophy of the spleen and liver in which death took place from suppuration of the blood. *Edinb Med Surg J*. 1845;64:413–23.

Cabot RC. A case of chronic cyanosis without discernible cause, ending in cerebral hemorrhage. *Boston Med Surg J*. 1899;141:574–5.

Craigie D. Case of disease of the spleen in which death took place consequent on the presence of purulent matter in the blood. *Edinb Med Surg J*. 1845;64:400–13.

§ Section 'Conclusion' adapted with permission from Mughal TI, et al. (2016). Chronic myeloid leukemia: reminiscences and dreams. *Haematologica*. 101(5):541–58. DOI:10.3324/haematol.2015.139337.

Daley GQ, van Etten RA, Baltimore D. Induction of chronic myelogenous leukemia in mice by the P210 BCR/ABL gene of the Philadelphia chromosome. *Science*. 1990;247:824–30.

Dameshek W. Some speculations on the myeloproliferative syndromes. *Blood*. 1951;6:372–5.

Di Guglielmo G. Richerche di ematologia. I. Un caso di eritroleucemia. megacariociti in circolo e loro funzione piastrinopoietico. *Folio Med (Pavia)*. 1917;13:386.

Drew J. Paul Ehrlich: magister mundi. *Nat Rev Drug Discov*. 2004;3:797–801.

Ehrlich P. Beitrag zur Kenntnis der Anilinfarbungen und ihrer Verwendung in der Microscopischen Technik. *Archives Mikrochirurgie Anatomischer*. 1877;13:263–77.

Elephanty AG, Hariharan IK, Cory S. Bcr-abl, the hallmark of chronic myeloid leukemia in man, induces multiple hemopoietic neoplasms in mice. *EMBO J*. 1990;9:1069–78.

Epstein E, Goedel A. Hamorrhagische thrombozythamie bei vascularer schrumpfmilz (Haemorrhagic thrombocythemia with a vascular, sclerotic spleen). *Virchows Archiv A Pathol Anat Histopathol*. 1934;293:233–48.

Fialkow PJ, Faguet GB, Jacobson RJ, Vaidya K, Murphy S. Evidence that essential thrombocythemia is a clonal disorder with origin in a multipotent stem cell. *Blood*. 1981;58:916–19.

Fialkow PJ, Garler SM, Yoshida A. Clonal origin of chronic myelocytic leukemia in man. *Proc Natl Acad Sci USA*. 1967;58:1468–71.

Groffen J, Stephenson JR, Heisterkamp N, et al. Philadelphia chromosome breakpoints are clustered within a limited region, bcr, on chromosome 22. *Cell*. 1984;36:93–9.

Gulliver G. *The Works of William Hewson*. London, UK: The Sydenham Society 1846; part III, 1vi: pp. 214–360.

Heisterkamp N, Stephenson JR, Groffen J, et al. Localization of the c-abl oncogene adjacent to a translocation break point in chronic myelocytic leukemia. *Nature*. 1983;306:239–42.

Heuck G. Zwei Falle von Leukamie mit eigenthumlichem Blutresp. nochenmarksbefund (two cases of leukemia with peculiar blood and bone marrow findings, respectively). *Arch Pathol Anat Physiol Virchows*. 1879;78:475–96.

Hirschfeld H. Die generalisierte aleukamische Myelose und ihre Stellung im System der leukamischen Erkrankungen. *Z Klin Med*. 1914;80:126–73.

Hooke R. *Micrographia: Or, Some Physiological Descriptions of Minute Bodies Made by Magnifying Glasses, 1st edition*. London, UK: J Martyn and J Allestry, 1665.

Jackson H Jr, Parker F Jr, Lemon HM. Agnogenic myeloid metaplasia of the spleen: a syndrome simulating other more definite hematological disorders. *N Engl J Med*. 1940;222:985–94.

James C, Ugo V, Couedic JP, et al. A unique clonal JAK2 mutation leading to constitutive signaling causes polycythaemia vera. *Nature*. 2005;434:1144–8.

Kralovics R, Passamonti F, Buser AS, et al. A gain-of-function mutation of JAK2 in myeloproliferative disorders. *N Engl J Med*. 2005;352:1779–90.

Levine RL, Wadleigh M, Cools J, et al. Activating mutation in the tyrosine kinase JAK2 in polycythemia vera, essential thrombocythemia, and myeloid metaplasia with myelofibrosis. *Cancer Cell*. 2005;7:387–97.

Lieutaud J. Elementa Physiologiae. Amsterdam, the Netherlands, 1749: pp. 82–4. [Translated and quoted in Dreyfus C. Milestones in the History of Hematology. New York, NY: Grune & Stratton, 1957: pp. 11–12].

Minot GR, Buckman TE, Isaacs R. Chronic myelogenous leukemia: age incidence, duration and benefit derived from irradiation. *JAMA*. 1924;82:1489–94.

Mughal TI, Radich JR, Dieninger MW at al. Chronic myeloid leukaemia: reminiscences and dreams. *Haematologica*. 2016;101:541–58

Nowell PC, Hungerford DA. A minute chromosome in human granulocytic leukemia. *Science*. 1960;132:1497.

Osler W. Chronic cyanosis with polycythemia and enlarged spleen. *Am J Med Sci*. 1903;126:187–201.

Parkes-Weber F. Polycythemia, erythrocytosis and erythraemia. *QJM*. 1908;2:85–134.

Piller G. Leukaemia – a brief historical review from ancient times to 1950. *Br J Haematol*. 2001;112:282–92.

Rowley JD. A new consistent chromosome abnormality in chronic myelogenous leukaemia identified by quinacrine fluorescence and Giemsa banding. *Nature*. 1973;243:290–3.

Turk W. Beitrage zur kenntnis des symptomenbildes polyzythamie mit milztumor and zyanose. *Wiener medizinische Wochenschrift*. 1904;17:153–60, 189–93.

van Leeuwenhoek A. More observations from Mr. Leewenhook, in a letter of Sept. 7. 1674. sent to the publisher. *Phil Trans R Soc*.1674;9:121–8.

Vaquez HM. Sur une forme speciale de cyanose s'accompagnant d'hyperglobulie excessive et persistente. *C R Soc Biol (Paris)*. 1892;44:384–8.

Vaughan JM, Harrison CV. Leuco-erythroblastic anaemia and myelosclerosis. *J Pathol Bacteriol.* 1939;48:339–3521939.

Velpeau A. Sur la resorption du puseat sur l' alteration du sang dans les maladies clinique de persection nenemant. Premier observation. *Rev Med.* 1827;2:216.

Virchow R. Weisses blut. *Froriep's Notzien.* 1845;36:151–6.

Wasserman LR. Polycythemia vera – its course and treatment: relation to myeloid metaplasia and leukaemia. *Bull NY Acad Med.* 1954;30:343–75.

Weber FP, Watson JH. Chronic polycythemia with enlarged spleen, probably a disease of the bone marrow. *Trans Clin Soc.* 1904;37:115.

Chapter 2

Genomic landscape of myeloproliferative neoplasms

Srinivas K. Tantravahi, Jamshid S. Khorashad, and Michael W. Deininger

Introduction to the genomic landscape of MPN *16*
Concepts of clonality *17*
Clonal diversity, evolution, and succession *17*
Types of mutations in MPN *19*
Chronic myeloid leukaemia *20*
Classical MPN: Polycythaemia vera, essential thrombocytosis, and primary myelofibrosis *22*
MPN predisposition alleles and germline mutations *24*
Chronic neutrophilic leukaemia, atypical chronic myeloid leukaemia *27*
Systemic mastocytosis *28*
Chronic myelomonocytic leukaemia *28*
Conclusions *29*

Introduction to the genomic landscape of MPN

Myeloproliferative neoplasms (MPN) are clonal haematopoietic stem cell disorders, characterized by expansion of myeloid progenitors in the bone marrow and excessive production of terminally differentiated cells in the peripheral blood (Table 2.1). William Dameshek coined the term 'myeloproliferative syndromes', recognizing that several of the diseases now termed MPN share common clinical manifestations including thrombosis, bleeding, and a risk of progression to acute myeloid leukaemia. He also speculated about the presence of an 'undiscovered stimulus' driving disease pathogenesis. The discovery of the Philadelphia chromosome (Ph) by Nowell and Hungerford in 1960 marks the beginning of the genomic age in MPN and cancer in general. After this splash, progress was slow initially and almost entirely driven by the study of karyotypic abnormalities. Laborious positional cloning was the basis for unrevealing the genomic structure of the t (9;22) and identifying the translocation partners *BCR* and *ABL1*, before polymerase chain reaction (PCR) and derivative technologies as well as automated sequencing significantly accelerated discovery efforts. Array-based platforms subsequently

Table 2.1 2016 WHO classification of myeloproliferative neoplasms

Myeloproliferative neoplasms (MPN)	Myeloid and lymphoid neoplasms with eosinophilia and abnormalities of *PDGFRA*, *PDGFRB*, or *FGFR1*	Myelodysplastic/ myeloproliferative neoplasms (MDS/MPN)
• Chronic myeloid leukaemia, *BCR-ABL1 positive* • Chronic neutrophilic leukaemia • Polycythaemia vera • Essential thrombocythaemia • Primary myelofibrosis • Chronic eosinophilic leukaemia, NOS • Systemic mastocytosis • Myeloproliferative neoplasms, unclassifiable	• Myeloid and lymphoid neoplasms with *PDGFRA* rearrangement • Myeloid neoplasms with *PDGFRB* rearrangement • Myeloid and lymphoid neoplasms with *FGFR1* abnormalities	• Chronic myelomonocytic leukaemia • Atypical chronic myeloid leukaemia, *BCR-ABL1* negative • Juvenile myelomonocytic leukaemia • Myelodysplastic/ myeloproliferative neoplasm, unclassifiable • Refractory anaemia with ring sideroblasts and thrombocytosis

Abbreviations: WHO, World Health Organization; NOS, not otherwise specified; *PDGFRA*, platelet derived growth factor A; *PDGFRB*, platelet derived growth factor B; *FGFR1*, fibroblast growth factor receptor 1.

Adapted from Arber DA, et al. The 2016 revision to the World Health Organization classification of myeloid neoplasms and acute leukemia. *Blood*. 127(20):2391–405. https://doi.org/10.1182/blood-2016-03-643544. Reprinted with permission from the American Society of Hematology.

allowed for genome-wide screening of mRNA expression and copy number variations. However, it is massively parallel next generation sequencing (NGS) that proved to be the truly disruptive technology to revolutionize the field of molecular genetics. It is likely that all major disease alleles in MPN have been discovered by now, but much more work remains to be done to characterize and functionally annotate the many less common variants identified by NGS, and even more to understand their complex interactions. Despite their phenotypic similarities MPN are genetically heterogeneous, consistent with their variable and frequently unpredictable clinical behaviour. Here we will give an overview of the mutational landscape in MPN, as it presents itself in the middle of 2015. In many respects this is a review of genomic alterations in myeloid malignancies, as many abnormalities found in MPN also occur in acute myeloid leukaemia (AML) or myelodysplastic syndromes (MDS), albeit with different frequencies.

Concepts of clonality

Clonal haematopoiesis in healthy individuals

It has been estimated that the adult human haematopoietic system may contain approximately 100 000 haematopoietic stem cells (HSCs). The accumulated progeny of each of these cells could be considered a clone. However, in the absence of a specific and unique genetic marker, these clones cannot be identified and therefore it is impossible to know precisely how many stem cells contribute to mature haematopoiesis at any given time. Once an HSC acquires a genetic abnormality its progeny can be identified as a unique clone and the detection limit is determined by the sensitivity of the detection assay. These considerations are not only theoretical. Recent studies have revealed that a fraction of older, haematologically normal individuals, harbour mutations associated with haematologic malignancies, a situation referred to as clonal haematopoiesis. This extends on previous observations of clonal haematopoiesis in older women detected by X-chromosome-based clonality assays. Estimates of clonal haematopoiesis in haematologically normal individuals vary, but it is certain that the prevalence of clonal haematopoiesis will increase with assay sensitivity. This suggests that the term 'clonal haematopoiesis' is not precise and may have to be replaced as we learn more about the physiological trends of clonal diversity with ageing.

Clonal diversity, evolution, and succession

Clonal evolution refers to the sequential acquisition of genetic abnormalities by a cell clone (Figure 2.1). This is a phenomenon well known in chronic myeloid leukaemia (CML), where it is indicative of disease progression and portends a poor prognosis even on tyrosine kinase inhibitor therapy. While metaphase cytogenetics is an old technology, it provides immediate resolution at the single cell level in contrast to the output of NGS and similar techniques that analyse bulk cells. Clonal evolution may be facilitated by genetic instability imparted by the initiating mutation or by the expansion of abnormal HSCs that increase the population at risk of additional mutations, both consistent with a hypermorphic (gain-of-function) mutation. Although inferences are possible from allelic ratios of NGS sequencing data, single cell or single colony analysis is required to precisely assess clonal diversity and achieve full deconvolution of clonal architecture. Coexistence of several independent abnormal clones (clonal diversity) suggests that more than one HSC has been transformed, much in the sense of the 'field carcinogenesis' of some solid tumours (Figure 2.1). Alternatively, seemingly unrelated diverse clones may have originated from a common ancestral cell with an as yet undetected underlying mutation. Until recently, testing this hypothesis relied on X-chromosome inactivation as a generic marker of clonal haematopoiesis with limited resolution, but this is now being superseded by NGS due to its comprehensive coverage of the genome. The term 'clonal succession' was originally used to describe the successive recruitment of HSCs to contribute to mature haematopoiesis, but is increasingly used to describe the succession of dominant malignant clones on therapy, irrespective of their clonal relationship (Figure 2.1).

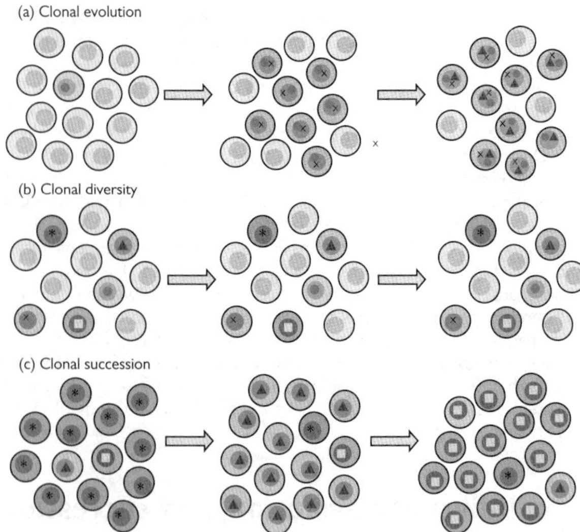

Figure 2.1 Concepts of clonality. (a) Clonal evolution. A single cell acquires a somatic mutation (mutation 1) and subsequently develops additional mutations during clonal expansion (mutations 2 and 3) resulting in a single clone with all three mutations. (b) Clonal diversity. Multiple diverse clones, each with a unique mutation (mutations 1, 2, 3, 4, or 5) coexist without significant change over time. (c) Clonal succession. Multiple diverse clones exist together with dominance of a single clone at different time points (mutation 3 or 4), e.g. related to selection on therapy (also see plate section).

Types of mutations in MPN

Structural chromosomal abnormalities are characteristic of CML, occur in 20–50% of cases of myelofibrosis (MF), aCML, and chronic myelomonocytic leukaemia (CMML), and are less common in essential thrombocytosis (ET) and polycythaemia vera (PV). Reciprocal translocations define several disease entities, such as CML and MPN associated with rearrangements of *PDGFRB* or *FGFR3*. Partial or complete deletions of chromosomes occur, for example, 20q– in PV, but have not defined entities. Numerical chromosomal abnormalities are typically associated with progression to the blast phase. Single nucleotide polymorphism (SNP) arrays have revealed many more copy number gains or losses than were previously appreciated by conventional cytogenetics or fluorescence *in situ* hybridization (FISH). Uniparental disomy (UPD) (Figure 2.2) is particularly common in MPN, for example in the case of the *JAK2*^{V617F} allele. This suggests that either the addition of another copy of the transforming allele or the loss of a suppressor function of the normal allele promote oncogenesis. Point mutations and insertions/deletions are the most common genetic alterations. Some point mutations are found predominantly (albeit not exclusively), in one or a small number of MPN phenotypes. For example, *KIT*^{D816V} is characteristic of systemic mastocytosis. However, the majority of MPN mutations are promiscuous and have no disease specificity. For example, *TET2* mutations have been found in literally all MPN. These observations beg the question of which factors drive the clinical MPN phenotype. A recent study showed that the sequence in which mutations are acquired in genetically complex

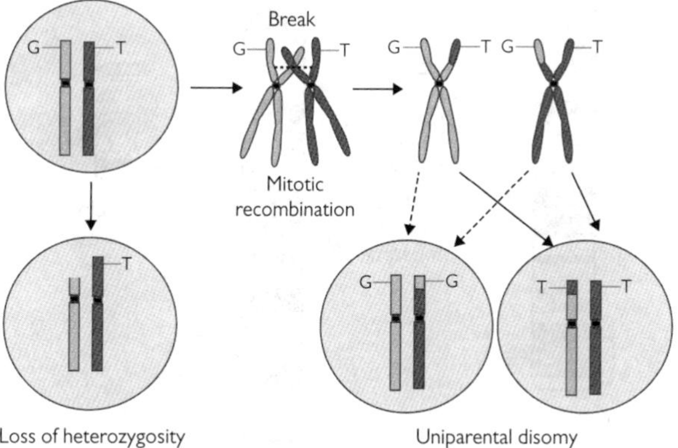

Figure 2.2 Schematic to illustrate loss of heterozygosity (LOH) and uniparental disomy (UPD). A human somatic cell is shown that contains paternal and maternal copies of a given chromosome and is heterozygous for a single nucleotide polymorphism (SNP). LOH results when one copy of the gene containing the SNP is lost. The cell shown is hemizygous for the genetic region in question. In contrast, in acquired UPD mitotic recombination leads to homozygosity for the SNP, but diploidy is maintained for the region in question.

diseases might inform the clinical phenotype. Another, as yet unproven, possibility is that the cell targeted by the initial mutation may dictate the phenotype. Lastly epigenetic alterations may contribute to the phenotype. These may be the result of somatic mutations in epigenetic regulators in the MPN cells, but it is also conceivable that microenvironmental factors contribute to the epigenetic imprint.

Chronic myeloid leukaemia

Molecular anatomy of the BCR-ABL translocation

In 1960 Peter Nowell and David Hungerford described an abnormally small chromosome 22 ('minute chromosome') in several patients with CML, thereby establishing that cancer was the result of abnormalities in the DNA. They termed the minute chromosome Philadelphia 1 (Ph^1) after the city of its discovery and anticipated it would be the first in a series of cancer-associated chromosomes. Thirteen years later Janet Rowley reported that Ph^1, nowadays usually referred to as Ph, was in fact the result of a reciprocal translocation between chromosomes 9 and 22. The 1980s identified the translocation partners as breakpoint cluster region (*BCR*), a previously unrecognized gene on 22q34 and *ABL1*, the human homologue of v-*abl*, a murine leukaemia virus first described by Abelson and Rabstein. Work from several groups clarified the molecular architecture of the *BCR-ABL1* fusion gene formed as a result of the Philadelphia translocation (Figure 2.3).

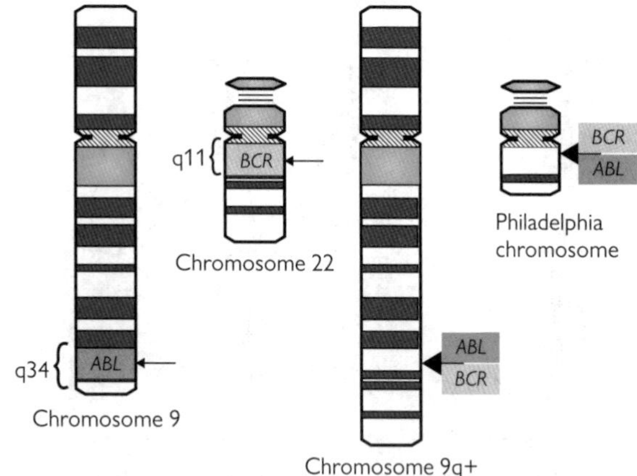

Figure 2.3 Schematic of the Philadelphia chromosome. A balanced reciprocal translocation between chromosome 9 containing the *ABL1* gene (region q34.1) and chromosome 22 containing the *BCR* gene (region q11.2) results in the formation of the Philadelphia chromosome (harbouring the *BCR-ABL1*) and derivative chromosome 9q+ (harbouring *ABL1-BCR*).

The breakpoints in *BCR* localize to three breakpoint cluster regions. Depending on whether the break occurs in the major (M-*bcr*), minor (m-*bcr*), or minimal (μ-*bcr*) breakpoint cluster regions, variable portions of *BCR* are preserved in the *BCR-ABL1* fusion gene (Figure 2.4). Most patients with CML and approximately one-third of patients with Ph+ acute lymphoblastic leukaemia (ALL) have breakpoints in the M-*bcr*. m-*bcr* breaks are typical of Ph+ ALL, but are very rare in CML. Lastly, breaks in the μ-*bcr* are associated with neutrophilic differentiation. In contrast to the clustering in *BCR*, the breakpoints in *ABL1* are spread out over a large genomic region and may occur 5' of exon 1b, between the two alternative exons 1b and 1a or between exons 1a and 2 (Figure 2.4). Despite the highly variable localization of the breakpoints, splicing of the primary mRNA transcript leads to fusion transcripts between *BCR* sequences and *ABL1* exon 2. Atypical *BCR-ABL1* transcripts are present in rare patients with CML or Ph+ ALL and can be missed by PCR assays designed to detect only the common transcripts.

Approximately 5% of CML patients present with more complex re-arrangements that involve chromosomes in addition to 9 and 22. Prior to the introduction of tyrosine kinase inhibitors (TKIs), these variant translocations were thought to be associated with an adverse prognosis, possibly related to loss of genetic material from the edges of the breaks. Therapy with TKIs abrogates the adverse prognostic impact, and the presence of a variant

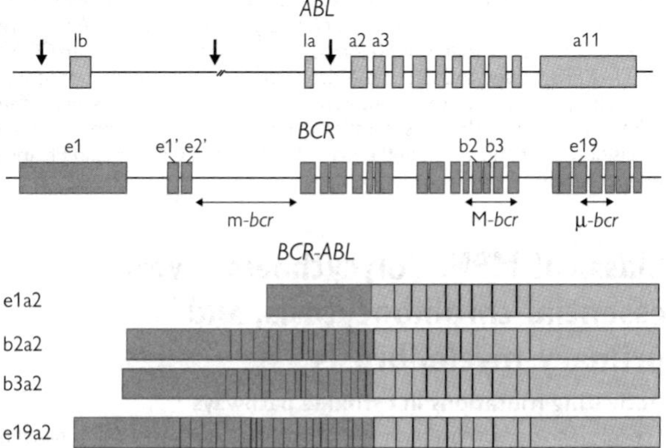

Figure 2.4 Molecular anatomy of the *BCR-ABL1* translocation. The upper panel shows the exon-intron organization of the *ABL1* (including the two alternative first exons, Ib and Ia) and *BCR* genes. Vertical arrows indicate the localization of the genomic breakpoints in *ABL1* and horizontal arrows the breakpoint cluster regions in *BCR*. The lower panel shows the structure of the chimeric mRNAs derived from fusion genes resulting from the different breakpoints in *BCR*.

Reproduced from Deininger MW, et al. (2010). The molecular biology of chronic myeloid leukemia. *Blood*. 96(10):3343–56. Reprinted with permission from the American Society of Hematology.

translocation should not influence clinical decisions. In a small proportion of CML patients the *BCR-ABL1* translocation is cytogenetically invisible (silent), but the clinical features and biology of these cases are identical to those with classical Ph.

Clonal cytogenetic evolution

Additional chromosomal abnormalities in the Ph$^+$ cell clone (CCA/Ph$^+$) are referred to as clonal evolution (CE). CCA/Ph$^+$ have long been recognized as a poor prognostic feature and are associated with progression to accelerated or blast phase. Classically the CCA/Ph$^+$ are grouped into major route abnormalities (additional copies of Ph, trisomy 8, trisomy 19, and isochromosome 17p) and minor route abnormalities (all others). CE present at diagnosis does not define accelerated phase, but has recently been shown to confer a poor outcome to patients on imatinib therapy. CCA/Ph$^+$ developing on TKI therapy indicates failure and define accelerated phase. Despite the relatively small number of typical CCA/Ph$^+$ abnormalities, little is known about the mechanisms by which they promote progression, perhaps with the exception of isochromosome 17p, which is associated with deletion of p53 in some cases. An alternative to a direct mechanistic explanation is that structural or numerical chromosomal abnormalities are a reflection of genetic instability that promotes progression, although this does not explain the non-random nature of CCA/Ph$^+$. Chromosomal abnormalities may also occur in Ph$^-$ cells (CCA/Ph$^-$), which should not be confused with CCA/Ph$^+$. The karyotypic abnormalities of CCA/Ph$^-$ are very similar to those found in myelodysplasia and some patients with CCA/Ph$^-$ have progressed to MDS and AML, particularly those with monosomy 7 or del(7q). In some cases, identical chromosomal abnormalities were seen in Ph$^+$ and Ph$^-$ metaphases, suggesting that a clonal Ph$^-$ state predated the acquisition of Ph; however, in the majority of cases CCA/Ph$^-$ and Ph arise independently.

Classical MPN: Polycythaemia vera, essential thrombocytosis, and primary myelofibrosis

Activating mutations in cytokine pathways

The long-known fact that haematopoietic progenitors from MPN patients form erythroid and megakaryocytic colonies *in vitro* with minimal or no cytokine support is an indication of the central role of aberrant cytokine signalling in MPN pathogenesis, and unsurprisingly mutations in cytokine pathways are very common.

JAK/STAT signalling

A common genetic basis for the classical MPN was discovered in 2005, when the laboratory of William Vainchencker and several other groups reported a somatic gain-of-function mutation in *JAK2* (*JAK2*^{V617F}). JAK2, a non-receptor tyrosine kinase of the Janus kinase family (along with JAK1,

JAK3, and TYK2), plays an important role in haematopoiesis. Binding of cytokines such as erythropoietin and thrombopoietin to their cognate receptors leads to recruitment and activation of JAK2, which in turn phosphorylates signal transduction and transcription activators 3 and 5 (STAT3 and STAT5). pSTAT3 and pSTAT5 form homodimers that translocate to the nucleus to regulate transcription of target genes, leading to increased proliferation and decreased apoptosis. *JAK2*^{V617F} is a constitutionally active tyrosine kinase whose expression imparts cytokine independent growth to cell lines and recapitulates an MPN phenotype in murine transplant models (discussed in Chapter 3). *JAK2*^{V617F} is present in ~96% of PV, and 50–60% ET and myelofibrosis (MF) patients. While the majority of PV and MF patients are at least partially homozygous due to mitotic recombination affecting chromosome 9p, most ET patients are heterozygous for *JAK2*^{V617F}. Subsequently, insertions and deletions in exon 12 of the *JAK2* gene were identified in the majority of *JAK2*^{V617F} negative PV patients. *JAK2* exon 12 mutations activate cytokine signalling, but for reasons that are not completely understood these patients typically present with isolated erythrocytosis and bone marrow morphological features that are distinct from the 'panmyelosis' of standard PV. The presence of *JAK2*^{V617F} or exon 12 mutations is one of the criteria for a diagnosis of PV. Mutations in the thrombopoietin receptor gene *MPL*, most commonly *MPL*^{W515L} and *MPL*^{W515K} were described in up to 5% of ET and 10% of MF patients, and are mutually exclusive with *JAK2*^{V617F} (Figure 2.5). *MPL* mutations impart cytokine independent growth to cell lines and produce an aggressive MPN phenotype resembling MF in murine transplant models. Loss of function mutations in exon 12 of *LNK*, an adaptor gene that negatively regulates thrombopoietin-MPL mediated JAK/STAT pathway, has been described in rare PV, ET, and PMF patients. The incidence of *LNK* mutations appears to be higher in the blast phase of MPN. *CBL* encodes a protein with E3 ubiquitin ligase activity and is involved in the degradation of cytokine receptors. Mutations in in the RING domain of *CBL* decrease ubiquitin ligase activity, thereby prolonging cytokine signalling by extending the half-life of receptor/ligand complexes. CBL mutations were described in variety of MPN including aCML, ET, PMF, CMML, and rarely chronic eosinophilic leukaemia (CEL).

Calreticulin mutations

The genetic basis of *JAK2* and *MPL* wild-type ET and MF patients had remained unclear for a number of years, until two groups independently reported recurrent somatic indels in exon 9 of the calreticulin (*CALR*) gene. *CALR* is highly conserved across species and encodes for a luminal endoplasmic reticulum chaperone protein involved in glycoprotein folding, calcium homeostasis, proliferation, and apoptosis. *CALR* mutations occur in 60–88% of *JAK2/MPL* wild-type ET and MF patients and are mutually exclusive with *JAK2* and *MPL* mutations (Figure 2.5). The two most common indels, a 52-base pair deletion (type 1) or a 5-bp insertion (type 2), account for 85% of *CALR* mutations. All *CALR* ins/del mutations lead to a one base pair shift in the mRNA reading frame, resulting in a mutant protein with a novel C-terminus and loss of Golgi-to-ER signalling motif (KDEL). *CALR* mutated cells exhibit constitutively active JAK/STAT signalling and cytokine independent growth, but the mechanism by which *CALR* activates JAK/STAT remains to be established.

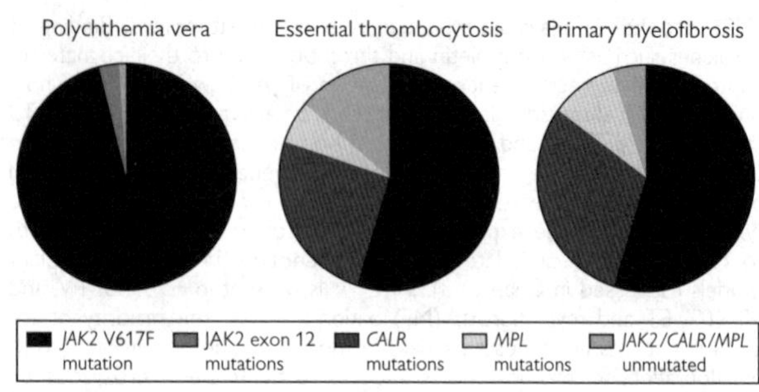

Figure 2.5 Schematic demonstrating frequency of mutually exclusive *JAK2*, *CALR*, and *MPL* mutations in classical myeloproliferative neoplasms.

Source: data from Pardanani AD, et al. (2016). MPL515 mutations in myeloproliferative and other myeloid disorders: a study of 1182 patients. *Blood*. 108(10):3472–6. DOI: 10.1182/blood-2006-04-018879; and Pikman Y, et al. (2016). MPLW515L is a novel somatic activating mutation in myelofibrosis with myeloid metaplasia. *PLoS Medicine*. 3(7):e370. https://doi.org/10.1371/journal.pmed.0030270.

MPN predisposition alleles and germline mutations

There are various degrees of familial predisposition in the MPN. Familial MPN refers to increased number of MPN cases in a family pedigree compared to the general population, typically affecting at least two members of the same family. In one study, the prevalence of familial MPN was 7.6% among apparently sporadic patients. The clinical phenotype was similar within the same pedigree in 60% of the families, while 40% of families had a different MPN. A predisposition is well established for *JAK2*^{V617F} positive MPN, referred to as *JAK2* 46/1 or 'GGCC' haplotype, a common very low penetrant predisposition allele in the *JAK2* gene. The *JAK2* 46/1 haplotype confers an odds ratio of developing an MPN 3–4-fold higher compared to non-carriers. The mechanistic basis for the increased MPN risk of *JAK2* 46/1 is unknown. In contrast, there is little if any familial predisposition in CML, which is thought to be the result of sporadic mutational events. Most MPN occur at comparable frequency around the world, in contrast to the much more significant geographic differences in some B cell malignancies, most prominently chronic lymphocytic leukaemia, which argues for mostly sporadic events.

Germ-line mutations in erythropoietin and thrombopoietin receptor genes, *EpoR* and *MPL* have been reported in hereditary MPN. In contrast to the very low penetrant predisposition alleles in familial MPN (e.g. *JAK2* 46/1 haplotype), mutations causing hereditary MPN are highly penetrant. Congenital erythrocytosis or primary familial congenital polycythaemia (PFCP) is an autosomal dominant disorder due to germ-line mutations in the *EpoR* gene. *EpoR* mutations were first described in a large Finnish family affecting 29 members, all of whom presented with erythrocytosis. Subsequently, over 22 additional heterozygous gain-of-function *EpoR* gene mutations were identified in congenital polycythaemia patients. *EpoR* mutations exclusively affect exon 8, and the majority generate a truncated protein deficient in the C-terminal negative regulatory domain, which leads to increased sensitivity of erythroid progenitors. Despite absolute erythrocytosis, congenital polycythaemia patients are not at increased risk of vascular complications or acute leukaemia. Similarly, germ-line mutations in the thrombopoietin gene (*THPO*) and *MPL* have been implicated in hereditary thrombocytosis. Mutations in the 5'-untranslated region of the *THPO* were identified in multiple pedigrees of hereditary thrombocytosis following an autosomal dominant pattern of inheritance. Most commonly, a G to C transversion in the splice donor site of intron 3 leads to an mRNA transcript with a shortened 5'-untranslated region and more efficient translation capability. Clinically these patients had elevated serum thrombopoietin (TPO) concentrations and experience both bleeding manifestations and vaso-occlusive symptoms that responded to aspirin treatment. MPL^{S505N}, a gain-of-function mutation in the transmembrane domain of the protein has been reported in several families of hereditary thrombocytosis. The mutation leads to TPO independent dimerization of MPL. Clinically patients developed thrombosis, splenomegaly, and bone marrow fibrosis, but without cytopenias or risk of progression to AML. *MPL* Baltimore is a single nucleotide substitution (1238 G > T) resulting in a K39N amino acid substitution that leads to incomplete MPL protein processing. This polymorphism was initially discovered in three African-American patients presenting with isolated thrombocytosis and is exclusive to African Americans, of whom 7% are heterozygotes. No increased risk of thrombosis was reported in these patients.

Mutations in epigenetic modifiers and transcription factors

Genes involved in epigenetic regulation are frequently mutated in MPN. These mutations are not specific to the classical MPN, but occur in a variety of myeloid neoplasms. *TET2, DNMT3A,* and *IDH1/2* are involved in DNA methylation, while *EZH2* and *ASXL1* regulate chromatin structure.

The TET (Ten-Eleven-Translocation) family of proteins hydroxylate 5-methylcytosine, the initial step in the process of DNA demethylation. The *TET2* mutations associated with MPN are loss of function mutations resulting in decreased 5-hydroxymethylcytsoine levels and DNA hypermethylation. *TET2* mutations occur in up to 20% of PV, ET, MF, including blast phase, but a higher frequency was observed in CMML and systemic mastocytosis (discussed in Chapter 11). In ET/PV/MF *TET2* mutations may be acquired prior to or after *JAK2* mutation, but the order of acquisition may affect clinical phenotype and clonogenic potential of the progenitors. For example, the occurrence of a mutation in *JAK2* prior to *TET2* increases the likelihood of a PV phenotype and is associated with higher risk of thrombosis and *in vitro* sensitivity of the progenitors to ruxolitinib. One study reported decreased overall survival and increased risk of transformation to AML in patients with *TET2* mutations, but this is not a universal finding. DNA methyltransferase 3A, *DNMT3A* carries out *de novo* DNA methylation of CpG islands of promoter regions. *DNMT3A* mutations were initially observed in AML. The most common mutation R882H exerts a dominant negative effect and mice null for *DNMT3A* develop a variety of myeloid neoplasms. *DNMT3A* mutations are observed in up to 15% of MF, 7% of PV, and 14% of blast phase MPN patients. The clinical significance of *DNMT3A* mutations in PV, ET, and MF is unknown.

The polycomb repressor complex 2 (PRC2) plays a critical role in posttranslational methylation of histone 3 at lysine residue 27 (H3K27), which leads to chromatin compaction and gene silencing. *ASXL1* (Addition of Sex Combs Like 1) is critical for recruitment of PRC2 to specific oncogenic target loci, while *EZH2* (enhancer of Zeste homologue) encodes for the catalytic subunit of PRC2. Loss of function mutations in *ASXL1* and *EZH2* result in impaired PRC2 mediated H3K27 methylation. *ASXL1* mutations are seen in ~7% of PV, 4% ET and 20% MF patients. In MF patients, *ASXL1* mutations are independently associated with inferior overall survival (OS). *EZH2* mutations occur in up to 13% of MF patients, and are also associated with inferior OS. Isocitrate dehydrogenase (*IDH1/2*) mutations are present in approximately 20% of blast phase MPN; and at a much lower frequency (1–4%) in PV, ET, and MF. IDH mutations in blast phase MPN are associated with poor prognosis and inferior OS. IDH1/2 enzymes catalyse the conversion of isocitrate to α-ketoglutarate in the citric acid cycle. The altered enzymatic activity of *IDH1/2* mutants leads to excessive production of 2-hydroxy glutarate that in turn impairs the function of *TET2* and blocks haematopoietic differentiation. As discussed earlier, clonal haematopoiesis and mutations in epigenetic regulator genes *TET2*, *DNMT3A*, and *ASXL1* occur in haematologically normal adults with increasing age and may precede haematological cancers. This data suggests that these mutations occur early in HSCs and confer an advantage to the mutated HSC, but additional genetic events are necessary to produce an MPN phenotype. Finally, transcription factor mutations are uncommon in chronic phase classical MPN. Runt-related transcription factor 1 (*RUNX1*) is essential for normal haematopoiesis and differentiation. *RUNX1* mutations can occur in association with transformation to blast phase. High-resolution SNP arrays identified *IKZF1* (Ikaros) deletions in rare patients with chronic phase PV, ET, and MF, but in up to 21% of blast phase patients, implicating *IKZF1* inactivation in blastic transformation.

Mutations in mRNA splicing genes

Spliceosome machinery genes involved in pre-mRNA splicing (*SF3B1*, *SRSF2*, *U2AF1* and *ZRSR2*) are frequently mutated in myeloid neoplasms, predominantly in those with dysplastic features. *SF3B1* mutations are highly prevalent in refractory anaemia with ringed sideroblasts (RARS) and RARS-thrombocytosis (RARS-T). *SRSF2* mutations frequently occur in 30–50% of CMML patients. While these mutations are rarely reported in PV and ET, *SRSF2* mutations are observed in up to 17% of MF patients. At this point it is unclear how splicing machinery gene mutations contribute to disease pathogenesis.

Mutations in genes regulating genome stability

TP53 mutations are rare in chronic phase PV, ET, and MF. Biallelic *TP53* loss, either due to acquisition of two separate mutations in both alleles or single allele mutation followed by 17p UPD occurs in approximately in 25% of PV, ET, and MF patients at blastic transformation. In patients without *TP53* mutations, amplification of chromosome 1p was frequently observed; as this region contains the gene coding for *MDM4*, a potent inhibitor of *TP53* function, this could reflect a functional equivalent of TP53 loss. Cohesin is a multimeric complex composed of four core subunits, the SMC1, SMC3, RAD21, and STAG proteins. Together with a number of other regulatory molecules, the cohesin complex promotes sister chromatid cohesion during metaphase. Somatic mutations in all four cohesin complex proteins occur in different myeloid neoplasms. The mutations are heterozygous, mutually exclusive, and observed in approximately 10% in CMML, 6% in CML, and 1% in MF.

Chronic neutrophilic leukaemia, atypical chronic myeloid leukaemia

Chronic neutrophilic leukaemia (CNL) and atypical chronic myeloid leukaemia (aCML) are two rare disorders belonging to the class of MPN and MDS/MPN overlap syndromes, respectively. Both diseases are characterized by the absence of *BCR-ABL1*, *PDGFRA*, *PDGFRB*, and *FGFR1* rearrangements as per the World Health Organization (WHO) 2008 diagnostic criteria. While the majority of CNL patients have normal cytogenetics, the reported frequency of chromosomal abnormalities in atypical CML is quite variable. Trisomy 8 and del (20q) are the two most common abnormalities observed in CNL and aCML at diagnosis or at progression. The genetic basis of chronic neutrophilic leukaemia and aCML was unknown for number of years, although *JAK2*^{V617F} mutation was observed in rare cases of CNL and aCML. Mutations in colony-stimulating factor-3 receptor (*CSF3R*) were recently reported in approximately 50–60% of patients with CNL and atypical CML. Two classes of mutations were reported: truncation mutations (nonsense and frameshift mutations leading to a truncated receptor) or membrane proximal mutations (point mutation in the extracellular domain of CSF3R; most commonly T618I). In a murine transplant model, mice expressing *CSF3R*^{T618I} developed an MPN phenotype with marked granulocytic expansion, which responded to JAK inhibitors. *SETBP1* mutations were reported in both CNL and aCML either or in association with *CSF3R* mutations. Up to 25% of aCML patients are positive for *SETBP1* mutations, and a lower frequency rate was observed in CMML (4%) and MDS/MPN (10%), but no SETBP1 mutations were identified in solid tumours. In aCML patients, *SETBP1* mutations are associated with higher white blood cell count at diagnosis and inferior OS. *ASXL1* and *TET2* are also frequently mutated in both aCML and CNL, while mutations in *EZH2*, *IDH1/2*, *SRSF2*, *CBL*, *KRAS*, and *NRAS* are less common.

Systemic mastocytosis

Gain-of-function somatic mutations in the tyrosine kinase domain of *KIT* occur in the majority of systemic mastocytosis (SM) patients. KIT^{D816V} mutation is the most common mutation, occurring in 95% of patients. Comprehensive mutational profiling of KIT^{D816V} positive mastocytosis identified recurrent somatic mutations in genes that are typically mutated in other myeloid neoplasms. The five most frequently mutated genes in SM were *TET2* (39%), *SRSF2* (36%), *RUNX1* (23%), *ASXL1* (20%), and *CBL* (20%). SM patients who are KIT^{D816V} positive plus at least one additional mutation had significantly inferior OS compared to KIT^{D816V} only patients. In patients with SM with associated haematologic non-mast cell disease (SM-AHNMD) *ASXL1* mutation is an independent predictor of inferior survival.

Chronic myelomonocytic leukaemia

In the WHO 2008 classification of myeloid neoplasms, CMML is grouped under the myelodysplastic/myeloproliferative neoplasms, reflecting the combination of dysplastic and proliferative features (Table 2.1). Clonal cytogenetic abnormalities are present in up to 30% of CMML patients and have a strong negative prognostic impact. The most frequent cytogenetic abnormalities are trisomy 8, loss of Y chromosome, and monosomy 7 or del(7q). The advent of NGS facilitated discovery of a number of somatic mutations in genes involved in various cellular pathways including signal transduction (*KRAS, NRAS, CBL, JAK2, FLT3*), epigenetic regulation (*TET2, DNMT3A, ASXL1, UTX, EZH2*), transcriptional regulation (*RUNX1*), mRNA splicing (*SRSF2, ZRSR2, U2AF1, SF3B1*), and metabolism (*IDH1/2*). *TET2* is the most frequently mutated gene in CMML patients (more than 50% of cases), followed by *SRSF2* and *ASXL1*. Recent data suggest that *TET2* mutations are often the first to occur and likely play a key role in disease initiation. *IDH1/2* mutations occur in ~10% of patients and are mutually exclusive of *TET2* mutations. In contrast, *DNMT3A* mutations, which occur less frequently in CMML, occur in association with *TET2* or *IDH1/2* mutations. *SRSF2* is the most commonly mutated splicing machinery gene in CMML (~50% of patients), and mutations occur frequently in association with *TET2* mutations. Other splicing machinery genes such as *ZRSR2, U2AF1*, and *SF3B1* are less frequently mutated in CMML. Not unexpectedly splicing gene mutations are mutually exclusive of each other. Loss of function mutations in histone modifying genes are also common, *ASXL1* being the most frequently mutated gene (up to 40%), while *EZH2* and *UTX* are mutated in up to 10% of patients. *ASXL1* mutations are associated with greater risk for progression to AML and reduced OS. In contrast to most other MPN, mutations in growth factor signalling genes are not a consistent feature of CMML, although mutations in *KRAS, NRAS, CBL, JAK2* all occur in ~10% of patients and are mutually exclusive. This likely reflects the dominance of the dysplastic features in many cases of CMML. Unlike in AML, *FLT3* mutations are infrequent in CMML occurring in approximately 5% of patients and do not exhibit similar prognostic effect. Lastly, *RUNX1* mutations occur in ~10% of CMML patients frequently associated with thrombocytopenia.

Conclusions

There has been enormous progress in unravelling the mutational landscape of MPN since the discovery of *JAK2*^{V617F} mutation in 2005. Mutations in genes *JAK2*, *CALR*, and *MPL* are mutually exclusive and aid in the diagnosis of PV, ET, and MF. *CSF3R* mutations may in the future define CNL and aCML. However, many somatic gene mutations reported in MPN are not specific to MPN, but also occur in other myeloid malignancies as well as healthy individuals, and their precise roles in disease initiation and progression remains to be established. Numerous disease alleles have been implicated, but only tyrosine kinase mutations have led to therapeutic breakthroughs. Lastly, deep sequencing is likely to reveal many more rare disease alleles, for which prognostic and functional annotation poses a major challenge. The work has only started (Table 2.2).

Table 2.2 Somatic mutations in myeloproliferative neoplasms

Genes	PV	ET	PMF	CMML	CNL	aCML	CEL	SM	BP MPN
Growth factor signalling pathways									
JAK2 V617F	95–97%	50–60%	50–60%	10%	10%	3–5%	rare	rare	50%
JAK2 exon 12	1–2%	rare	rare	rare	rare	rare	rare	rare	unknown
Calreticulin	rare	25%	30%	rare	rare	rare	rare	rare	unknown
MPL	rare	6%	10%	rare	rare	rare	rare	rare	8%
LNK	rare	2–6%	3–6%	rare	rare	rare	rare	rare	10%
CBL	rare	rare	6%	20%	rare	10%	rare	20%	rare
KIT	rare	rare	rare	rare	rare	rare	rare	98%	rare
CSF3R	rare	rare	rare	rare	60%	40%	rare	rare	unknown
FLT3	rare	rare	rare	5%	rare	rare	rare	rare	rare
RAS signalling*									
KRAS	rare	rare	rare	5–10%	rare	35%	rare	rare	rare
NRAS	rare	rare	rare	10%	rare	35%	rare	rare	rare
Epigenetic modifiers and transcription factors									
TET2	17%	5%	15%	40–60%	30%	40%	rare	40%	20%
DNMT3A	5–10%	2–5%	15%	5%	rare	rare	rare	rare	15%
ASXL1	7%	4%	20%	50%	57%	66%	rare	20%	20%
EZH2	3%	rare	13%	5%	rare	13%	rare	5%	rare
IDH1/2	2%	1%	4%	5–10%	rare	rare	rare	rare	20%

Table 2.2 *(contd.)*

Genes	PV	ET	PMF	CMML	CNL	aCML	CEL	SM	BP MPN
RUNX1	rare	rare	rare	15%	rare	rare	rare	23%	rare
IKZF1	rare	rare	rare	rare	rare	rare	rare	rare	20%
UTX	rare	rare	rare	10%	rare	rare	rare	rare	rare
mRNA splicing									
SF3B1	rare	rare	7%	5–10%	rare	rare	rare	rare	4%
SRSF2	rare	rare	17%	30–50%	21%	40%	rare	40%	19%
U2AF1	rare	rare	16%	5%	rare	rare	rare	rare	6%
ZRSR2	rare	rare	rare	5–10%	rare	rare	rare	rare	unknown
Genome stability									
SETBP1	rare	rare	2%	5–10%	40%	30%	rare	rare	rare
TP53	rare	rare	4%	1%	rare	rare	rare	rare	10%
Cohesin family	1%	1%	1%	6%	rare	rare	rare	rare	rare

*Mutations affecting other genes of the RAS pathway, *NF1*, and *PTPN11* are rare in MPN. *NF1* mutations are observed in rare cases of PV and MF. *PTPN11* mutations are infrequent in adult CMML, despite being a major molecular event juvenile myelomonocytic leukaemia. PV, polycythaemia vera; ET, essential thrombocythaemia; PMF, primary myelofibrosis; CMML, chronic myelomonocytic leukaemia; CNL, chronic neutrophilic leukaemia; aCML, atypical chronic myeloid leukaemia; CEL, chronic eosinophilic leukaemia; SM, systemic mastocytosis; BP MPN, blast phase myeloproliferative neoplasm.

Further reading

Arber DA, Orazi A, Hasserjian R, et al. The 2016 revision to the World Health Organization (WHO) classification of myeloid neoplasms and acute leukemia. *Blood*. 2016;127(20):2391–405.

Baccarani M, Deininger MW, Rosti G, et al. European LeukemiaNet recommendations for the management of chronic myeloid leukemia: 2013. *Blood*. 2013;122(6):872–84.

Campbell PJ, Griesshammer M, Dohner K, et al. V617F mutation in JAK2 is associated with poorer survival in idiopathic myelofibrosis. *Blood*. 2006;107(5):2098–100.

Cross NC, Melo JV, Feng L, Goldman JM. An optimized multiplex polymerase chain reaction (PCR) for detection of BCR-ABL fusion mRNAs in haematological disorders. *Leukemia*.1994;8(1):186–9.

Dameshek W. Some speculations on the myeloproliferative syn-dromes. *Blood*. 1951;6(4):372–5.

Deininger MW, Goldman JM, Melo JV. The molecular biology of chronic myeloid leukemia. *Blood*. 2000;96(10):3343–56.

Fleischman AG, Maxson JE, Luty SB, et al. The CSF3R T618I mutation causes a lethal neutrophilic neoplasia in mice that is responsive to therapeutic JAK inhibition. *Blood*. 2013;122(22):3628–31.

Gotlib J, Maxson JE, George TI, Tyner JW. The new genetics of chronic neutrophilic leukemia and atypical CML: implications for diagnosis and treatment. *Blood*. 2013;122(10):1707–11.

Groffen J, Stephenson JR, Heisterkamp N, de Klein A, Bartram CR, Grosveld G. Philadelphia chromosomal breakpoints are clustered within a limited region, bcr, on chromosome 22. *Cell*. 1984, 36(1):93–9.

Itzykson R, Kosmider O, Renneville A, et al. Clonal architecture of chronic myelomonocytic leukemias. *Blood*. 2013;121(12):2186–98.

Itzykson R, Kosmider O, Renneville A, et al. Prognostic score including gene mutations in chronic myelo-monocytic leukemia. *J Clin Oncol*. 2013;31(19):2428–36.

James C, Ugo V, Le Couedic JP, et al. A unique clonal JAK2 mutation leading to constitutive signalling causes polycythaemia vera. *Nature*. 2005;434(7037):1144–8.
Jelinek J, Oki Y, Gharibyan V, et al. JAK2 mutation 1849G>T is rare in acute leukemias but can be found in CMML, Philadelphia chromosome-negative CML, and megakaryocytic leukemia. *Blood*. 2005;106(10):3370–3.
Klampfl T, Gisslinger H, Harutyunyan AS, et al. Somatic mutations of calreticulin in myeloproliferative neoplasms. *N Engl J Med*. 2013;369(25):2379–90.
Kralovics R, Passamonti F, Buser AS, et al. A gain-of-function mutation of JAK2 in myeloproliferative disorders. *N Engl J Med*. 2005;352(17):1779–90.
Lasho TL, Pardanani A, Tefferi A. LNK mutations in JAK2 mutation-negative erythrocytosis. *N Engl J Med*. 2010;363(12):1189–90.
Melo JV. The diversity of BCR-ABL fusion proteins and their relationship to leukemia phenotype. *Blood*. 1996;88(7):2375–84.
Nangalia J, Massie CE, Baxter EJ, et al. Somatic CALR mutations in myeloproliferative neoplasms with nonmutated JAK2. *N Engl J Med*. 2013;369(25):2391–405.
Nowell P, Hungerford D. A minute chromosome in human chronic granulocytic leukemia. *Science*. 1960;132:1497.
Rowley JD. A new consistent chromosomal abnormality in chronic myelogenous leukaemia identified by quinacrine fluorescence and Giemsa staining. *Nature*. 1973;243(5405):290–3.
Scott LM, Scott MA, Campbell PJ, Green AR. Progenitors homozygous for the V617F mutation occur in most patients with polycythemia vera, but not essential thrombocythemia. *Blood*. 2006;108(7):2435–7.
Tyner JW, Erickson H, Deininger MW, et al. High-throughput sequencing screen reveals novel, transforming RAS mutations in myeloid leukemia patients. *Blood*. 2009;113(8):1749–55.

Chapter 3

Pathogenesis of myeloproliferative neoplasms

Angela G. Fleischman and Richard A. Van Etten

Introduction to pathogenesis of MPN *33*
The Philadelphia (Ph) chromosome and BCR-ABL1 *34*
Atypical CML and CNL *35*
Systemic mastocytosis and hypereosinophilic syndrome *35*
The classic Ph-negative MPN *35*
MPN signalling and insights from mouse models *38*
Conclusion *43*

Introduction to pathogenesis of MPN

The myeloproliferative neoplasms (MPN) include chronic myeloid leukaemia (CML, also known as chronic myelocytic or myelogenous leukaemia), polycythaemia vera (PV), essential thrombocythaemia (ET), primary myelofibrosis (PMF), and several other closely related conditions. This group of diseases is characterized by several shared features:

- MPN are clonal disorders of haematopoiesis that arise in a haematopoietic stem or early progenitor cell.
- MPN are characterized by overproduction of a particular lineage of mature myeloid-erythroid cells with fairly normal differentiation.
- MPN exhibit a variable tendency to progress to acute leukaemia, usually acute myeloid leukaemia (AML).
- MPN patients exhibit abnormalities of haemostasis and thrombosis.

The individual MPN predominantly affect a single myeloid or erythroid cell type, resulting in an excess of neutrophils and their precursors in CML, erythrocytes in PV, and platelets in ET. However, there is considerable overlap between the clinical features. The current revised World Health Organization (WHO) classification (2016) of the MPN also includes categories for neoplasms with features that overlap between MPN and myelodysplastic syndromes, and for myeloid/lymphoid neoplasms with eosinophilia and mutations in *PDGFRA* or *FGFR1* (Figure 3.1). In this chapter,

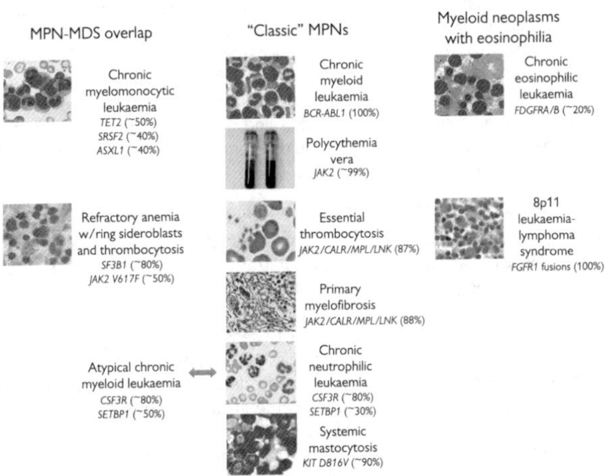

Figure 3.1 Molecular pathogenesis of MPN. The 'classic' MPN together with the MPN-MDS overlap syndromes and myeloid neoplasms with eosinophilia are depicted, with representative histopathology of blood, marrow, or lymph node. Specific mutations and their approximate frequencies in each disease are given in red. Note that atypical chronic myeloid leukaemia and chronic neutrophilic leukaemia are similar and overlapping diseases (also see plate section).

we will touch briefly upon the key pathologic and molecular genetic features of each MPN and then provide a more comprehensive review of our current understanding of the molecular pathogenesis of MPN.

The Philadelphia (Ph) chromosome and BCR-ABL1

The protein product of the Philadelphia chromosome, the BCR-ABL1 fusion protein, is unique to the neoplastic cells and is the fundamental cause of the abnormalities observed in the Ph-positive leukaemias. Understanding the functions of this protein and those encoded by the normal cellular genes involved in the Ph translocation, c-ABL1 and BCR, is essential to elucidate the molecular pathophysiology of these leukaemias. While much is known regarding the structure of the *BCR* and *c-ABL1* genes that come together to form the *BCR-ABL1* fusion gene, there is limited information on their normal function. The protein products of these genes have no intrinsic oncogenic properties. However, together they produce the BCR-ABL1 fusion protein, which is essential for the development of CML.

BCR-ABL1 induces leukemogenesis through kinase-dependent and kinase-independent signalling pathways. Presumably, the specific cellular abnormalities observed in CML are the consequence of aberrant intracellular signalling. Through the use of chemical inhibitors, dominant-negative mutants, and genetically deficient cells and mice, it has been possible to demonstrate that some of the signalling pathways are required for transformation and/or leukemogenesis by BCR-ABL1, validating these downstream pathways as targets for rational therapy of Ph-positive leukaemia. However, there is considerable overlap and redundancy between the different pathways and activation of multiple pathways is probably required for the complete leukaemic phenotype *in vivo*.

Tyrosine kinase activity of BCR-ABL

BCR-ABL1 is a constitutively active tyrosine kinase. The tyrosine kinase activity of ABL1 is absolutely required for transformation by BCR-ABL1, as evidenced by the observation that mutations in the catalytic domain that inactivate kinase activity also abolish transformation. Similarly, mutations in ABL1 that render the catalytic activity sensitive to temperature inactivate transformation at the non-permissive temperature. BCR-ABL1 induces tyrosine phosphorylation of a large number of cellular proteins in haematopoietic cells. As a result, a diverse group of intracellular signalling pathways is activated by BCR-ABL1, in part through induction of protein complexes between tyrosine-phosphorylated proteins and SH2-containing proteins. Some of these pathways overlap with signalling induced by haematopoietic cytokines such as IL-3. A central role for the BCR-ABL1 tyrosine kinase in the pathogenesis of CML has been established by the therapeutic efficacy of small molecule inhibitors of the ABL1 tyrosine kinase. Specific BCR-ABL1 tyrosine kinase inhibitors decrease cellular proliferation of BCR-ABL1-expressing cells *in vitro* by more than 90% but have minimal effects on normal cells. Tyrosine kinase inhibitors have become the standard therapy for most patients with CML. While these agents have a high rate of long-term disease control, they are not able to cure CML. The inability of tyrosine kinase inhibitors to cure CML is thought to reflect a natural resistance of at least a population of leukaemia stem cells to these agents.

Atypical CML and CNL

While the vast majority of patients with CML have acquired the BCR-ABL translocation, a small percentage (about 1–2%) do not. These CML patients without the BCR-ABL translocation are classified as atypical CML (aCML). A closely related but distinct clinical entity is chronic neutrophilic leukaemia (CNL). Recently, mutations in colony stimulating factor 3 (*CSF3R; GCSFR*) and Set binding protein (*SETBP1*) have been identified in patients with CNL and aCML. The most common CSF3R mutation in CNL/aCML is a membrane proximal mutation (T618I) which strongly activates the JAK/signal transducer and activator of transcription (STAT) pathway. The JAK1/2 inhibitor ruxolitinib is currently being investigated therapeutically in clinical trials for CNL/aCML.

Systemic mastocytosis and hypereosinophilic syndrome

Expansion of mast cells or eosinophils characterize systemic mastocytosis (SMCD) and hypereosinophilic syndrome (HES), respectively. Many of the molecular defects associated with mastocytosis involve gain-of-function mutations in *KIT*, the gene encoding the receptor for stem cell factor (SCF), also called kit ligand. SCF is an essential growth factor for normal development and expansion of mast cells from haematopoietic progenitors. Translocations involving platelet-derived growth factor receptor (PDGFR) α/β or fibroblast growth factor receptor 1 (FGFR1) are seen in myeloproliferative HES variants and the former individuals respond quite well to the tyrosine kinase inhibitor imatinib.

The classic Ph-negative MPN

Philadelphia-negative MPN are haematopoietic stem cell (HSC) diseases characterized by an expansion of one or more of the myeloid lineages and include the classical entities PV, ET, and PMF. A number of somatically acquired mutations which activate myeloid growth factor signalling pathways have been identified in Ph-negative MPN. The majority of Ph-negative MPN patients have an identifiable clonal mutation (Figure 3.2).

JAK2 mutations

In 2005 a single gain-of-function point mutation in the Janus kinase 2 (*JAK2*) gene was identified in the majority of patients with Ph-negative MPN concurrently by several groups. This mutation is present in 95–97% of patients

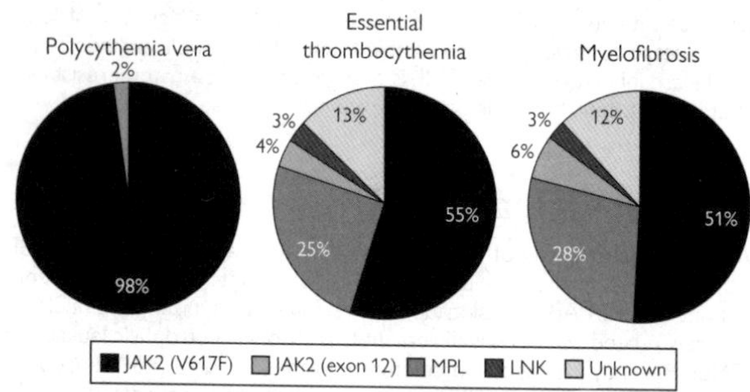

Figure 3.2 Mutational landscape of the Ph-negative MPN. The proportion of mutations in the indicated genes for polycythaemia vera, essential thrombocythaemia, and primary myelofibrosis is indicated.

with PV, 23–75% with ET, and 43–57% with PMF. JAK2 is a cytoplasmic tyrosine kinase that is critical in intracellular signalling by cytokine receptors such as erythropoietin (EPO), thrombopoietin (TPO), interleukin-3 (IL-3), granulocyte colony stimulating factor (G-CSF), and granulocyte macrophage colony stimulating factor (GM-CSF). Mutations in exon 12 of JAK2 are also seen less frequently in MPN and are exclusive to PV. At least eight different somatic missense, deletion, and insertion mutations in *JAK2* exon 12 have been identified in *JAK2*^{V617F}-negative PV. *JAK2*^{V617F} as well as exon 12 mutations confer growth factor independence of Ba/F3 cells when co-expressed with a homodimeric Type I cytokine receptor such as the EPO receptor, the TPO receptor, or the GM-CSF receptor. These mutations result in a constitutively active JAK2, with continual activation of downstream intracellular signalling cascades driving the production of mature myeloid cells even in the absence of ligand.

The presence of *JAK2*^{V617F} haematopoietic cells does not inevitably result in MPN. Haematopoietic cells with the *JAK2*^{V617F} are found in some normal individuals without any evidence of haematologic malignancy. The frequency of detectable *JAK2*^{V617F} mutations in normal individuals increases with age, rising to about 3% of normal elderly people over age 80. Why a *JAK2*^{V617F} clone leads to a clinical MPN in some but not others remain to be determined.

Calreticulin mutations

Mutations in the calreticulin (*CALR*) gene are present in the majority of MPN patients who do not harbour the *JAK2*^{V617F} mutation. The mechanism by which mutated calreticulin contributes to the pathogenesis of MPN is unclear. The most common MPN-associated calreticulin mutations are a 5 bp insertion or a 52 bp deletion. These are frameshift mutations that lead to the loss of most of the C-terminal acidic domain and the KDEL signal replaced by a novel 36 amino acid peptide. Loss of the KDEL sequence suggests that the mutant CALR may have compromised retention or retrieval in the endoplasmic reticulum.

MPL mutations

Mutations in the juxtamembrane region of the TPO receptor *MPL* (MPL-W515L/K) are present in about 6% myelofibrosis (MF) patients and 4% of ET patients, these mutations are not seen in PV patients. The MPN-associated MPL mutations cause constitutive activation of the TPO receptor (MPL) pathway. These mutations endow Ba/F3 cells with cytokine independence and result in a robust myeloproliferative phenotype in mice. MPL^{W515L} or MPL^{W515K} mutations are present in patients with MF or ET at a frequency of approximately 6% and 3%, respectively, but are not observed in patients with PV or other myeloid disorders. *MPL* mutations generally occur in patients without the $JAK2^{V617F}$ mutation, but *MPL* mutations have been reported in patients with the $JAK2^{V617F}$ mutation.

Cooperating mutations in MPN

Cooperating mutations could afford $JAK2^{V617F}$ mutant HSCs an advantage over their wild-type counterparts. Mutations in epigenetic regulators such as *TET2, DNMT3A, ASXL1, EZH2*, and *IDH1/2* have been reported in chronic phase MPN. Loss of TET2, a methylcytosine dioxygenase that converts 5-methylcytosine to 5-hydroxymethylcytosine (5-hmC), causes decreased levels of 5-hmC in MPN patients, which leads to an increase the *in-vivo* repopulating capacity of HSCs. Homozygous loss of TET2 hydroxylase activity does not appear to augment the competitive advantage. *TET2* mutations in MPN may occur either before or after acquisition of the $JAK2^{V617F}$ mutation and can also occur in a distinct clone from the $JAK2^{V617F}$ mutant clone.

Somatic mutations of *ASXL1, DNMT3A, RUNX1*, and *TET2* have also been identified in patients with CML, demonstrating that cooperating mutations can occur in addition to BCR-ABL1. The majority of these cooperating mutations were part of the Ph-positive clone, demonstrating that these cooperating mutations generally occur subsequent to BCR-ABL. However, one patient was found to have a DNMT3A mutation in Ph-negative cells that was also present in Ph-positive cells at diagnosis, implying that the mutation preceded the BCR-ABL1 rearrangement.

One mutation, three diseases

How the $JAK2^{V617F}$ mutation leads to three distinct clinical entities is a central question in MPN. There is evidence that the 'dosage' of $JAK2^{V617F}$ has an effect on disease phenotype (Figure 3.3). Homozygous $JAK2^{V617F}$ erythroid colonies are present in almost all PV patients but are rare in ET patients. To identify disease-specific gene expression profiles, Chen et al. compared the signature of genes upregulated by $JAK2^{V617F}$ in PV versus ET. To reduce interindividual variation, they plucked erythroid colonies from PV and ET patients, genotyped each for $JAK2^{V617F}$ mutational status, pooled the mutant and wild-type colonies from each patient, then compared gene expression in $JAK2^{WT}$ versus $JAK2^{V617F}$ colonies from each patient. A total of 5302 BFU-E colonies from 36 MPN patients (20 ET and 16 PV) were plucked. $JAK2^{V617F}$ was associated with enhanced interferon (IFN) signalling, predominantly involving the IFNγ pathway, in erythroblasts from patients with ET but not in those from patients with PV. STAT1 was preferentially phosphorylated

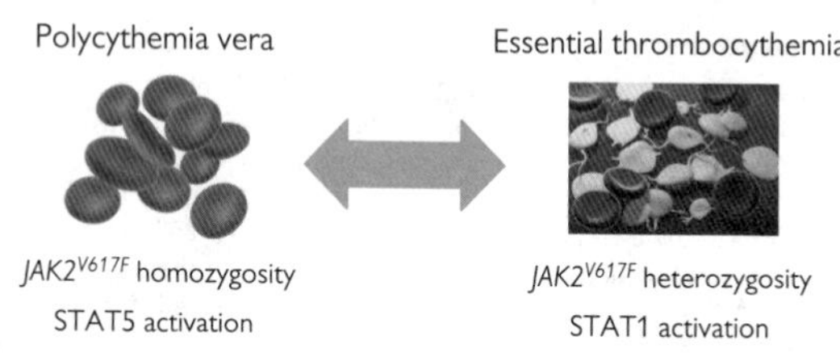

Figure 3.3 Model for determination of phenotype in *JAK2*^{V617F}-positive MPN. Several lines of evidence from studies in human MPN progenitors and mouse models suggest that the phenotype of *JAK2*^{V617F}–positive MPN may be determined by the gene dosage of the *JAK2*^{V617F} mutation, and the balance between STAT1 and STAT5 signalling in the progenitors, which may in turn be influenced by other genetic and non-cell-autonomous factors.

in ET but not PV patients, providing an explanation for the increased IFN signalling in ET but not PV. Lentiviral expression of STAT1 in K562 cells as well as purified CD34$^+$ cord blood cells promoted megakaryocyte differentiation and inhibited erythroid differentiation, supporting an instructive role for STAT1 in megakaryocyte differentiation. Downregulation of STAT1 by ectopic expression of a dominant-negative STAT1 (STAT1DN) in CD34$^+$ progenitors from ET patients resulted in a skewing away from erythroid development and favoured megakaryocyte development. Taken together, these results suggest that the relative strength of STAT1 versus STAT5 signalling induced by *JAK2*^{V617F} may dictate whether an ET or PV phenotype results (Figure 3.3).

Inflammatory cytokines in MPN

Severe constitutional symptoms, such as weight loss, night sweats, and fever are common in MF. These symptoms are related to increased inflammatory cytokines, such as TNF, IL-6, and interferon-γ (IFN-γ). In clinical trials treatment of MPN patients with JAK inhibitors improves constitutional symptoms and reduces plasma inflammatory cytokines.

MPN signalling and insights from mouse models

Murine models of *JAK2*^{V617F}-mutated MPN have been instrumental in advancing our understanding of the disease. Several murine models have been developed to recapitulate *JAK2*^{V617F}-positive MPN *in vivo*. Ectopic expression of mutated calreticulin in haematopoietic cells results in thrombocytosis and splenomegaly. This demonstrates mutated calreticulin can directly induce an MPN phenotype and that murine models will likely prove to be a useful tool to elucidate the pathogenesis of calreticulin-mutated MPN just as they have been for *JAK2*^{V617F}-mutated MPN.

All models develop an MPN but there is variation in the phenotype depending on mouse strain background and type of system used. A PV-like disease with secondary MF arises in lethally irradiated mice transplanted with bone marrow infected with *JAK2*^{V617F} retrovirus. Mice transgenic for *JAK2*^{V617F} develop an ET or PV-like MPN demonstrating that the *JAK2*^{V617F} mutation is sufficient to cause a myeloproliferative phenotype. Knock-in models have been developed in which physiologic levels of either murine or human *JAK2*^{V617F} are produced from the endogenous JAK2 allele. In both models a myeloproliferative phenotype develops, although expression of human *JAK2*^{V617F} results in a much milder disease as compared with expression of murine *JAK2*^{V617F}. In an inducible *JAK2*^{V617F} knock-in model, homozygous *JAK2*^{V617F} results in increased reticulocytes, leukocytes, neutrophils, and platelets with increased expansion of EPO independent colonies, more splenomegaly, and more fibrosis as compared to mice heterozygous for the *JAK2*^{V617F} mutation. To investigate the requirement for individual genes in the development of *JAK2*^{V617F} mediated MPN, various MPN models have been crossed onto knockout backgrounds with the gene of interest.

Use of MPN models to assess response to novel therapies

Mouse MPN models have been useful in providing preclinical rationale for the evaluation of therapeutic agents for the treatment of MPN. Treatment with tyrosine kinase inhibitors (TKIs) rescue mice from a lethal BCR-ABL mediated MPN, consistent with their ability to efficiently reduce the neoplastic burden in humans treated with TKIs. The utility of therapeutic agents for Ph-negative MPN has also been tested in mouse models. Because the molecular pathogenesis of Ph-negative MPN is more complicated than simply *JAK2*^{V617F}, the concordance between mouse models and humans with Ph-negative is somewhat more limited. Nevertheless, the effects of JAK inhibitors in humans recapitulate the effects seen in human MPN patients with JAK inhibitors with respect to normalization of inflammatory cytokines and reduction of spleen size.

Influence of STATs on the MPN phenotype

The use of knockout mouse strains deficient for individual Stats have allowed investigators to define the role of each Stat in the pathogenesis of *JAK2*^{V617F}-mediated MPN (Table 3.1). Intact Stat5 is necessary for the development of erythrocytosis and splenomegaly in two separate *JAK2*^{V617F} MPN mouse models. Using a conditional *JAK2*^{V617F} knock-in crossed with a *Stat5* (*Stat5*$^{fl/fl}$) and *Mx*-Cre transgenic, Mohi and coworkers simultaneously induced expression of *JAK2*^{V617F} and deletion of *Stat5* at 4 weeks after birth. In *Stat5* null mice *JAK2*^{V617F} did not induce abnormal peripheral blood counts, splenomegaly, or fibrosis. Van Etten and coworkers used *Stat5a/b* conditional knockouts to assess the impact of *Stat5a/b* on retrovirally induced *JAK2*^{V617F} MPN. In this model, loss of *Stat5a/b* resulted in the inability of *JAK2*^{V617F} to induce erythrocytosis and splenomegaly, but fibrosis was still present. In both models, loss of *Stat5* in adult HSCs did not impact normal haematopoiesis, suggesting that STAT5 may be a viable therapeutic target in MPN.

Table 3.1 Impact of loss of STATs on disease phenotype in mouse models of *JAK2*^{V617F}-induced MPN

Stat gene knockout	Effect on MPN phenotype
Stat1	↑ erythrocytes ↓ platelets
Stat3	↑ platelets ↑ or no Δ in neutrophils (depending on model)
Stat5	↓ erythrocytes ↓ splenomegaly

In contrast, loss of *Stat3* accentuates the *JAK2*^{V617F} induced MPN phenotype. Skoda et al. crossed transgenic *Scl*-Cre; *JAK2*^{V617F} mice with a conditional *Stat3* knockout and used these as donors for transplantation into lethally irradiated wild-type recipient mice. Loss of *Stat3* reduced the survival of *JAK2*^{V617F} mice. They found that the loss of *Stat3* increased platelet counts but normalized neutrophilia. Moreover, megakaryocytes were actually increased in the spleen and bone marrow of *Stat3* knockout mice and there was a slight increase in MF. Loss of *Stat3* leads to an increase in Stat1. Mohi et al. have also found that crossing of the *JAK2*^{V617F} conditional knock-in onto a conditional *Stat3* knockout background does not impact erythrocytosis, worsened neutrophilia, and reduced survival of mice. HSC and GMP compartments were expanded in *JAK2*^{V617F} mice on a *Stat3* null background; moreover the *Stat3* null background resulted in increased cycling of HSCs. *Stat3* knockout mice have an inflammatory phenotype characterized by inflammatory bowel disease. Although the inflammatory bowel disease was mild in the mice with *Stat3* knocked out in only haematopoietic cells, it is possible that the increased inflammatory milieu played a role in enhancing disease development in the *Stat3* knockout.

The role of *Stat1* in the MPN phenotype has also been investigated. Crossing of *JAK2*^{V617F} transgenic with *Stat1* knockout mice resulted in higher red blood cells and lower platelets than *JAK2*^{V617F} transgenic on a *Stat1* wild-type background. This effect was haematopoietic cell intrinsic, as transplantation of *Stat1* knockout bone marrow cells into a wild-type host resulted in the same increased red blood cells and decreased platelets. These results are consistent with the notion that STAT1 activation drives expansion of platelets resulting in an ET-like phenotype.

Thrombopoietin signalling pathway in MPN mouse models

The TPO receptor (MPL) signalling pathway is not only critical for megakaryocyte development but also plays an important role in haematopoietic stem maintenance. Activation of the MPL pathway is the common thread of MPN driver mutations including *MPL*, *JAK2*, *CALR*, and *LNK*. The observation that TPO mimetics induce reversible marrow fibrosis demonstrates that excessive signalling through MPL is in itself capable of mediating bone marrow fibrosis.

Intact MPL signalling is critical *JAK2*^{V617F} to induce MPN in mouse models. Hitchcock and coworkers crossed *JAK2*^{V617F} transgenic mice onto a *Mpl*$^{-/-}$ background. These mice had thrombocytopenia and lower neutrophils compared to *JAK2*^{V617F} transgenic on a *Mpl* wild-type background. *JAK2*^{V617F} transgenic in a TPO deficient (*Tpo*$^{-/}$) background however had a different effect. *JAK2*^{V617F} restored platelets to a normal level in these mice which are normally thrombocytopenic.

Spivak and coworkers also identified the critical role for a functional TPO receptor in the development of PV in a mouse model. They crossed *JAK2*^{V617F} transgenic mice onto the following backgrounds: homozygous for MPL C40R (a mutation affecting the extracellular domain that disrupts the receptor-ligand interaction, *Tpo*$^{-/-}$, and *Mkl1*$^{-/-}$, which has impaired megakaryopoiesis). Loss of TPO production (*Tpo*$^{-/-}$) delayed erythrocytosis, decreased spleen size, and reversed fibrosis. They found that loss of functional MPL decreased haematocrit, decreased leukocytosis, decreased platelet count, and reduced fibrosis. A single functional *Mpl* gene restored the PV phenotype. The *Mkl1* knockout mice had a slowed rate of increased platelets and haematocrit but no effect on the spleen or fibrosis.

Effect of JAK2^{V617F} on HSCs

It is currently thought that Ph-negative MPN arises from the transformation of an HSC. The HSC origin of the disease was first suggested over 30 years ago with a study showing all haematopoietic cells carried the same polymorphic variant of the X-linked G6PD gene in two female patients with PV. The *JAK2*^{V617F} mutation can be found in granulocytes as well as lymphoid cells from patients with PV, suggesting that the disease originates in a progenitor with lympho-myeloid potential. In addition, HSCs isolated by fluorescence-activated cell sorting from patients with MPN carry the *JAK2*^{V617F} mutation. In mouse MPN models only HSCs are capable of transplanting disease. Together, these data define the disease-initiating cell in MPN as a multipotent progenitor or HSC.

Ectopic expression of *JAK2*^{V617F} fails to confer a competitive advantage over normal HSCs in mouse models, suggesting that non-cell autonomous factors may be required to allow for the clonal expansion of *JAK2*^{V617F} cells in MPN patients. Conditional *hJAK2*^{V617F} knock-in mice have reduced numbers of LKS (Lin^{neg}c-Kit^{+}Sca-1^{+}) cells, increased DNA damage and reduced cell cycling at 26 weeks but not at 6 weeks following pIpC induction of *JAK2*^{V617F}. Apoptosis was decreased in HSC from *JAK2*^{V617F} mice at both 6 and 24 weeks following pIpC induction. In a subsequent paper Kent et al. performed a detailed analysis of the effect of *JAK2*^{V617F} on HSCs. In contrast to normal aged mice, HSC do not expand in aged *JAK2*^{V617F} knock-in mice. In addition, HSC from aged *JAK2*^{V617F} mice have inferior repopulation ability in secondary recipients as well as delayed entry into the cell cycle.

A similar study by Lundberg et al. used an inducible *hJAK2*^{V617F} transgenic model to evaluate the effect of *JAK2*^{V617F} on the function and competitive abilities of HSC. They found that at a ratio of 1:10, *JAK2*^{V617F} cells were able to out-compete wild-type bone marrow with increased numbers of LKS and LT-HSC. However, when limiting dilution transplantation was performed, mice that reconstituted with *JAK2*^{V617F} haematopoietic cells did not have an increased LKS compartment at 20 weeks post-transplant.

Interestingly, of the mice that were transplanted with a single *JAK2*^{V617F} HSC and had subsequent engraftment only a fraction developed an MPN phenotype. This finding reiterates that presence of haematopoietic cells with the *JAK2*^{V617F} mutation does not invariably lead to development of an MPN.

TET2 mutations in MPN

The impact of concurrent loss of *Tet2* and *JAK2*^{V617F} has been explored using mouse models. Kameda et al. used fetal liver cells from *JAK2*^{V617F} transgenic in a *Tet2* wild-type, *Tet2*-knockdown heterozygous, or *Tet2* homozygous background to transplant wild-type lethally irradiated hosts. In the context of wild-type *JAK2*, mice transplanted with *Tet2* deficient cells had normal blood counts, no splenomegaly, and minimal extramedullary haematopoiesis of lung and liver. *JAK2*^{V617F} on a *Tet2*-deficient background had prolonged leukocytosis, increased LKS cells in the bone marrow and spleen, increased splenomegaly, and increased extramedullary haematopoiesis over *JAK2*^{V617F} mice on a wild-type background. *In vitro* serial colony plating assays demonstrated that *JAK2*^{V617F} HSC had decreased self-renewal capabilities, but this was rescued by knockdown of *Tet2*. In addition, *JAK2*^{V617F} (*Tet2* wild-type) cells had lower chimerism and did not develop an MPN phenotype (but developed leukopenia) upon secondary transplantation whereas double mutant cells were able to sustain engraftment in secondary recipients and produced an MPN phenotype.

Chen and colleagues also found that concomitant *JAK2*^{V617F} and loss of *Tet2* accentuates the MPN phenotype in mice. They crossed conditional *JAK2*^{V617F} mice with *Tet2* conditional knockout mice (*Vav*-Cre to knockout *Tet2* in the haematopoietic compartment). Loss of *Tet2* increased *JAK2*^{V617F} driven splenomegaly and leukocytosis in mice greater than 6 months old but did not impact haematocrit or platelet numbers. *Tet2* loss accentuated the number of megakaryocytes with increased atypia. They did not see any evidence of leukaemic transformation in compound mutant mice, nor did they see any impact of loss of *Tet2* on survival of mice. They also found that loss of *Tet2* confers a strong advantage in competitive repopulation assays, both alone as well as in concert with *JAK2*^{V617F}. *Tet2* homozygous null HSC have an increased *in vitro* replating ability, which is slightly enhanced by the addition of *JAK2*^{V617F} (whereas *JAK2*^{V617F} alone does not increase serial replating ability). *Tet2* loss may drive clonal expansion of HSCs, and *JAK2*^{V617F} drives expansion of downstream precursor cell populations; these two effects may result in disease progression. *TET2* mutations in human MPN can be acquired temporally either before or after the *JAK2*^{V617F} mutation. To determine whether the order in which mutations are acquired affects the disease phenotype, Kent et al. compared characteristics of MPN patients who had acquired *TET2* mutations first with those who had acquired *JAK2*^{V617F} mutations first. Patients who acquired a *TET2* mutation first presented on average 12.3 years later than patients who acquired *JAK2*^{V617F} first and had a lower proportion of *JAK2*^{V617F} homozygous erythroid colonies, suggesting that the order of acquisition affected both cellular composition and disease evolution. They analysed the haematopoietic stem cell compartments from these MPN patients and found that acquisition of a *JAK2*^{V617F} mutation reduces the competitiveness of *TET2* single mutant HSCs. In contrast, acquisition of a *TET2* mutation enhances the competitiveness of *JAK2*^{V617F} single mutant HSCs.

Conclusion

MPN are clonal haematologic disorders characterized by the unrestrained expansion of mature myeloid cells resulting from somatically acquired activating mutations in myeloid development signalling pathways. Each MPN has a unique molecular pathogenesis that drives its distinct clinical features. Targeted therapies with TKIs are extremely effective in reducing the neoplastic clone (such as imatinib in CML), whereas targeted therapies in other MPN do not impact the neoplastic burden (such as ruxolitinib in MF). A comprehensive understanding of the key drivers of disease pathogenesis in MPN will facilitate the development of therapeutic agents with curative potential.

Further reading

Adamson JW, Fialkow PJ, Murphy S, Prchal JF, Steinmann L. Polycythemia vera: stem-cell and probable clonal origin of the disease. *N Engl J Med*. 1976;295(17):913–16.

Akada H, Yan D, Zou H, Fiering S, Hutchison RE, Mohi MG. Conditional expression of heterozygous or homozygous Jak2V617F from its endogenous promoter induces a polycythemia vera-like disease. *Blood*. 2010;115(17):3589–97.

Bumm TG, Elsea C, Corbin AS, et al. Characterization of murine JAK2V617F-positive myeloproliferative disease. *Cancer Res*. 2006;66(23):11156–65.

Chen E, Beer PA, Godfrey AL, et al. Distinct clinical phenotypes associated with JAK2V617F reflect differential STAT1 signaling. *Cancer Cell*. 2010;18(5):524–35.

Chou FS, Mulloy JC. The thrombopoietin/MPL pathway in hematopoiesis and leukemogenesis. *J Cell Biochem*. 2011;112(6):1491–8.

Duek A, Lundberg P, Shimizu T, et al. Loss of Stat1 decreases megakaryopoiesis and favors erythropoiesis in a JAK2-V617F-driven mouse model of MPNs. *Blood*. 2014;123(25):3943–50.

Grisouard J, Shimizu T, Duek A, et al. Deletion of Stat3 in hematopoietic cells enhances thrombocytosis and shortens survival in a JAK2-V617F mouse model of MPN. *Blood*. 2015;125(13):2131–40.

Jamieson CH, Gotlib J, Durocher JA, et al. The JAK2 V617F mutation occurs in hematopoietic stem cells in polycythemia vera and predisposes toward erythroid differentiation. *Proc Natl Acad Sci USA*. 2006;103(16):6224–9.

Kim E, Abdel-Wahab O. Focus on the epigenome in the myeloproliferative neoplasms. *Hematology Am Soc Hematol Educ Program*. 2013;2013:538–44.

Klampfl T, Gisslinger H, Harutyunyan AS, et al. Somatic mutations of calreticulin in myeloproliferative neoplasms. *N Engl J Med*. 2013;369(25):2379–90.

Lacout C, Pisani DF, Tulliez M, Gachelin FM, Vainchenker W, Villeval JL. JAK2V617F expression in murine hematopoietic cells leads to MPD mimicking human PV with secondary myelofibrosis. *Blood*. 2006;108(5):1652–60.

Li J, Kent DG, Chen E, Green AR. Mouse models of myeloproliferative neoplasms: JAK of all grades. *Dis Model Mech*. 2011;4(3):311–17.

Li J, Spensberger D, Ahn JS, Anand S, et al. JAK2 V617F impairs hematopoietic stem cell function in a conditional knock-in mouse model of JAK2 V617F-positive essential thrombocythemia. *Blood*. 2010;116(9):1528–38.

Marty C, Harini N, Pecquet C, et al. Calr mutants retroviral mouse models lead to a myeloproliferative neoplasm mimicking an essential thrombocythemia progressing to a myelofibrosis. *Blood*. 2014;124(21):157a.

McKerrell T, Park N, Moreno T, et al. Leukemia-associated somatic mutations drive distinct patterns of age-related clonal hemopoiesis. *Cell Rep*. 2015;10(8):1239–45.

Mullally A, Lane SW, Ball B, et al. Physiological Jak2V617F expression causes a lethal myeloproliferative neoplasm with differential effects on hematopoietic stem and progenitor cells. *Cancer Cell*. 2010;17(6):584–96.

Nangalia J, Massie CE, Baxter EJ, et al. Somatic CALR mutations in myeloproliferative neoplasms with nonmutated JAK2. *N Engl J Med*. 2013;369(25):2391–405.

Ortmann CA, Kent DG, Nangalia J, et al. Effect of mutation order on myeloproliferative neoplasms. *N Engl J Med*. 2015;372(7):601–12.

Schmidt M, Rinke J, Schafer V, et al. Molecular-defined clonal evolution in patients with chronic myeloid leukemia independent of the BCR-ABL status. *Leukemia*. 2014;28(12):2292–9.

Scott LM, Scott MA, Campbell PJ, Green AR. Progenitors homozygous for the V617F mutation occur in most patients with polycythemia vera, but not essential thrombocythemia. *Blood*. 2006;108(7):2435–7.

Shide K, Shimoda HK, Kumano T, et al. Development of ET, primary myelofibrosis and PV in mice expressing JAK2 V617F. *Leukemia*. 2008;22(1):87–95.

Spivak JL, Merchant A, Williams DM, et al. A functional thrombopoietin receptor is required for full expression of phenotype in a JAK2 V617F transgenic mouse model of polycythemia vera. *Blood*. 2012;120(21):427a.

Tiedt R, Coers J, Ziegler S, Wiestner A, et al. Pronounced thrombocytosis in transgenic mice expressing reduced levels of Mpl in platelets and terminally differentiated megakaryocytes. *Blood*. 2009;113(8):1768–77.

Tiedt R, Hao-Shen H, Sobas MA, et al. Ratio of mutant JAK2-V617F to wild-type Jak2 determines the MPD phenotypes in transgenic mice. *Blood*. 2008;111(8):3931–40.

Vannucchi AM, Rotunno G, Bartalucci N, et al. Calreticulin mutation-specific immunostaining in myeloproliferative neoplasms: pathogenetic insight and diagnostic value. *Leukemia*. 2014;28(9):1811–18.

Walz C, Ahmed W, Lazarides K, et al. Essential role for Stat5a/b in myeloproliferative neoplasms induced by BCR-ABL1 and JAK2(V617F) in mice. *Blood*. 2012;119(15):3550–60.

Wernig G, Mercher T, Okabe R, Levine RL, Lee BH, Gilliland DG. Expression of Jak2V617F causes a polycythemia vera-like disease with associated myelofibrosis in a murine bone marrow transplant model. *Blood*. 2006; 107:4274–81.

Xing S, Wanting TH, Zhao W, et al. Transgenic expression of JAK2V617F causes myeloproliferative disorders in mice. *Blood*. 2008;111(10):5109–17.

Yan D, Hutchison RE, Mohi G. Critical requirement for Stat5 in a mouse model of polycythemia vera. *Blood*. 2012;119(15):3539–49.

Zaleskas VM, Krause DS, Lazarides K, et al. Molecular pathogenesis and therapy of polycythemia induced in mice by JAK2 V617F. *PLoS One*. 2006; 1:e18.

Chapter 4

Haematopathology of classic myeloproliferative neoplasms

Hans Michael Kvasnicka and Jürgen Thiele

Introduction *46*
Impact of the 2016 WHO myeloid classification in classic MPN *46*
Reproducibility of the 2016 WHO morphological criteria *47*
Standardization of morphological MPN diagnosis *50*
Initial stages of MPN *51*
Clinical impact of prefibrotic/early PMF *52*
Overt (classical) primary myelofibrosis *55*
Essential thrombocythaemia *56*
Polycythaemia vera *58*
Summary *60*

Introduction

A principal objective of the revised 2016 Fourth Edition of the World Health Organization (WHO) classification of myeloid neoplasms is to enable pathologists and physicians to reduce diagnostic uncertainty by improving the accuracy of the diagnostic criteria to help optimize clinical management of patients. In most patients, this requires an analysis of the morphology of peripheral blood and bone marrow (BM), immunophenotyping, cytogenetics, molecular genetics, and clinical features of patients. The 2016 WHO classification of myeloproliferative neoplasms (MPN) entities comprise of the 'classic' MPN (a historical reference to William Dameshek's original classification, discussed in Chapter 1), which includes BCR/ABL1-positive chronic myeloid leukaemia (CML), primary myelofibrosis (PMF), essential thrombocythaemia (ET), polycythaemia vera (PV), and 'non-classic' MPN, which include chronic neutrophilic leukaemia (CNL), chronic eosinophilic leukaemias not otherwise specified (CEL, NOS) and an unclassifiable MPN group (MPN-U). In this chapter we discuss the haematopathological characteristics of the classic Ph-negative MPN, PMF, ET, and PV. CML, while the non-classic MPN are discussed in Chapters 7 and 12, respectively.

Impact of the 2016 WHO myeloid classification in classic MPN

For patients with PMF, ET, and PV, the revised criteria require an assessment of the MPN-associated genetic driver mutations, JAK2V617F, JAK2 exon 12, MPLW515L/K and calreticulin (CALR). Furthermore, the diagnostic haemoglobin thresholds for PV were reduced to 16.5 g/dL in males and 16.0 g/dL in females following the recognition of 'masked' prepolycythaemic PV, previously diagnosed as ET. It also underscores the importance of BM morphology in MPN patients, particularly in the distinction of 'masked' PV and ET, and also 'early' or 'prefibrotic' PMF (pre-PMF) and ET. Megakaryocytic morphology associated with variable amounts of granulocytic and erythroid proliferation represents the histopathological denominator in MPN. Diagnosis of classical MPN requires absence of significant dysgranulopoiesis or dyserythropoiesis to separate these cases from myelodysplastic syndromes (MDS) or MDS/MPN overlaps.

The accurate diagnosis of MPN subtypes depends on a representative and treatment-naive BM trephine biopsy with a minimal length of 1.5 cm taken at a right angle from the cortical bone. Discrimination between MPN subtypes (i.e. histopathological diagnosis), should be based on standardized morphological features. The spatial distribution of the megakaryocytes within the BM, their nuclear abnormalities as well as maturation defects are important, for example to differentiate ET from pre-PMF. Standardization of diagnosis is significantly improved by the 2016 WHO criteria (Box 4.1 and Figure 4.1). Parenthetically, it is important to emphasize that the WHO classification is not aimed to guarantee a complete diagnostic specificity or to identify all biological true cases of MPN, rather it is a work in progress and further refinements may well be required. In this regard, it is important

Box 4.1 Key features of pre-PMF according to WHO

- Increased cellularity (age-matched) with predominant neutrophil granulopoiesis
- Increased megakaryopoiesis, small to large
- Atypical histotopography of megakaryocytes
  - endosteal translocation
  - formation of dense clusters*
- Distinctive nuclear features of megakaryocytes
  - hypolobulation (bulbous/cloud-like)
  - maturation defects

*WHO definition of a megakaryocyte cluster: three or more megakaryocytes lying strictly adjacent—without other haematopoietic cells lying in between.

Source: data from Arber DA, et al. (2016). The 2016 revision to the World Health Organization classification of myeloid neoplasms and acute leukemia. *Blood*. 127(20):2391–405. https://doi.org/10.1182/blood-2016-03-643544.

to incorporate both morphology and molecular genetics for optimal classification. Recent work on the unfolding genomic landscape highlights the importance of integrating these findings with BM morphology. Along these lines, the order of acquisition of the somatic mutations has observed to influence the biology and clinical features in MPN. For example, the order in which JAK2V617F and TET2 mutations were acquired can determine the phenotype of the MPN, risk of thrombosis, and might also be predictive for therapy. Further studies are required to elucidate these and other factors, such as the precise role of inflammatory cytokines.

Reproducibility of the 2016 WHO morphological criteria

Over the past few years, the reproducibility of the histological characteristics defining MPN subtypes has been critically discussed. Controversy is in particular focused on pre-PMF presenting with thrombocythaemia and the crucial discrimination from ET. Along these lines, the clinical usefulness of the WHO approach for daily routine has been challenged. Conversely, an increasing number of investigators were able to validate the diagnostic accuracy of the WHO-defined morphological BM features. These reports strongly support the definition of an early/prefibrotic stage of PMF which can to be separated from ET by histological and haematological features. Furthermore, an interobserver agreement of more than 80% (Table 4.1 and Table 4.2) was reported in subsequently performed studies involving many patients and local pathologists from different institutions and central review. This result is comparable or even better than the reported level of diagnostic concordance presented by international panel evaluations for assessing dysplasia in MDS or classification of lymphomas. However, other studies based on the old Polycythemia Vera Study Group (PVSG) definition of ET challenged the accuracy of these confirmatory data. Notably,

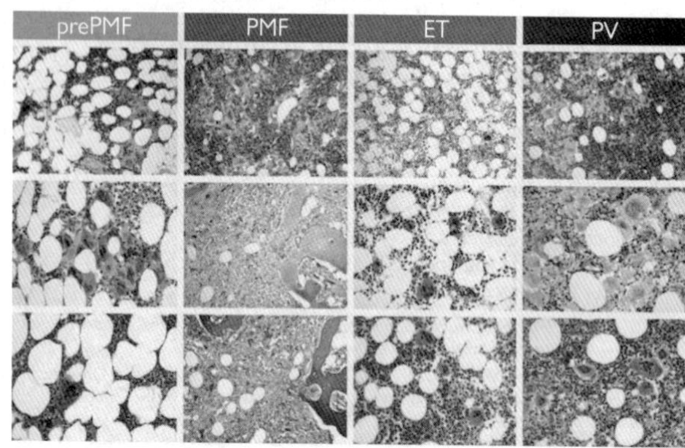

Figure 4.1 Bone marrow morphology in WHO-defined prefibrotic/early primary myelofibrosis (prePMF), advanced primary myelofibrosis (PMF), essential thrombocythaemia (ET), and polycythaemia vera (PV). **Prefibrotic/early primary myelofibrosis (prePMF):** remarkable hypercellularity for advanced age revealing large clusters of megakaryocytes abnormally dislocated towards the trabecular bone. In addition to megakaryocyte proliferation, there is a conspicuous increase in neutrophil granulopoiesis accompanied by reduction of nucleated erythroid precursors. Clustered small to giant megakaryocytes show a prevalence of striking maturation defects including cloud-like, hypolobulated, and hyperchromatic nuclei with only some irregular foldings. No significant increase in reticulin fibres. **Advanced primary myelofibrosis (PMF):** streaming-like pattern of haematopoiesis including atypical megakaryocytes in addition to initial osteosclerosis. Densely clustered megakaryocytes surrounded by neutrophil granulopoiesis but only a very few erythrocyte precursors. Clustered megakaryocytes are lying along a dilated sinus and reveal severe aberrations of maturation including cloud-like, dense, or abnormally lobulated nuclei. Overt myelofibrosis showing bundles of collagen between a dense network of reticulin and osteosclerosis. **Essential thrombocythaemia (ET):** age-matched cellularity, except for a prominent increase in large to giant megakaryocytes loosely clustered or dispersed throughout the bone marrow space. No proliferation or significant left shift of neutrophil granulopoiesis or erythropoiesis surrounding giant mature megakaryocytes. Conspicuous increase in large megakaryocytes without maturation defects showing hyperlobulated, occasionally staghorn-like nuclei. No increase in reticulin fibres, but giant megakaryocytes with deep foldings of their nuclei. **Polycythaemia vera (PV):** conspicuous hypercellularity for age with increase of all three cell lineages (panmyelosis) including extended islets of nucleated erythroid precursors and dispersed mature megakaryocytes. Prominent enlargement of erythropoiesis surrounded by left-shifted neutrophil granulopoiesis. Megakaryocytes of different size ranging from small to giant ones are increased and may be clustered, but fail to show maturation defects. No increase in reticulin fibres (also see plate section).

Reproduced courtesy of Prof. Dr. Hans Michael Kvasnicka, University Cancer Centre, Frankfurt, Germany.

Table 4.1 Reproducibility of the WHO criteria for prePMF and ET (studies with formal assessment of concordance between pathologists)

Study	Consensus	N	Study	Consensus	N
Barbui T, et al. Survival and disease progression in essential thrombocythemia are significantly influenced by accurate morphologic diagnosis: an international study of 1,104 patients. *J Clin Oncol.* 2011;29(23):3179–84.	81%	1104	Wilkins BS, et al. Bone marrow pathology in essential thrombocythemia: interobserver reliability and utility for identifying disease subtypes. *Blood.* 2008;111(1):60–70.	53%	370
Thiele J, et al. Essential thrombocythemia versus early primary myelofibrosis: a multicenter study to validate the WHO classification. *Blood.* 2011;117(21):5710–8.	88%	295	Brousseau M, et al. Practical application and clinical impact of the WHO histopathological criteria on bone marrow biopsy for the diagnosis of essential thrombocythemia versus prefibrotic primary myelofibrosis. *Histopathology.* 2010;56(6):758–67.	65%	127
Gisslinger H, et al. Anagrelide compared with hydroxyurea in WHO-classified essential thrombocythemia: the ANAHYDRET Study, a randomized controlled trial. *Blood.* 2013;121(10):1720–8.	83%	259	Koopmans SM, et al. Reproducibility of histologic classification in nonfibrotic myeloproliferative neoplasia. *Am J Clin Pathol.* 2011 Oct;136(4):618–24. DOI:10.1309/AJCP2UG9SGGWAHUA.	70%	56
Madelung AB, et al. WHO-defined classification of myeloproliferative neoplasms: morphological reproducibility and clinical correlations—The Danish experience. *Am J Hematol.* 2013;DOI:10.1002/ajh.23554.	83%	272	Buhr T, et al. European Bone Marrow Working Group trial on reproducibility of World Health Organization criteria to discriminate essential thrombocythemia from prefibrotic primary myelofibrosis. *Haematologica.* 2012;97(3):360–5.	62%	102
Gianelli U, et al. The European Consensus on grading of bone marrow fibrosis allows a better prognostication of patients with primary myelofibrosis. *Mod Pathol.* 2012;25(9):1193–202.	76%	103			
Overall consensus	82%	2033	Overall consensus	63%	655

Table 4.2 Additional studies supporting validity of the WHO criteria (n=736)

Study	N
Florena AM, et al. Value of bone marrow biopsy in the diagnosis of essential thrombocythemia. *Haematologica*. 2004;89(8):911–9.	142
Kreft A, et al. The incidence of myelofibrosis in essential thrombocythaemia, polycythaemia vera and chronic idiopathic myelofibrosis: a retrospective evaluation of sequential bone marrow biopsies. *Acta Haematol*. 2005;113(2):137–43.	275
Gianelli U, et al. Essential thrombocythemia or chronic idiopathic myelofibrosis? A single-center study based on hematopoietic bone marrow histology. *Leuk Lymphoma*. 2006;47(9):1774–81.	116
Gianelli U, et al. The significance of bone marrow biopsy and JAK2V617F mutation in the differential diagnosis between the 'early' prepolycy-themic phase of polycythaemia vera and essential thrombocythemia. *Am J Clin Pathol*. 2008;130(3):336–42.	50
Vener C, et al. Prognostic implications of the European consensus for grading of bone marrow fibrosis in chronic idiopathic myelofibrosis. *Blood*. 2008;111(4):1862–5.	113
Ejerblad E, et al. Diagnosis according to World Health Organization determines the long-term prognosis in patients with myeloproliferative neoplasms treated with anagrelide: results of a prospective long-term follow-up. *Hematology*. 2013;18(1):8–13.	40

in a conspicuously wide range of included cases high levels of BM fibrosis (37–76% among the panellists) as well as osteosclerosis were reported in these series although the included patients were explicitly categorized as ET according to the diagnostic guidelines of the PVSG. Following strictly the WHO criteria of MPN, however, (minor) reticulin fibrosis (MF-1) is extremely rare at onset of ET and observed in less than 5% of cases. Furthermore, the diagnostic specificity of haematological features in early/prefibrotic PMF has been recently questioned. However, results from a large series underscore the WHO postulate that integration of histological and haematological parameters is essential for subtyping MPN. Altogether, the diagnosis of specific MPN subtypes is directed by a strong consensus of clinical, morphological, and molecular genetic findings according to the WHO guidelines.

Standardization of morphological MPN diagnosis

The standardization of relevant BM features is mandatory to recognize characteristic and to assess patterns that enable an accurate discrimination between the MPN subtypes. Characteristic constellations of important features like cellularity, distinctive features of megakaryocytes as well as erythropoiesis and neutrophil granulopoiesis in context with the grade of BM fibrosis are key to the differential diagnosis of MPN subtypes, especially in initial disease stages that might mimic ET because of elevated platelet counts. In order to evaluate haematopoietic cellularity, age-associated changes must be considered, especially when evaluating the subcortical marrow spaces. Furthermore, for the accurate assessment of BM fibrosis, the simplified three-graded system proposed by the WHO should be applied because it has shown clinical relevance.

Although the level of unclassifiable cases (MPN-U) significantly correlates with the experience of the investigator, the amount of unclear cases generally should not exceed a range between 5% and 10%. In this regard, diagnostic reproducibility can be improved by a representative, properly sized BM trephine biopsy obtained at diagnosis. Sometimes clinicians may not be fully conversant of the clinical utility of BM morphology, or might require additional BM biopsy procedure training. Consequently, their cooperating pathologists are not familiar with an elaborate processing and evaluation of the specimens that include advanced techniques and the use of standardized features that facilitate the histopathological diagnosis of MPN.

Initial stages of MPN

The diagnosis of initial MPN raises several clinical issues, particularly because typical haematological features and symptoms generally found in overt stages of MPN may not be present at this disease stage. The overlap in clinical presentation is in some cases challenging for the haematologist; however, scrutinized assessment of BM features and integration of molecular data (*JAK2, CALR*, and *MPL*) guides the differential diagnosis in early disease stage. In this regard, recent studies emphasized the stepwise evolution of pre-PMF with lower overall survival, increased risk of myelofibrotic transformation, and significantly more complications as compared to ET. Although evolution to overt myelofibrosis and blastic transformation might also occur in ET patients, the overall risk is significantly lower than in pre-PMF patients. Furthermore, identification of initial stage MPN enables early therapeutic intervention to prevent disease-related complications. It is important to recognize that major thrombotic and other complications can sometime precede a definite clinical diagnosis of MPN. Along these lines, several studies have described patients with positive driver mutation status and cerebral or splanchnic vein thrombosis including Budd–Chiari syndrome but without clinical features of overt MPN. Unfortunately, in most series a detailed description of BM findings is missing and therefore it is not clear how many of these occult cases represent initial stages of MPN. Furthermore, the heterogenous group of MDS/MPN overlaps with ring sideroblasts and thrombocytosis (MDS/MPN-RS-T) must be excluded, particularly when myelodysplastic features are not very conspicuous. The occurrence of ring sideroblasts is not uncommon in overt MPN and therefore the demonstration of an MPN-associated driver mutation may cause differential diagnostic problems, as has been previously outlined.

Clinical impact of prefibrotic/early PMF

The differentiation between ET and pre-PMF with thrombocythaemia is clinically relevant and impacts treatment. In the majority of patients with pre-PMF the clinical presentation may include mild anaemia, few circulating immature white blood cells, and splenomegaly (Table 4.3). Table 4.3 depicts the major and minor diagnostic criteria in the new WHO edition.

Following conventional therapy, studies such as a large international effort assessing over 1000 patients (891 ET and 180 pre-PMF) have demonstrated significant lower survival rates in pre-PMF when diagnosed according to the 2016 WHO MPN diagnostic criteria. These data confirmed a significant shorter overall and event-free survival, and an increased risk of overt myelofibrotic progression as well as transformation to blast phase in pre-PMF patients. As compared with ET, a significantly higher rate of haemorrhagic complications was shown in pre-PMF. These data indicate a higher risk of major bleeding in patients with pre-PMF, which, in some cases, was considered to be related to aspirin medication. Finally, it has been reported that increased white blood cell counts in pre-PMF exert a significant impact on the incidence of arterial and venous thrombotic events.

The importance of BM histopathology for discriminating ET from pre-PMF as well as the impact on overall outcome has been confirmed in a prospective, long-term observational study. In addition, randomized studies enrolling patients with WHO-defined ET treated with anagrelide or hydroxyurea revealed no significant differences regarding the incidence of arterial and venous thrombosis (minor and major), severe bleeding, or transformation into overt MF or blast phase between both groups during an observation time of 12 and 36 months. In pre-PMF the BM is hypercellular, with substantial neutrophil granulocytic and megakaryocytic proliferation, and reduced nucleated red cell precursors in the absence of overt fibrosis (Box 4.1, Figure 4.1, and Figure 4.2). In this regard, although characteristic, significant BM reticulin fibrosis is not a specific feature for the diagnosis of PMF. Morphology of megakaryocytes in PMF usually demonstrated a higher degree of cytological atypia (megakaryocytic dysplasia) than in any other subtype of MPN, particularly ET. It is important to underline, that early stages of PMF without significant reticulin fibrosis may not be identified and separated from ET by clinical features alone.

In terms of clinically relevant complications, such as myelofibrotic transformation, the morphological assessment of increasing fibre grades (reticulin/collagen) should be clearly separated from the evolution, with clinical features of PMF with extramedullary haematopoiesis. The calculated overall incidence of overt myelofibrotic progression in pre-PMF after 5 and 10 years of follow-up is 2.3% and 12.3%, respectively. In contrast, in WHO-defined ET cases the calculated risk was only 0.2% and 0.8% at 5 and 10 years. For the transformation to blast phase, similar differences were reported. The 10- and 15-years cumulative incidences for ET were calculated as 0.7% and 2.1%, contrasting a significant higher risk of blastic transformation in pre-PMF (10 years: 5.8%; 15 years: 11.7%). In summary, when applying the diagnostic guidelines of the WHO, progression to overt myelofibrosis and/or blast phase is rarely seen in ET in the first 5 years of follow-up. Conversely, patients with PMF may present initially with few disease features, and thereafter, following a poorly defined period, develop signs and symptoms of ineffective hemopoiesis, with the BM showing features of myelodysplasia and blast phase.

Table 4.3 The 2016 edition of the WHO criteria for the diagnosis of primary myelofibrosis (PMF), essential thrombocythaemia (ET), and polycythaemia vera (PV)

prePMF	Overt PMF	ET	PV
Major criteria Megakaryocytic proliferation and atypia, without reticulin fibrosis >grade 1 and accompanied by increased age-adjusted bone marrow cellularity, granulocytic proliferation and often decreased erythropoiesis Not meeting WHO criteria for ET, PV, BCR-ABL1+ CML, MDS, or other myeloid neoplasms Presence of JAK2, CALR, or MPL mutation or in the absence of these mutations, presence of another clonal marker* or absence of minor reactive myelofibrosis** **Minor criteria***** Anaemia not attributed to a comorbid condition	**Major criteria** Presence of megakaryocytic proliferation and atypia, usually accompanied by either reticulin and/or collagen fibrosis grades 2 or 3 Not meeting WHO criteria for ET, PV, BCR-ABL1+ CML, MDS, or other myeloid neoplasms Presence of JAK2, CALR, or MPL mutation or in the absence of these mutations, presence of another clonal marker* or absence of reactive myelofibrosis** **Minor criteria***** Anaemia not attributed to a comorbid condition Leukocytosis >11K/uL Palpable splenomegaly LDH increased to above upper normal limit of institutional reference range Leukoerythroblastosis	**Major criteria** Platelet count equal to or greater than 450 x 10^9/uL Bone marrow biopsy showing proliferation mainly of the megakaryocyte lineage with increased numbers of enlarged, mature megakaryocytes with hyperlobulated nuclei. No significant increase or left shift of neutrophil granulopoiesis or erythropoiesis and very rarely minor increase in reticulin fibres. Not meeting WHO criteria for BCR-ABL1+ CML, PV, PMF, MDS, or other myeloid neoplasms Presence of JAK2, CALR, or MPL mutation **Minor criteria** Presence of a clonal marker or absence of evidence for reactive thrombocytosis	**Major criteria** Hb >16.5 g/dL in men, Hb >16.0 g/dL in women OR, Hct > 49% in men, Hct >48% in women OR, Increased red cell mass Bone marrow biopsy showing hypercellularity for age with trilineage growth (panmyelosis) including prominent erythroid, granulocytic, and megakaryocytic proliferation with pleomorphic megakaryocytes (differences in size) Presence of JAK2 mutation **Minor criteria** Subnormal serum EPO level

(Continued)

Table 4.3 *(contd.)*

prePMF	Overt PMF	ET	PV
Palpable splenomegaly lactate dehydrogenase (LDH) increased to above upper normal limit of institutional reference range			
Diagnosis of prePMF requires meeting all three major criteria, and minor criteria	Diagnosis of overt PMF requires meeting all three major criteria, and minor criteria	Diagnosis of ET requires meeting all four major criteria or the first three major criteria and one of the minor criteria	Diagnosis of PV requires meeting either all three major criteria, or the first two major criteria and the minor criterion
			In cases with sustained absolute erythrocytosis (Hb levels >18.5 g/dL, Hct >55.5% in men or >16.5 g/dL, 49.5% in women), bone marrow biopsy may not be necessary for diagnosis if major criterion 3 and the minor criterion are present

* In the absence of any of the three major clonal mutations, the search for the most frequent accompanying mutations (ASXL1, EZH2, TET2, IDH1/IDH2, SRSF2, SF3B1) is of help in determining the clonal nature of the disease.

**Bone marrow fibrosis, secondary to infection, autoimmune disorder, or other chronic inflammatory condition, hairy cell leukaemia or other lymphoid neoplasm, metastatic malignancy, or toxic (chronic) myelopathies.

*** Confirmed in two consecutive determinations.

Adapted from Arber DA, et al. The 2016 revision to the World Health Organization classification of myeloid neoplasms and acute leukemia. *Blood*. 127(20):2391–2405. https://doi.org/10.1182/blood-2016-03-643544. Reprinted with permission from the American Society of Hematology.

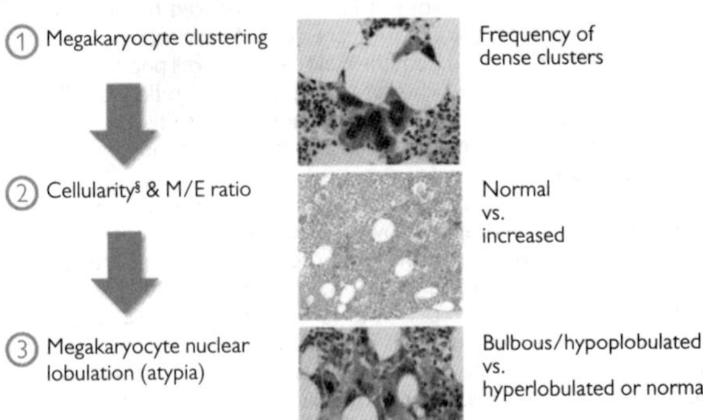

Figure 4.2 Relative importance of distinctive morphological features for the diagnosis of prefibrotic/early primary myelofibrosis (pre-MF) (also see plate section).
Reproduced courtesy of Prof. Hans Michael Kvasnicka, University Cancer Centre, Frankfurt, Germany.

Overt (classical) primary myelofibrosis

Advanced stages of PMF are consistent with classical MF with myeloid metaplasia. The clinical picture of overt PMF includes a leukoerythroblastic peripheral blood smear with teardrop poikilocytosis, splenomegaly, and anaemia of varying degree (Table 4.3). BM cellularity may be variable and often patchy separated by adipose tissue or grossly developed fibrosis generating a streaming effect. Neutrophil granulopoiesis as well as erythropoiesis are usually reduced in areas revealing still existing haematopoiesis; foci of immature cells, with <10% myeloblasts, are notable. Similar, but often more pronounced compared to the early stages, abnormalities of megakaryocytes are prevalent including a prominent clustering and deployment along the dilated large BM vessels or together with other precursors an intraluminal dislocation. An overtly expressed myelofibrosis displaying a tight network of reticulin and dense bundles of collagen fibres is recognizable, often associated with initial to gross osteosclerosis conforming with grades 2 and 3 of the WHO-adopted scoring system (Figure 4.2). Progression of myelofibrosis is significantly associated with a significant alteration of the vascular architecture including not only a remarkable increase in quantity of the microvasculature but also a conspicuous luminal dilatation and tortuosity. Profound myelofibrosis is a secondary phenomenon associated with the clonal proliferation of haematopoietic stem cells. Collagen type 3, also known as reticulin, and collagen type 1 are the predominant extracellular components of marrow fibrosis in PMF and produced by marrow fibroblasts that do not belong to the malignant clone. Abnormal megakaryocytes and monocytes are derived from the malignant stem cell population release of fibrogenic cytokines, which cause a deposition of reticulin/collagen in the marrow space. However, accumulation of fibres is observed in diverse conditions, both benign and malignant, and therefore cannot be considered a specific feature of PMF.

In the terminal osteosclerotic phase of PMF, the BM marrow haematopoiesis is progressively replaced by a broad and irregular appositional bud-like endophytic new bone formation. Accelerated phase of the disease is indicated by increased blood and/or marrow blasts (<20%), as well as a high frequency of CD34+ cells with formation of small clusters and/or an endosteal dislocation, whereas 20% or more blasts is defined as blastic transformation (i.e. acute leukaemia). In some rare cases with overt reticulin or collagen fibrosis, the marrow space is almost devoid of haematopoietic cells and only small groups of haematopoietic precursors located mostly within the vascular sinuses can be observed.

Essential thrombocythaemia

Principal features of ET comprise of sustained elevated platelet counts, often $>1000 \times 10^9$/L, with distinct morphological features, such as anisocytosis, ranging from tiny forms to atypical large, giant platelets with bizarre shapes, pseudopods, and agranularity. The other haematopoietic lineages are usually not affected. In patients with persistent 'borderline' thrombocytosis (below the WHO-defined threshold of 450×10^9/L), and other 'difficult' cases, including pre-PMF and reactive thrombocytosis, the demonstration of clonality by demonstration of one of the molecular genetic mutations (JAK2, CALR, MPL) and the strict application of the 2016 WHO ET morphological criteria is often helpful in making a definitive diagnosis, which impacts treatment (Table 4.3 and Figure 4.2). The marrow morphology usually shows an age-matched cellularity without a significant erythroid or neutrophilic proliferation, but a predominant megakaryopoiesis; atypia in megakaryocyte topography like extensive dense clustering or prominent lining along the bony trabeculae is usually absent. Megakaryocytes are randomly distributed or very loose grouped within the BM space. Key features of this cell lineage are the large to giant cell forms with extensively folded (hyperlobulated) nuclei surrounded by well differentiated (mature) cytoplasm. The absence of reticulin fibrosis is in patients with (early stage) ET is noteworthy. Conversely, in cases with pre-PMF presenting with significant thrombocytosis, an increase in age-matched cellularity accompanied by a significantly left-shifted neutrophil granulopoiesis is observed. In the rare patients where a firm discrimination of ET and pre-PMF remains a diagnostic problem, a working diagnosis of MPN-U and close monitoring of the patient to capture any relevant progression is recommended. In patients with a mild to moderate granulocytic and erythroid proliferation (panmyelosis) and an erythropoietin (EPO) level below the reference range, masked PV mimicking ET should be excluded by a careful BM examination.

The impact of an accurate classification including BM morphology on the overall risk of complications as well as prognosis in ET has been confirmed in several studies. In line with these data, strict adherence to the WHO definition of ET reveals nearly normal survival including a very low risk of transformation into blast phase and overt myelofibrotic progression compared to other MPN that might mimic ET at initial clinical onset. Consequently, in patients who have transformed to post-ET MF or, very rarely, acute leukaemia, initial BM biopsy samples should be re-evaluated (Table 4.4).

Table 4.4 WHO criteria for the diagnosis of post-essential thrombocythaemia myelofibrosis (post-ET MF) and post-polycythaemia myelofibrosis (post-PV MF)

Post-ET MF	Post-PV MF
Required criteria	
Documentation of a previous diagnosis of WHO-defined essential thrombocythaemia Bone marrow fibrosis grade MF-2 or MF-3	Documentation of a previous diagnosis of WHO-defined polycythaemia vera Bone marrow fibrosis grade 2–3 (on 0–3 scale) or grade 3–4 (on 0–4 scale)
Additional criteria (2 are required)	
Anaemia and a more than 2 g/dL decrease from baseline haemoglobin level Leukoerythroblastic peripheral blood picture Increasing splenomegaly defined as either an increase in splenomegaly (>5 cm from baseline) or the appearance of a newly palpable splenomegaly Increase in lactate dehydrogenase level (LDH) above reference level Development of more than one of these constitutional symptoms: >10% weight loss in 6 months, night sweats, unexplained fever (>37.5 °C)	Anaemia* or sustained loss of either phlebotomy (in the absence of cytoreductive therapy) or cytoreductive treatment requirement for erythrocytosis Leukoerythroblastic peripheral blood smear Increasing splenomegaly defined as either an increase in palpable splenomegaly of >5 cm (distance from the left costal margin) or the appearance of a newly palpable splenomegaly Development of > 1 of 3 constitutional symptoms: >10% weight loss in 6 months, night sweats, unexplained fever (>37.5°C)

*Below the reference range for appropriate age, sex, gender, and altitude considerations

Adapted from Arber DA, et al. The 2016 revision to the World Health Organization classification of myeloid neoplasms and acute leukemia. *Blood*. 127(20):2391–2405. https://doi.org/10.1182/blood-2016-03-643544. Reprinted with permission from the American Society of Hematology.

Finally, in cases presenting simultaneously with myelodysplastic and myeloproliferative features in the BM and more than 15% ring sideroblasts in the aspirate, the diagnosis of MDS/MPN-RS-T should be rendered (Chapter 12). It is important to emphasize that the diagnostic criteria for MDS/MPN-RS-T include the presence of ring sideroblasts and morphologically abnormal megakaryocytes in the marrow in association with an elevated platelet count as major haematological finding.

Polycythaemia vera

Regarding PV, the diagnostic WHO guidelines take specific molecular (JAK2V617F and Exon 12), biological, and haematological features into account that are not present in reactive conditions. In the former edition of the WHO classification, BM morphology analysis was generally considered of less diagnostic importance and consequently listed among the minor diagnostic criteria. However, following a systematically performed evaluation of BM biopsies, more insight has been gained concerning early stage PV. These investigations were predominantly focused on patients presenting with borderline erythrocytosis and thrombocytosis not conforming to the former WHO criteria. Furthermore, assessment of initial (minor) reticulin fibrosis turned out to be important for clinical outcome, especially progression to post-PV myelofibrosis. Thus, performance of core biopsies is not only encouraged in doubtful cases, but especially in masked PV, representing one of the extreme endpoints in the evolution of disease. Altogether, the natural history of PV may be grossly divided into three more or less distinctive phases including a prepolycythaemic or masked, a polycythaemic (classical) and a so-called spent phase, consistent with post-PV MF (Table 4.4).

The recognition of the wider disease spectrum of PV, including masked (i.e. prepolycythaemic PV), was a major trigger for the 2016 WHO PV diagnostic criteria to lower the diagnostic haemoglobin/haematocrit thresholds (Hb >16.5 g/dL in men, Hb >16.0 g/dL in women; Hct >49% in men, Hct >48% in women). Historically these measurements were considered as surrogate markers of an increased red cell mass. However, the correlation between absolute erythrocytosis assessed by red cell mass and haemoglobin and haematocrit levels is uncertain and remains a topic of considerable debate. Indeed, at present, at least in the real world, there is very little clinical utility of red cell mass measurement. Additionally, the diagnostic relevance of low serum erythropoietin values (<4 mU/mL) has also been re-assessed critically. Although a low serum erythropoietin is very typical in PV and indeed a useful clinical parameter, up to 20% of patients have normal values at time of diagnosis. Clearly, an accurate and prompt diagnosis of PV is important for the optimal clinical management and prevention of complications, in particular thrombotic events. In this regard, several recent efforts underscore the usefulness of BM morphology, in particular for patients with masked PV, some of whom were classified previously as ET (Figure 4.2). Even in early phase, an age-adjusted hypercellular marrow with increased trilineage proliferation (panmyelosis) is observed. In this regard, BM morphology may serve as a potential surrogate of an increased red cell mass since all patients with increased values also presented with a

BM morphology typical for the broader spectrum of PV. Of interest, the evaluation of a diagnostic BM biopsy is helpful in assessing reticulin content, as slightly increased BM fibres might indicate potential higher risk of disease progression. Overall, at presentation of 2016 WHO-defined PV, the incidence of minor BM fibrosis ranges between 10% to 20%, and is associated with splenomegaly and a significantly higher risk of progression to post-PV MF at 10 years of follow-up. In this context, the correlation between minor BM fibrosis at time of diagnosis and overall thrombotic risk needs to be validated by additional studies.

In addition to some clinical similarities between masked PV and ET, recent work has also defined overlapping features between overt JAK2-associated PV and JAK-2 mutated (but not CALR-mutated) ET, suggestive of a biological continuum. In this regard, the extent of erythrocytosis would be reflected by physiological and genetic factors. In a recent series of JAK2-mutated ET, transformation to PV was reported with a cumulative risk of 29% at 15 years. In contrast, results obtained in strictly WHO-defined cohorts of JAK-positive ET demonstrated significantly lower risk of transformation of about 1.4–5%. In balance, it is likely that these observations support the notion of distinctive MPN subtypes, rather than the evolution of a single MPN clone.

Barbui and colleagues studied over 1000 patients with PV and observed thrombotic events to precede the clinical diagnosis of PV in up to 14%, and in 20% thrombotic events were the presenting symptom of disease. These observations underscore the importance of recognizing the presence of vascular complications in a significant number of cases during the prodromal stage, preceding the clinically recognized (overt) polycythaemic manifestation. So far it remains unclear how many of the JAK2-positive patients initially presenting with splanchnic vein thrombosis, Budd–Chiari syndrome, or cerebral thrombosis clinically and morphologically represent early stage or masked PV. Interestingly, even in cases which at onset clinically mimicked ET and presented without significant erythrocytosis, dynamics of JAK2 allele burden during follow-up correlates with transformation to overt PV.

In initial-prodromal stages of PV, that have been eventually termed latent, occult, or smouldering PV, histological BM features are characterized by a slight to moderate increase in age-matched haematopoietic cellularity expanding in elderly patients into the adipose tissue of the subcortical marrow spaces. There is always a prominent proliferation of the nucleated erythroid precursor cells accompanied by a varying amount of large to small megakaryocytes and a moderate increase in neutrophil granulopoiesis. In PV megakaryocytes are characterized by a pleomorphous aspect without gross abnormalities of maturation due to a striking variability in size ranging from small to giant forms (Figure 4.2). In cases with a high platelet count clinically suggesting ET or so-called overlapping MPN, megakaryopoiesis is very prominent with loose clustering of giant megakaryocytes revealing hyperlobulated nuclei. In secondary conditions (i.e. reactive/secondary erythrocytosis) there is a predominance of smaller to medium-sized megakaryocytes, which is accompanied by a characteristic stromal reaction pattern (i.e. perivascular plasmacytosis), many cell debris-laden macrophages, and mature eosinophils. The degree of granulocytic and erythropoietic proliferation is quite variable in these cases and associated with the underlying disorder like inflammatory conditions or hypoxia.

Polycythaemic (classical) PV is characterized by a conspicuously hypercellular BM expanding towards the superficial marrow spaces due to a trilineage proliferation (panmyelosis) of erythroid and granulocytic precursors in variable proportions, associated with increased megakaryopoiesis. It is of importance that an age-matched subnormal or even normal amount of haematopoietic tissue is hardly compatible with the diagnosis of treatment-naive PV. For a reliable assessment and quantification of granulopoiesis and erythropoiesis (M:E ratio) special stains like naphthol-A-SD chloroacetate esterase or immunohistochemical staining with myeloperoxidase are helpful. In contrast to the normal BM with small and rounded groups of nucleated erythroid precursors, the erythropoietic islets in PV are significantly enlarged and often merged into large sheets. Megakaryopoiesis reveals some peculiar features not only by showing a variable increase in number with either a random distribution or loose clustering but also a pleomorphous aspect including small, medium-sized, and large to giant cells (Figure 4.2). It has to be emphasized that megakaryocytes in PV do not display abnormalities like maturation defects. Iron-laden macrophages are rarely observable (less than 6%) in the BM and should be preferably recognized on smears of aspirates.

Post-PV myelofibrosis (spent phase)—which is consistent with an advanced-terminal PV—is clinically characterized by a leukoerythroblastic blood smear, poikilocytosis with teardrop-shaped red blood cells, and splenomegaly due to extramedullary haematopoiesis (Table 4.4). The morphological hallmark is overt reticulin and collagen BM fibrosis, and osteosclerosis may also occur. Contrasting overt polycythaemic stages cellularity varies in this terminal stage and hypocellular specimens are common. Frequently a patchy distribution of haematopoiesis is seen, probably associated with applied cytoreductive regimens. Erythropoiesis and granulopoiesis are decreased, and generally there is a prevalence of left-shifted neutrophils. Clusters of megakaryocytes, often with hyperchromatic and very dysmorphic, bizarre-looking nuclei are prominent. The abundant BM fibrosis shows coarse bundles of collagen with a terminal scarring of the BM and effacement of haematopoiesis. This stage of disease is clinically regarded as a possible prelude to blast phase (i.e. acute leukaemia). For this reason, special staining (CD34, CD117) for an easy recognition of immature cells including distribution (clustering) of blasts are recommended.

Summary

Although the 2016 WHO classic MPN classification accurately distinguishes the principal subtypes, PMF, PV, and ET, the diagnostic criteria are enhanced by the addition of expert hematopathology analysis. Morphological details are also important in distinguishing masked prepolycythaemic PV and ET, and pre-PMF and ET. Morphology also impact risk assessment for thrombosis and prognosis. Recent experience, in particular in the assessment of triple-negative MPN, suggest emerging correlations between molecular genetics information and morphological characteristics, such as cellularity, vascularity, and osteosclerosis. These findings underscore the importance of haematopathology for the optimal diagnosis, risk assessment, and treatment of MPN.

Further reading

Arber DA, Orazi A, Hasserjian R, et al. The 2016 revision to the World Health Organization (WHO) classification of myeloid neoplasms and acute leukemia. *Blood*. 2016;127(20):2391–405.

Barbui T, Thiele J, Carobbio A, et al. Discriminating between essential thrombocythemia and masked polycythemia vera in JAK2 mutated patients. *Am J Hematol*. 2014;89(6):588–90.

Barbui T, Thiele J, Carobbio A, et al. Disease characteristics and clinical outcome in young adults with essential thrombocythemia versus early/prefibrotic primary myelofibrosis. *Blood*. 2012;120(3):569–71.

Barbui T, Thiele J, Carobbio A, et al. Masked polycythemia vera diagnosed according to WHO and BCSH classification. *Am J Hematol*. 2014;89(2):199–202.

Barbui T, Thiele J, Passamonti F, et al. Initial bone marrow reticulin fibrosis in polycythemia vera exerts an impact on clinical outcome. *Blood*. 2012;119(10):2239–41.

Barbui T, Thiele J, Passamonti F, et al. Survival and disease progression in essential thrombocythemia are significantly influenced by accurate morphologic diagnosis: an international study of 1,104 patients. *J Clin Oncol*. 2011;29(23):3179–84.

Barbui T, Thiele J, Vannucchi AM, Tefferi A. Problems and pitfalls regarding WHO-defined diagnosis of early/prefibrotic primary myelofibrosis versus essential thrombocythemia. *Leukemia*. 2013;27(10):1953–8.

Ejerblad E, Kvasnicka HM, Thiele J, et al. Diagnosis according to World Health Organization determines the long-term prognosis in patients with myeloproliferative neoplasms treated with anagrelide: results of a prospective long-term follow-up. *Hematology*. 2013;18(1):8–13.

Gianelli U, Iurlo A, Vener C, et al. The significance of bone marrow biopsy and JAK2V617F mutation in the differential diagnosis between the 'early' prepolycythemic phase of polycythemia vera and essential thrombocythemia. *Am J Clin Pathol*. 2008;130(3):336–42.

Gianelli U, Vener C, Bossi A, et al. The European Consensus on grading of bone marrow fibrosis allows a better prognostication of patients with primary myelofibrosis. *Mod Pathol*. 2012;25(9):1193–202.

Gisslinger H, Gotic M, Holowiecki J, et al. Anagrelide compared with hydroxyurea in WHO-classified essential thrombocythemia: the ANAHYDRET study, a randomized controlled trial. *Blood*. 2013;121(10):1720–8.

Grinfeld J, Nanglia J, Baxter EJ, et al. Classification and personalized prognosis in myeloproloferative neoplasms. *N Engl J Med*. 2018;379:1416–30.

Kvasnicka HM, Orazi A, Thiele J, et al. European LeukemiNet study of reproducibility of bone marrow features in masked polycythemia vera and differentiation from essential thrombocythemia. *Am J Hematol*. 2017;92(10):1062–7.

Kvasnicka HM, Thiele J. Bone marrow angiogenesis: methods of quantification and changes evolving in chronic myeloproliferative disorders. *Histol Histopathol*. 2004;19(4):1245–60.

Kvasnicka HM, Thiele J. Classification of Ph-negative chronic myeloproliferative disorders—morphology as the yardstick of classification. *Pathobiology*. 2007;74(2):63–71.

Kvasnicka HM, Thiele J. Prodromal myeloproliferative neoplasms: the 2008 WHO classification. *Am J Hematol*. 2010;85(1):62–9.

Kvasnicka HM, Thiele J. The impact of clinicopathological studies on staging and survival in essential thrombocythemia, chronic idiopathic myelofibrosis, and polycythemia rubra vera. *Semin Thromb Hemost*. 2006;32(4):362–71.

Thiele J, Kvasnicka HM. Clinicopathological criteria for differential diagnosis of thrombocythemias in various myeloproliferative disorders. *Semin Thromb Hemost*. 2006;32(3):219–30.

Thiele J, Kvasnicka HM. Diagnostic impact of bone marrow histopathology in polycythemia vera (PV). *Histol Histopathol*. 2005;20(1):317–28.

Thiele J, Kvasnicka HM. Grade of bone marrow fibrosis is associated with relevant hematological findings-a clinicopathological study on 865 patients with chronic idiopathic myelofibrosis. *Ann Hematol*. 2006;85(4):226–32.

Thiele J, Kvasnicka HM. Myelofibrosis—what's in a name? Consensus on definition and EUMNET grading. *Pathobiology*. 2007;74(2):89–96.

Thiele J, Kvasnicka HM, Diehl V. Initial (latent) polycythemia vera with thrombocytosis mimicking essential thrombocythemia. *Acta Haematol*. 2005;113(4):213–19.

Thiele J, Kvasnicka HM, Diehl V. Standardization of bone marrow features—does it work in hematopathology for histological discrimination of different disease patterns? *Histol Histopathol*. 2005;20(2):633–44.

Thiele J, Kvasnicka HM, Facchetti F, Franco V, Van der Walt J, Orazi A. European consensus for grading of bone marrow fibrosis and assessment of cellularity. *Haematologica*. 2005;90(8):1128–32.

Thiele J, Kvasnicka HM, Mullauer L, Buxhofer-Ausch V, Gisslinger B, Gisslinger H. Essential thrombocythemia versus early primary myelofibrosis: a multicenter study to validate the WHO classification. *Blood*. 2011;117(21):5710–18.

Thiele J, Kvasnicka HM, Schmitt-Graeff A, Diehl V. Bone marrow histopathology following cytoreductive therapy in chronic idiopathic myelofibrosis. *Histopathology*. 2003;43(5):470–79.

Thiele J, Kvasnicka HM, Schmitt-Graeff A, Zankovich R, Diehl V. Follow-up examinations including sequential bone marrow biopsies in essential thrombocythemia (ET): a retrospective clinicopathological study of 120 patients. *Am J Hematol*. 2002;70(4):283–91.

Kvasnicka HM, Thiele J, Werden C, Zankovich R, Diehl V, Fischer R. Prognostic factors in idiopathic (primary) osteomyelofibrosis. *Cancer*. 1997;80(4):708–19.

Silver RT, Chow W, Orazi A, Arles SP, Goldsmith SJ. Evaluation of WHO criteria for diagnosis of polycythemia vera: a prospective analysis. *Blood*. 2013;122(11):1881–6.

Swerdlow S, Campo E, Harris N, et al. Tissues. Lyon, France: IARC Press, 2008.

Chapter 5

Prognostic factors of chronic myeloid leukaemia

Michele Baccarani, Fausto Castagnetti, Gabriele Gugliotta, Francesca Palandri, Simona Soverini, and Gianantonio Rosti

Introduction to chronic myeloid leukaemia *64*
The prognostic scores (Sokal, EURO, EUTOS, ELTS) *64*
Cytogenetics *68*
Transcript type and transcript level *69*
Pharmacokinetics, pharmacodynamics, and pharmacogenomics *71*
Age and comorbidities *71*
Prognosis on second-line treatment *72*
Conclusions *73*
Acknowledgements *75*

Introduction to chronic myeloid leukaemia

Prior to the introduction of the ABL tyrosine kinase inhibitors (TKIs) in the clinics, in 1998, for patients with chronic myeloid leukaemia (CML), the prognosis was, in general, poor with a median survival of 3 to 4.5 years. The historical and current treatments of CML are reviewed in Chapters 1 and 7, and herein we address the prognosis and the methods available to assess it. The first principal method was developed in 1984 by Sokal and Baccarani, in the chemotherapy era. It divided patients into three risk categories based on a mathematical formula that took into account the patient's age, blast cell percentage in peripheral blood, spleen size and platelet count.Thereafter, the prognostic value of Sokal score was clinically validated first in patients treated with interferon-alpha (IFNα)-based regimes, and second in those treated with TKIs. The next important prognostic method proposed by a European collaborative group, known as 'EURO', and including basophil and eosinophil percentage in peripheral blood, in addition to the Sokal variables, was developed in 1998 for CML patients being treated with IFNα and validated in a large data set of over 1500 patients. Then in 2011, the European LeukemiaNet (ELN) proposed a new prognostic score specifically designed to predict outcome to the first generation TKI, imatinib mesylate (imatinib), the EUTOS (European Treatment and Outcome Study), which required only an assessment of the spleen size and percentage of basophils in peripheral blood. This simple method has been published in 2011 and successfully validated in large cohorts of CML patients, but it has not been adopted widely. A new score, the EUTOS Long Term Survival Score (ELTS), has been recently developed to predict the disease-specific death. The variables included in this new score are: age at diagnosis (in years), maximum spleen size (in cm from costal margin), peripheral blood blast percentage, and platelet count. The ELTS score has been recently recommended by the ELN panel for risk assessment of CML patients at diagnosis. It is of some interest, and somewhat puzzling, that in the era of molecular haematology the prognosis of a disease like CML, where the molecular bases are so well known, the CML community has been reliant on such old-fashioned scores that are based on few, simple, haematologic data and on the subjective assessment of spleen size by manual palpation. In this chapter, we will present a critical review of the various risk scores and we will discuss which other baseline characteristics have a prognostic value.

The prognostic scores (Sokal, EURO, EUTOS, ELTS)

Characteristically, CML is a biphasic or triphasic disease that is usually diagnosed in the initial chronic phase (CP). This CP used to last 3 to 6 years but is today very significantly longer for patients treated with TKIs. A small minority of patients (< 5%) present with advanced phase, which can be accelerated phase (AP) or blast crisis (BC). Importantly most of the prognostic methods, including the Sokal, the EURO, the EUTOS and the ELTS were specifically developed and validated for patients in the first CP. All four prognostic scores are based on a few simple baseline characteristics, that must be recorded at diagnosis, before any treatment, and depicted in Table 5.1. The main difference between the Sokal, EURO, EUTOS and ELTS scores concerns age. Age was significant, both as a continuous variable (Sokal), and at a cut-off value of 50 years (EURO), in patients treated with conventional chemotherapy (Sokal) or with IFNα (EURO). Age showed inferior significance when patients were treated with TKIs and was not included in the EUTOS score and was differently weighted (reduced importance) in the ELTS score; the reason is that in older people the response to TKIs is only slightly inferior. However, a recent analysis of an international multicentre series of newly diagnosed CP CML patients suggested that age may be still important for survival, both for overall survival (OS), and for leukaemia-related survival (LRS), where deaths in remission are counted as competitive events. An analysis of more than 500 newly diagnosed CP-CML patients in the GIMEMA (Gruppo Italiano Malattie Ematologiche dell'Adulto) data set, who were treated front-line with imatinib, compared Sokal, EURO and EUTOS scores confirming that all three scores were able to distinguish low from high-risk patients, while intermediate risk patients behaved more as low risk ones (Table 5.2). Since the risk score may influence treatment choice, treatment results, and the interpretation of treatment results, the choice of the risk score may not be neutral; however, an answer to the question of which risk score is more convenient is difficult. Sokal risk is more sensitive and less specific than EURO and EUTOS risk; not all the patients who are high risk by Sokal are high risk also by EURO and EUTOS, while almost all the patients who are high risk by EURO or EUTOS are high risk also by Sokal. For Sokal, the separation in three risk groups was proposed on empirical bases;

Table 5.1 Baseline variables for the prognostic scores (to be recorded before any antileukemic treatment, including hydroxyurea)

	Sokal	EURO	EUTOS	ELTS
Age	Yes (continuous)	Yes (≥ 50 years)	No	Yes (continuous)
Spleen*	Yes (continuous)	Yes (continuous)	Yes (continuous)	Yes (continuous)
Platelet count	Yes (continuous)	Yes (≥1500 x 10^9/L)	No	Yes (continuous)
Myeloblasts, %	Yes (continuous)	Yes (continuous)	No	Yes (continuous)
Basophils, %	No	Yes (≥3%)	Yes (continuous)	No
Eosinophils	No	Yes (continuous)	No	No

*Cm below costal margin, maximum distance, evaluated by manual palpation

Source: data from Sokal JE, et al. (1984). Prognostic discrimination in 'good-risk' chronic granulocytic leukemia. *Blood.* 63(4):789–799; Hasford J, et al. (2011). Predicting complete cytogenetic response and subsequent progression-free survival in 20160 patients with CML on imatinib treatment: the EUTOS score. *Blood.* 118(3):686–692. DOI: 10.1182/blood-2010-12-319038; and Hoffman VS, et al. (2017). Treatment and outcome of 2904 CML patients from the EUTOS population-based registry. *Leukemia.* 31(3):593–601. DOI: 10.1038/leu.2016.246.

Table 5.2 Response and outcome by risk

	Sokal				EURO				EUTOS		
	Low	Int	High	P	Low	Int	High	P	Low	High	P
3-mo EMR	83%	79%	84%	0.481	83%	81%	79%	0.812	82%	75%	0.268
1-year MMR	72%	68%	52%	0.001	70%	67%	41%	0.002	68%	48%	0.010
6-year MR 4.0	68%	65%	44%	0.001	65%	61%	41%	0.019	62%	45%	0.031
1-year CCyR	83%	81%	69%	0.006	93%	78%	59%	0.002	80%	63%	0.009
6-year PFS	93%	84%	82%	0.003	92%	84%	76%	0.005	88%	79%	0.132
6-year LRS	97%	95%	88%	0.002	96%	95%	80%	0.001	95%	85%	0.039

EMR = early molecular response (BCR-ABL1 ≤ 10% at 3 months).

MMR = major molecular response (BCR-ABL1 ≤ 0.1%).

MR 4.0 = BCR-ABL1 ≤ 0.01%.

CCyR = complete cytogenetic response (Ph+ 0).

PFS = progression (transformation)-free survival.

LRS = leukaemia-related survival (not counting as events the deaths in remission).

Source: data from Sokal JE, et al. (1984). Prognostic discrimination in 'good-risk' chronic granulocytic leukemia. *Blood.* 63(4):789–799; Hasford J, et al. (2011). Predicting complete cytogenetic response and subsequent progression-free survival in 20160 patients with CML on imatinib treatment: the EUTOS score. *Blood.* 118(3):686–692. DOI: 10.1182/blood-2010-12-319038; and Hoffman VS, et al. (2017). Treatment and outcome of 2904 CML patients from the EUTOS population-based registry. *Leukemia.* 31(3):593–601. DOI: 10.1038/leu.2016.246.

Table 5.3 Cumulative probability of achieving MR 4.5 by 5 years of treatment with imatinib 400 mg once daily, nilotinib 300 mg twice daily, and nilotinib 400 mg twice daily.

Sokal risk	Imatinib 400 mg once daily	Nilotinib 300 mg twice daily	Nilotinib 400 mg twice daily
Low	37%	53%	61%
Intermediate	32%	60%	50%
High	23%	45%	42%

Source: data from Saglio G, et al. (2010). Nilotinib versus Imatinib for Newly Diagnosed Chronic Myeloid Leukemia. *N Engl J Med.* 362(24):2251–9. DOI: 10.1056/NEJMoa0912614; and Hochhaus A, et al. (2016). Long-term benefits and risks of frontline nilotinib vs imatinib for chronic myeloid leukemia in chronic phase: 5-year update of the randomized ENESTnd trial. *Leukemia.* 30(5):1044–54. DOI: 10.1038/leu.2016.5.

the patients were divided into three groups of approximate identical size. For EURO and EUTOS, the minimal p-value approach was used, a statistical procedure that maximizes the difference among the resulting groups and the relevant variables. Therefore, the EUTOS score may be privileged, both for methodologic reasons, and because it was based on imatinib-treated patients. However, the EUTOS score was designed to predict the probability of being in complete cytogenetic response (CCyR) at 18 months, that is an important surrogate marker of survival, but it is not survival. Therefore, it is not so surprising that Sokal score predicted 6-year progression-free survival (PFS) and OS better than EUTOS (Table 5.2). Moreover, Sokal risk, which is still more familiar to many investigators, was used in the majority of the principal recent studies, and is still the reference score for the prognostic evaluation of CML. It is worth noticing that the retrospective application of Sokal score was able to predict also the probability of achieving a deep molecular response (MR 4.5, BCR-ABL1 ≤0.0032) in patients treated front-line with either imatinib or nilotinib (Table 5.3), and that again Sokal score was able, retrospectively, to predict the probability of remaining in MR 4.5 after treatment discontinuation. In the GIMEMA series of newly diagnosed CP-CM, patients treated front-line with imatinib, no score was shown, so far, to predict early molecular response (EMR, BCR-ABL1 transcript level ≤10% at 3 months) (Table 5.2), suggesting that the risk of not achieving an EMR may depend also, or even more, on other factors, that are not related only to leukaemia itself, like compliance and dose reduction for side effects. The ELTS score seems to have superior ability to discriminate high risk patients if compared with other scores, particularly in elderly patients (> 65 years old), but further confirmations are required.

Following the remarkable success of the TKIs, it was increasingly recognized that many patients died as a result of causes unrelated to CML. In order to address this point, an analysis was carried out by the EUTOS group on almost 2300 patients with CML in CP treated with imatinib on six trials. Older age, higher peripheral blast counts, larger splenomegaly and low platelet count were noted to be significantly associated with a greater probability of death due to CML. Consequently, a new prognostic score (ELTS) was developed in 2016 and validated clinically. This score is essentially a first effort to predict prognosis of long-term survival considering disease-specific death in patients with CML. The ELTS is calculated by using a mathematical formula: $0.0025 \times \text{age}/10)^3 + 0.06 \times \text{spleen size} + 0.1052 \times \text{peripheral blood blasts} + 0.4104 \times \text{platelet count} \times 10^9/\text{L})^{-0.5}$ (http://www.leukemianet.org/content/leukemias/cml/cml_score/index_eng.html) and divides patients into three risk groups: low (<1.5680), intermediate (>1.5680, <2.2185), and high (>2.2185).

The usefulness of the Sokal, the EURO, the EUTOS, or the ELTS prognostic scores had been assessed in patients with the advanced phases, data from the EUTOS database, in which patients were defined to have AP or BC by the 2013 ELN criteria. A total of 283 patients, which comprised of 203 in AP and 80 in BC, were analysed in 2019. It was established that prognosis of CML patients in AP or BC was defined by a blast count >20% in peripheral blood, older age, additional cytogenetic abnormities (ACA), and a low haemoglobin (<9.9 g/dL). The ELTS score seems to have superior ability to discriminate high risk patients if compared with other scores, particularly in elderly patients (> 65 years old), but further confirmations are required. The clinical utility of the ELTS has been incorporated into the ELN 2020 guidelines.

Cytogenetics

Cytogenetic abnormalities can be identified by chromosome banding analysis (CBA) of marrow cell metaphases, and by fluorescence-*in-situ* hybridization (FISH) of marrow or blood cell nuclei. CBA is required to identify the presence of other or additional clonal chromosome abnormalities (CCA; in Ph+ cells [CCA/Ph+]). To be relevant, it is recommended that the abnormality should be detected in at least two cells in two consecutive tests, but it is not always clear if this definition was used in all reports. Since CCA/Ph+ represent macroscopic genomic abnormalities, and since it is believed that in cancer the greater the abnormalities the poorer the response to therapy and the outcome, it is highly likely that in CML CCA/Ph+ identify subgroups of patients with a poorer prognosis. As a matter of fact, already in the antique era of conventional chemotherapy, it was shown that patients with CCA/Ph+ had a shorter survival, but CCA/Ph+ were not included in any prognostic classifications, because the amount and the quality of the data were not sufficient. However, CCA/Ph+ were already considered as a marker of advanced phase, because they are detected more and more frequently at progression to AP and BC.

Today, the acquisition of CCA/Ph+ during TKIs treatment must be considered as a marker of treatment failure and of progression to AP. Several studies of patients treated second line with imatinib, mainly 400 mg once daily, reported that the presence of CCA/Ph+ before initiating imatinib predicted for a poorer response and outcome, both in CP and in advanced phases, and that the occurrence of ACA during imatinib treatment heralded progression. Less data are available in patients treated with imatinib front-line. Luatti et al. found CCA/Ph+, including Y loss, in 21/378 (5.6%) patients who were treated with imatinib 400 mg once or twice daily, and reported a significant difference in the cumulative probability of achieving a CCyR (67% vs. 89%, $p < 0.006$), but no difference in PFS and in OS. Lee et al found CCA/Ph+ in 13/281 patients (4.6%) treated with imatinib 400 mg once daily and reported a significant worse PFS, but not OS, in such patients. Fabarius et al.

analysed 1151 patients treated with several imatinib-based regimes (400 mg once daily, 400 mg twice daily, 400 mg once daily and IFNα, 400 mg once daily and low-dose arabinosyl cytosine), and reported CCA/Ph+ in 6.9% of patients (3.3% Y loss, 2.2% 'minor route', and 1.4% 'major route'). 'Major route' included trisomy 8 alone or with other abnormalities, trisomy Ph (der(22) t(9;22)(q34;q11), trisomy 19, and ider (22) (q10 or q11)t(9;22)(q34;q11). The cumulative probability of achieving a CCyR and a major molecular response (MMR) was lower only in patients with 'major route' CCA/Ph+. In such patients, 5-year PFS (69%) and 5-year OS (73%) were also lower than in all other patients. Y loss and 'minor route' abnormalities were not found to affect response and outcome. A subsequent report from the same group, on 1346 patients, showed that not only 'major route' CCA/Ph+, but also other unbalanced karyotypes had a negative prognostic effect. Lipper et al. compared 30 patients with Y loss with 30 matched patients without Y loss, and found a significant poorer outcome in patients with Y loss, so the significance of Y loss is uncertain. Variant or atypical translocations (VT) and the deletions of the long arm of chromosome 9 (9q-) can be detected by FISH. VT, where the fusion bcr-abl1 gene is located outside chromosome 22, have been reported in 3% to 8% of patients. A prognostic value of VT was not detectable in any study. A detectable deletion in the long arm of chromosome 9 (9q- or del9q) is found in about 15% of patients. In patients treated with chemotherapy (CHT) or with IFNα that deletion was associated with a poorer outcome, but in patients treated with imatinib no prognostic value was found.

In summary, there is sufficient evidence to conclude that CCA/Ph+ are a marker of high risk when they are detected at diagnosis, and that they are markers of progression when they are detected during treatment of CP. Whether the prognostic value of CCA/Ph+ is limited to so-called major route abnormalities and to unbalanced karyotypes, or if also minor abnormalities and Y loss are significant, it is not yet clear. According to the 2020 ELN recoommendations, high rish baseline CCA/Ph+ predicting poorer response to TKIs and higher risk of progression are: +8, a second Ph-chromosome (+Ph), i(17q), +19, −7/7q-, 11q23, or 3q26.2 aberrations, and complex aberrant karyotypes. On the contrary, 9q- and VT have no detectable prognostic value. Therefore, the use of FISH, baseline, can be limited to the rare cases of so-called masked Ph, to distinguish Ph+ from Ph– neoplasms.

This summary of cytogenetic abnormalities is still provisional, since more data and longer follow-up are needed, particularly in patients treated frontline or second-line with second-generation TKIs, where data are very scanty. Also, it is not known if a cytogenetic abnormality can affect the probability of achieving a condition of treatment-free remission (TFR).

Transcript type and transcript level

The BCR-ABL1 transcript can result from several BCR-ABL1 genes that differ depending on the breakpoint in the BCR gene in chromosome 22. The major breakpoint cluster region (M-*bcr*) includes exons b2 (e13) and b3 (e14), and the resulting fusion gene is transcribed into either a b2a2 (e13a2) or a b3a2 (e14a2) transcript coding for two similar proteins of slightly different size ($p210^{BCR\text{-}ABL1}$). The synthesis of either proteins can vary also for post-transcriptional, splicing processes. About 45% of patients harbor the b3a2, about 35% the b2a2, and about 15% have both transcripts. In some CML patients, the breakpoint occurs at the so-called minor bcr (m-*bcr*), giving rise to a shorter transcript (e1a2) coding for the $p190^{BCR\text{-}ABL1}$ protein that is usually associated with Ph+ acute lymphoblastic leukaemia, or at the so-called micro bcr (μ-*bcr*) giving rise to a longer transcript (e19a2) coding for the $p230^{BCR\text{-}ABL1}$ protein, that is usually associated with a picture of so-called chronic neutrophilic leukaemia. Although the data are mainly anecdotal, it is believed that the few patients presenting with p190 or with p230, as well as the rare patients who present with other transcripts, respond less well to TKIs, and have a poorer prognosis. Instead, there are several data on the prognostic evaluation of the two CML-typical transcript type, namely b2a2 (e13a2) and b3a2 (e14a2). The b3a2 transcript, that is more frequent than the b2a2 one, has been reported to predict for a slightly better response, but survival differences have not been clearly demonstrated.

Recent efforts to accord patients who have had an optimal response the potential for TFR and a normal OS without life-long therapy, has identified disease persistence, to be a principal challenge. Though the precise causes currently remain unelucidated, it has been "hypothesized that the variability in breakpoint position within the M-bcr, resulting in two $p210^{BCR\text{-}ABL1}$ proteins that differ by 25 amino acids, may be a cause of persistence: the relationships between the BCR-ABL1 transcript types, the response to TKIs, the outcome, and the immune response, suggest that the e14a2 transcript is associated with more and deeper molecular responses, with a higher probability of achieving TFR'.[1]

Some other genomic alterations that are more frequent in acute myeloid leukaemia and in the myelodysplastic syndrome, and have been found also in healthy elderly people, may be detected, sometimes, also in CML, but their frequency is likely to be low, and their prognostic value is unknown. The study of gene expression profile (GEP) can help identifying the patients who are less sensitive to TKIs, both baseline and during the treatment, because it has been reported that there is a small cluster of genes that are overexpressed to a similar extent in the Ph+ cells of the patients who fail imatinib as well as in the cells of BP, but these data require confirmation before a screening of GEP can be added to the diagnostic workup of CML, and can be used to monitor the response. Other genes that are linked to the proliferation and the differentiation of stem and progenitor cells, like *PTCH1*, are candidate to a prognostic value. The application of more sensitive techniques, like ultra-deep sequencing and single nucleotide polymorphism analysis, will help us to understand better which other genes are relevant to the pathogenesis and to the evolution of CML, to develop a genomically-based risk assessment.

In conclusion, early response to TKI treatment has been recognized as a major prognostic factor, and management guidelines based on the *BCR-ABL1* transcript levels at 3, 6, or 12 months following the initiation of TKI treatment were developed by the ELN and recently updated in 2020. Optimal molecular responses are now defined as *BCR-ABL1* transcript levels <10% at 3 months, <1% at 6 months, and <0.1% from 12 months. There remain some challenges in measuring the absolute levels of transcripts and the harmonization of results in accordance to the International Scale (IS).

Pharmacokinetics, pharmacodynamics, and pharmacogenomics

The concentration of imatinib outside and inside target cells depends at least in part by the expression and the function of some proteins that are involved in drug transportation. Some proteins belonging to the multidrug resistance family, have an effect on the efflux of imatinib outside the cells. Their expression and their function affect not only imatinib concentration in leukaemic cells, to some extent, but also imatinib absorption and distribution in body tissues. It has been reported that the overexpression of some multidrug resistance proteins affected sometimes the response to imatinib. It has been reported that some particular polymorphisms of these genes modify the absorption and the pharmacokinetic profile of imatinib and have an effect on plasma drug concentration and on response. None of these findings was used so far to predict prospectively the response and the outcome. Measuring and monitoring plasma drug concentration of imatinib is expected to be useful, as in many other cases of chronic drug treatment. As a matter of fact, several studies have shown a relationship between plasma imatinib concentration and response, and have also shown that measuring the concentration may help optimizing imatinib dose and response. However, the attention on pharmacokinetic data is falling, and measuring plasma level is no longer widely recommended. More information is available on the human organic cation transporter 1 (OCT1). It has been shown that OCT1 regulates the influx of imatinib into the cells, and that OCT1 affects the response to imatinib; a high OCT1 was associated with a better and a faster response. However, it is not the amount, nor the quantitative expression, of OCT1 that is important, but its functional activity that counts, which is measured with a method that is not available worldwide and is not standardized, regrettably, because the importance of this piece of information would not be limited to predict the response, but also, and more importantly, to adjust the dose of imatinib or to select the proper TKI.

There are very few data on pharmacokinetics, pharmacodynamics, and pharmacogenomics of second-generation TKIs. The drug transporters were not found, so far, to affect the intracellular concentration of nilotinib and dasatinib, but there are no studies comparing OCT1 function with the response to these, and to other, TKIs. The therapeutic effect of TKIs may depend also on different mechanisms, affecting the ability of TKIs to suppress Ph+ cells. It has been reported that a particular polymorphism of a gene, *BIM*, that is implicated in apoptosis, and that is present in about 15% of Asian people, prevents imatinib-induced apoptosis and is correlated with a poorer response to imatinib. A particular genotype (KIR2DS1) of the killer immunoglobulin-like receptor family, that has a role in the natural killer-mediated immune response, was reported to affect the response to imatinib but not to dasatinib.

Age and comorbidities

Age was recognized as a negative prognostic factor in almost all studies of CML patients treated with conventional CHT or with IFNα. As a matter of fact, the response to imatinib was reported to be only marginally affected by old age. However, the relationship between age and outcome may be more complex, and bidirectional. On one hand, older people are fragile, but on another hand they may have a less aggressive disease. Also the baseline characteristics of the disease are different in different age groups. In children, CML is more aggressive (more splenomegaly, bigger spleen, more myeloblasts, etc.). In adolescents and in young adults, splenomegaly is also frequent, while in older people the spleen is more rarely palpable, and big spleens are rare. Since splenomegaly is the most important, recognized and confirmed, prognostic factor, the inferior leukemia burden may explain why in elderly people the response to TKIs is as good as in young and adult patients: the leukaemic risk is higher in young patients than in older people. However, including age in the calculation of the risk, does not help much to select the proper treatment for individual patients, because old patients have different problems and different life expectancy, as compared to young and adult ones. In other words, including an old patient into a high-risk group may not be useful, because an old patient may not be eligible for a more intensive, more aggressive, or different treatment because of comorbidities. It should not be overlooked that the median age at presentation is close to 60 years, consequently in CML patients, comorbidities are frequent. Comorbidities affect treatment toxicity and compliance. Therefore, comorbidities affect survival, both leukaemia related and unrelated. The Charlson comorbidity index can be useful to stratify older patients within each risk group.

Prognosis on second-line treatment

There are three main possible scenarios on second-line treatment. The first scenario is that of second-line second-generation TKIs treatment after imatinib. In such patients, the baseline risk, the Hb level, the percentage of basophils in blood, recurrent neutropenias during prior imatinib treatment, and particularly the cytogenetic response to prior imatinib treatment, have been reported to affect response and outcome. Based on these data, two prognostic models were proposed, and can be used in practice (Table 5.4). The second scenario is that of patients resistant to second-generation TKIs first line. These patients are rather rare. Until more data are available, it is wise to consider all such patients as high risk. The third scenario is that of second line imatinib after hydroxyurea or IFNα, a scenario that today is highly uncommon in western countries, but is still relatively common in other countries where the access to TKIs is limited. In this scenario, it is reasonable to assume that risk and CCA/Ph+ continue to be important, but it must be pointed out that the response to prior therapy, particularly to IFNα, is also important, maybe even more.

Table 5.4 Predicting the response to second-generation TKIs in second line

Prior CyR to imatinib	Complete	Point 0
Hammersmith model		
	1–94% Ph+	Point 1
	≥95% Ph+	Point 3
Sokal risk	Low	Point 0
	Int/High	Point 0.5
Prior neutropenia on imatinib	Grade <3	Point 0
	Grade 3–4	Point 1
Low risk	Score <1.5	2-year OS 100%
Intermediate risk	Score 1.5–2.5	2-year OS 90%
High risk	Score >2.5	2-year OS 75%
MD Anderson model		
Mutations poorly sensitive to nilotinib	Present	point 1
Less than MCyR to prior imatinib	Yes	point 1
Hb <120 g/L	Yes	point 1
Basophils ≥4%	Yes	point 1
Low risk	Score 0	2-year PFS 89%
Intermediate risk	Score 1	2-year PFS 50%
High risk	Score ≥3	2-year PFS <20%

Source: data from Milojkovic D, et al. (2010). Early prediction of success or failure of treatment with second generation tyrosine kinase inhibitors in patients with chronic myeloid leukemia. *Haematologica*. 95(2):224–31. DOI: 10.3324/haematol.2009.012781; Jabbour E, et al. (2013). Prediction of outcomes in patients with Ph+ chronic myeloid leukemia in chronic phase treated with nilotinib after imatinib resistance/intolerance. *Leukemia*. 27(4):907–13. DOI: 10.1038/leu.2012.305.

Conclusions

Several factors and baseline characteristics were reported to have a prognostic value, but the more robust and internationally shared prognostic factor of newly diagnosed CP-CML patients in the TKIs era is still the risk score (Box 5.1). Although there are no studies comparing prospectively the usefulness of the four available risk scores, according to the ELN panel the preferred risk score is ELTS.

There are sufficient data to support the prognostic value of ACA, although it is not yet clear if all abnormalities have the same value. High risk and ACA have been listed in the 2020 ELN recommendations as baseline 'warning' factors, requiring a more careful and frequent monitoring. It is time to consider high risk and ACA more than a 'warning' factor, but as factors identifying patients who require a different, risk-adapted, treatment.

Box 5.1 Summary of confirmed and putative or possible prognostic factors and baseline characteristics

High-risk score (Sokal, EURO, EUTOS)

- 'High risk' ACAs: +8, +Ph, i(17q), +19, −7/7q-, 11q23, or 3q26.2 aberrations
- Complex aberrant karyotypes
- Variant translocations
- *BCR-ABL1* transcript type
- *BCR-ABL1* transcripts level
- Gene polymorphisms (*BIM*, *KIR*, *MDR1*, etc.)
- Expression and function of the human organic cationic transporter 1 (OCT-1)
- Overexpression of multidrug resistance family genes
- Gene expression profile (gene clusters, *PTCH1*, etc.)

Source: data from Sokal JE, et al. (1984). Prognostic discrimination in 'good-risk' chronic granulocytic leukemia. *Blood.* 63(4):789–99; Hasford J, et al. (2011). Predicting complete cytogenetic response and subsequent progression-free survival in 20160 patients with CML on imatinib treatment: the EUTOS score. *Blood.* 118(3):686–692. DOI: 10.1182/blood-2010-12-319038; and Hoffman VS, et al. (2017). Treatment and outcome of 2904 CML patients from the EUTOS population-based registry. *Leukemia.* 31(3):593–601. DOI: 10.1038/leu.2016.246.

Unfortunately, what is a specific, risk-adapted treatment is still a matter of investigation or speculation. High-dose imatinib failed to show a superiority on standard dose imatinib in Sokal high-risk patients. The use of second-generation TKIs is expected to do better, but it is already known that also with second-generation TKIs the response of high-risk patients is inferior to the response of non-high-risk ones. All these considerations apply to adults. As far as ACA patients are concerned, no data are available on the value of alternative treatments. In children, Ph+, BCR-ABL1+ CML is rare, is more aggressive, and is worth of specific studies and analyses.

The problem is that these factors, risk and ACA, help identifying the patients who have a poorer response and outcome, but cannot help understanding why response and outcome are poorer. This is the case also in so many leukaemias and other cancers, when high-risk patients, once identified, become eligible for 'more' therapy, although it is quite clear that 'more' is not always 'better' than standard, and may not be cost-effective. In CML, is 'more' also 'better'? And what is 'more'? It was already noticed that 'more' imatinib was not clearly better than 'standard' imatinib. Also 'more' nilotinib (400 mg twice daily) was not better than 'standard' nilotinib (300 mg twice daily), as well as 'more' dasatinib (70 mg twice daily) versus 'standard' dasatinib (100 mg once daily). Maybe all second-generation TKIs are 'more' than imatinib, and can perform better in high-risk patients, but are they cost-effective? What about the impact on unrelated deaths? Allogeneic stem cell transplantation (SCT) is believed to be 'more' than TKIs, but the very well-known problems of age, donor, and particularly of transplant-related morbidity and mortality, limit the application of SCT.

Since 'more' is not always better, the identification of the poor responders is not sufficient to improve treatment and outcome, and should include the identification of the causes of poor response, so that the cause can be specifically targeted, guiding the choice of the treatment. This principle is already applied at least in part in second-line treatment, when the choice of the TKI is helped by the identification of a BCR-ABL1 mutation. This principle could be applied also baseline, if one could validate the findings about BIM, about drug transporters, particularly OCT-1, and about other genes, making it possibly a specific, targeted choice of treatment. Emerging novel agents may help TKIs to suppress Ph+ cells, including the stem ones, but the step from lab to bed is difficult, and progress in this area were limited, so far.

Finally, two considerations are important. First, the results of TKIs treatment are already so good that it is more and more difficult to predict response and outcome and to identify the few patients who will die of leukaemia. Second, a careful monitoring during treatment is of utmost importance, whatever it may be the baseline risk.

Acknowledgements

This work was supported by European LeukemiaNet, by the EUTOS project, and by the European LeukemiaNet Foundation. The authors wish to thank Chiara Ferri and Michela Apolinari for excellent technical assistance, and Professor Tariq I. Mughal for editorial assistance.

Reference

1. Baccarani M, Rosti G, Soverini S. Chronic myeloid leukemia: the concepts of resistance and persistence and the relationship with the BCR-ABL transcript type. *Leukemia*. 2019;33:2358–64.

Further reading

Ali S, Sergeant R, O'Brien SG, et al. Dasatinib may overcome the negative prognostic impact of KIR2DS1 in newly diagnosed patients with chronic myeloid leukemia. *Blood*. 2012;120(3):697–8.

Alonso-Dominguez JM, Grinfeld J, Alikian M, et al. PTCH1 expression at diagnosis predicts imatinib failure in chronic myeloid leukemia patients in chronic phase. *Am J Hematol*. 2015;90(1):20–6.

Andolina JR, Neudorf SM, Corey SJ. How I treat childhood CML. *Blood*. 2012;119:1821–30.

Angelini S, Soverini S, Ravegnini G, et al. Association between imatinib transporters and metabolizing enzymes genotype and response in newly diagnosed chronic myeloid leukemia patients receiving imatinib therapy. *Haematologica*. 2013;98(2):193–200.

Apperley JF. Part I: mechanisms of resistance to imatinib in chronic myeloid leukemia. *Lancet Oncol*. 2007; 8:1018–29.

Apperley JF. Part II: management of resistance to imatinib in chronic myeloid leukaemia. *Lancet Oncol*. 2007; 8:1116–29.

Baccarani M, Deininger MW, Rosti G, et al. European LeukemiaNet recommendations for the management of chronic myeloid leukemia: 2013. *Blood*. 2013;122(6):872–84.

Baccarani M, Rosti G, Castagnetti F, et al. A comparison of imatinib 400 mg and 800 mg daily in the first-line treatment of high risk, Philadelphia-positive, chronic myeloid leukemia. A European LeukemiaNet study. *Blood*. 2009;113:4497–504.

Baccarani M, Rosti G, Soverini S. Chronic myeloid leukemia: the concepts of resistance and persistence and the relationship with the BCR-ABL transcript type. *Leukemia*. 2019;33:2358–64.

Baccarani M, Russo D, Rosti G. Interferon-alfa for chronic myeloid leukemia. *Semin Hematol*. 2003;40:22–33.

Branford S, Kim DDH, Apperly JF, et al. Laying the Foundation for Genomically-Based Risk Assessment in Chronic Myeloid Leukemia. *Leukemia*. 2019;33(8):1835–1850.

Castagnetti F, Gugliotta G, Baccarani M, et al. Differences among young adults, adults, and elderly chronic myeloid leukemia patients. *Ann Oncol*. 2015;26;185–92.

Castagnetti F, Testoni N, Luatti S, et al. Deletions of the derivative chromosome 9 do not influence the response and the outcome of chronic myeloid leukemia in early chronic phase treated with imatinib mesylate: GIMEMA CML working party analysis. *J Clin Oncol*. 2010;28:2748–54.

Dulucq S, Bouchet S, Turcq B, et al. Multidrug resistance gene (MDR1) polymorphisms are associated with major molecular responses to standard-dose imatinib in chronic myeloid leukemia. *Blood*. 2008;112:2024–7.

Fabarius A, Leitner A, Hochhaus A, et al. Impact of additional cytogenetic aberrations at diagnosis on prognosis of CML: long-term observation of 1151 patients from the randomized CML Study IV. *Blood*. 2011;118:6760–8.

Fausto C, Gugliotta G, Soverini S, Baccarani M, Rosti G. Current treatment approaches in CML. *Hemsphere*. 2019;3(S2):54–6.

Gong Z, Medieros J, Cortes JE, et al. Cytogenetic-based risk prediction of blast transformation of CML in the era of TKI therapy. *Blood Adv*. 2017;1:2541–52.

Gugliotta G, Castagnetti F, Palandri F, et al. Frontline imatinib treatment of chronic myeloid leukemia: no impact of age on outcome, a survey by the GIMEMA CML Working Party. *Blood*. 2011;117(21):5591–9.

Guilhot F, Hughes TP, Cortes J, et al. Plasma exposure of imatinib and its correlation with clinical response in the Thyrosine Kinase Inhibitor Optimization and Selectivity Trial. *Haematologica*. 2012;97(5):731–8.

Hanfstein B, Lauseker M, Hehlmann R, et al. Distinct characteristics of e13a2 versus e14a2 BCR-ABL1 driven chronic myeloid leukemia under first-line therapy with imatinib. *Haematologica*. 2014;99(9):1441–7.

Hasford J, Baccarani M, Hoffman V, et al. Predicting complete cytogenetic response and subsequent progression-free survival in 20160 patients with CML on imatinib treatment: the EUTOS score. *Blood*. 2011;118:686–92.

Hasford J, Pfirmann M, Hehlmann R, et al. A new prognostic score for survival of patients with chronic myeloid leukemia treated with interferon alfa. *J Natl Cancer Inst*. 1998;90:850–8.

Hehlmann R, Hochhaus A, Baccarani M, et al. Chtonic myeloid lekaemia. *Lancet*. 2007;370:342–50.

Hochhaus A, Baccarani M, Silver RT, et al. European LeukemiaNet 2020 recommendations for treating chronic myeloid leukemia. *Leukemia*. 2020. https://doi.org/10.1038/s41375-020-0776-2

Hochhaus A, Larson RA, Guilhot F, et al. Long-term outcomes of imatinib treatment for chronic myeloid leukemia. *N Engl J Med*. 2017;376:917–27.

Hoffman VS, Baccarani M, Hasford J, et al. Treatment and outcome of 2904 CML patients from the EUTOS population-based registry. *Leukemia*. 2017;31:593–601.

Jabbour E, le Coutre PD, Cortes J, et al. Prediction of outcomes in patients with Ph+ chronic myeloid leukemia in chronic phase treated with nilotinib after imatinib resistance/intolerance. *Leukemia*. 2013;27(4):907–91.

Kalmanti L, Saussele S, Lauseker M, et al. Younger patients with chronic myeloid leukemia do well in spite of poor prognostic indicators: results from the randomized CML study IV. *Ann Hematol*. 2014;93:71–80.

Lauseker M, Bachl K, Turkina A, et al. Prognosis of patients with chronic myeloid leukemia presenting in advanced phase is defined mainly by blast count, but also by age, chromosomal berrations and hemoglobin. *Am J Hematol*. 2019;94(11):1236–43.

Lippert E, Etienne G, Mozziconacci M-J, et al. Loss of the Y chromosome in Philadelphia-positive cells predicts a poor response of chronic myeloid leukemia patients to imatinib mesylate therapy. *Haematologica*. 2010;95(9):1604–7.

Luatti S, Castagnetti F, Marzocchi G, et al. Additional chromosome abnormalities in Philadelphia-positive clone: adverse prognostic influence on frontline imatinib therapy: a GIMEMA Working Party on CML analysis. *Blood*. 2012;120(4):761–7.

Mahon FX, Rea D, Guilhot J, et al. Discontinuation of imatinib in patients with chronic myeloid leukaemia who have maintained complete molecular remission for at least 2 years: the prospective, multicentre Stop Imatinib (STIM) trial. *Lancet Oncol*. 2010;11:1029–35.

Marin D, Gabriel IH, Ahmad S, et al. KIR2DS1 genotype predicts for complete cytogenetic response and survival in newly diagnosed chronic myeloid leukemia patients treated with imatinib. *Leukemia*. 2012;26:296–302.

Marzocchi G, Castagnetti F, Luatti S, et al. Variant Philadelphia translocations: molecular-cytogenetic characterization and prognostic influence on frontline imatinib therapy, a GIMEMA working party on CML analysis. *Blood*. 2011;117(25):6793–800.

McWeeney SK, Pemberton LC, Loriaux MM, et al. A gene expression profile of CD34+ cells to predict major cytogenetic response in chronic-phase chronic myeloid leukemia patients treated with imatinib. *Blood*. 2010;115:315–25.

Melo JV. The diversity of BCR-ABL. Fusion proteins and their relationship to leukemia phenotype. *Blood*. 1996;88(7):2375–84.

Milojkovic D, Nicholson E, Apperley JF, et al. Early prediction of success or failure of treatment with second generation tyrosine kinase inhibitors in patients with chronic myeloid leukemia. *Haematologica*. 2010;95:224–31.

Mughal TI, Dieninger MW, Radich JP, et al. Chronic myeloid leukemia: reminiscences and dreams. *Haematologica*. 2016;101:541–58.

Mughal TI, Radich JR, Deininger MW, et al. Chronic myeloid leukemia: reminiscences and dreams. *Haematologica*. 2016;101:541–58.

Ng KP, Hillmer AM, Chuah CTH, et al. A common BIM deletion polymorphism mediates intrinsic resistance and inferior responses to tyrosine kinase inhibitors in cancer. *Nature Med*. 2012;18(4):521–8.

O'Brien SG, Guilhot F, Larson R, et al. Imatinib compared with interferon and low-dose cytarabine for newly diagnosed chronic-phase chronic myeloid leukemia. *N Engl J Med*. 2003;348:994–1004.

Pavlu J, Szydlo RM, Goldman JM, Apperley JF. Three decades of transplantation for chronic myeloid leukemia: what have we learned? *Blood*. 2011;117(3):755–63.

Pfirmann M, Baccarani M, Sauselle S, et al. Prognosis of long-term survival considering disease-specific death in patients with chronic myeloid leukemia. *Leukemia*. 2016;30:48–56.

Preudhomme C, Guilhot J, Nicolini FE, et al. Imatinib plus Peginterferon alfa-2a in chronic myeloid leukemia. *N Engl J Med*. 2010;363:2511–21.

Radich JR, Dai H, Mao M, et al. Gene expression changes associated with progression and response in chronic myeloid leukemia. *PNAS*. 2006;103(8):2794–9.

Rosti G, Castagnetti F, Gugliotta G, Baccarani M. Tyrosine kinase inhibitors in chronic myeloid leukemia: which, when, for whom? *Nat Clin Oncol Rev*. 2017;14:141–54.

Rosti G, Iacobucci I, Bassi S, et al. Impact of age on the outcome of patients with chronic myeloid leukemia in late chronic phase: results of a phase II study of the GIMEMA CML Working Party. *Haematologica*. 2007;92(01):101–5.

Saglio G, Kim DW, Issaragrisil S, et al. Nilotinib versus imatinib for newly diagnosed chronic myeloid leukemia. *N Engl J Med*. 2010, 362:2251–9.

Sokal JE, Baccarani M, Russo D, Tura S. Staging and prognosis in chronic myelogenous leukemia. *Semin Hematol*. 1988;25(1):49–61.

Sokal JE, Baccarani M, Tura S, et al. Prognostic discrimination among younger patients with chronic granulocytic leukemia: relevance to bone marrow transplantation. *Blood*. 1985;66(6):1352–7.

Sokal JE, Cox EB, Baccarani M, et al. Prognostic discrimination in 'good-risk' chronic granulocytic leukemia. *Blood*. 1984;63:789–99.

Sokal JE, Gomez GA, Baccarani M, et al. Prognostic significance of additional cytogenetic abnormalities at diagnosis of Philadelphia chromosome-positive chronic granulocytic leukemia. *Blood*. 1988;72(1):294–8.

Sovereini S, Mancini M, Bavaro L, Cavo M, Martinelli G. Chronic myeloid leukemia: the paradigm of targeting and counteracting resistance for successful cancer therapy. *Molecular Cancer*. 2018;17:49–64.

Soverini S, Gnani A, Colarossi S, et al. Philadelphia-positive patients who already harbour imatinib-resistant Bcr-Abl kinase domain mutations have a higher likelihood of developing additional mutations associated with resistance to second- or third-line tyrosine kinase inhibitors. *Blood*. 2009;114:2168–71.

Soverini S, Hochhaus A, Nicolini FE, et al. BCR-ABL kinase domain mutations analysis in chronic myeloid leukemia patients treated with tyrosine kinase inhibitors. Recommendations from an expert panel on behalf of European Leukemia Net. *Blood*. 2011;118(5):1208–15.

The Italian Cooperative Study Group on Chronic Myeloid Leukemia. Chronic myeloid leukemia, BCR-ABL transcript, response to alfa-interferon and survival. *Leukemia*. 1995;9:1648–52.

Thomas J, Wang L, Clark RE, Pirmohamed L. Active transport of imatinib into and out of cells: implications for drug resistance. *Blood*. 2004;104(12):3739–45.

Tura S, Baccarani M, Corbelli G, et al. Staging of chronic myeloid leukaemia. *Br J Haematol*. 1981;47:105–19.

Tura S, Baccarani M, Zaccaria A. Chronic myeloid leukemia. *Haematologica*. 1986;71:168–76.

Verma D, Kantarjian H, Shan J, et al. Survival outcomes for clonal evolution in chronic myeloid leukemia patients on second generation tyrosine kinase inhibitor therapy. *Cancer*. 2010;116:2673–81.

Vigneri P, Stagno F, Stella S, et al. High BCR-ABL/GUSIS levels at diagnosis are associated with unfavourable responses to imatinib. *Haematologica*. 2014;99(S1):74.

White DL, Dang P, Engler J, et al. Functional activity of the OCT-1 protein is predictive of long-term outcome in patients with chronic-phase chronic myeloid leukemia treated with imatinib. *J Clin Oncol*. 2010;28:2761–7.

White DL, Radich J, Soverini S, et al. Chronic phase chronic myeloid leukemia patients with low OCT-1 activity randomised to high-dose imatinib achieve better responses, and lower failure rates, than those randomized to standard-dose. *Haematologica*. 2012;97(6):907–14.

Chapter 6

Molecular risk stratification of myeloproliferative neoplasms

Paola Guglielmelli and Alessandro M. Vannucchi

Molecular risk stratification and Ph-negative chronic myeloproliferative neoplasms *80*
Mutations in phenotypic driver genes: *JAK2*, *MPL*, *CALR* *80*
Subclonal mutations: Less common, more complex, but prognostically meaningful *87*
Conclusions *91*

Molecular risk stratification and Ph-negative chronic myeloproliferative neoplasms

The term myeloproliferative neoplasms (MPN) has been attributed by the World Health Organization (WHO) in 2016 to those relatively common haematologic neoplasia also known as Philadelphia chromosome-negative, classic, chronic myeloproliferative diseases, including polycythaemia vera (PV), essential thrombocythaemia (ET), and primary myelofibrosis (PMF), as initially described by W. Dameshek in 1951. In 2005, several investigators concurrently described the presence of a point mutation in exon 14 of the Janus kinase 2 (*JAK2*) gene in the large majority of patients with PV and about 50–60% of those with ET and PMF. Additional genetic mutations have been described since, including mutations in the thrombopoietin receptor (MPL) gene in ET and PMF, and mutations in exon 12 of *JAK2* in *JAK2*V617F-negative PV. More recently, mutations in the gene encoding the endoplasmic protein calreticulin (*CALR*) have been discovered in about 20% of ET and PMF patients. The current 2016 WHO classification includes these genetic findings as major criteria (Table 6.1). Collectively, these mutations in *JAK2, MPL*, and *CALR* are now recognized as 'phenotypic driver mutations'. Recent studies have also observed a number of additional mutations occur in a subset of patients, particularly those with PMF, that are usually harboured by subclones of variable size. These abnormalities, found in diverse myeloid malignancies, target genes involved in the epigenetic gene regulations, the spliceosome, or oncogenes, impact on the prognosis of patients with MPN.

Mutations in phenotypic driver genes: *JAK2, MPL, CALR*

The V617F mutation, a 'gain-of-function' mutation, located in exon 14 of *JAK2*, encodes for the pseudokinase domain of the protein and exerts an auto-inhibitory regulation of the kinase activity of JAK2. It autonomously (i.e. in the absence of cytokines bound to cognate receptors) leads to downstream target activation through deregulated protein phosphorylation, ultimately resulting in sustained JAK/STAT signalling. Expression of mutated JAK2 in mice results in a myeloproliferative disease characterized by erythrocytosis, varying degree of leukocytosis and thrombocytosis, splenomegaly, and eventual progression to myelofibrosis; transformation to leukaemia is not clearly documented. Mutations in exon 12 of *JAK2* have been identified in about 40–50% of patients with a PV phenotype who are negative for the *JAK2*V617F mutation. Over 20 variants have been reported to date, the most common being N542-E543del, found in 30% of cases. Clinically, these cases present with erythrocytosis but less marked leukocytosis and thrombocytosis compared with V617F mutated PV, although the rate of thrombosis, transformation to myelofibrosis or leukaemia, and overall survival, are comparable to *JAK2*V617F mutated PV.

Table 6.1 The 2016 WHO classification for MPN

	Polycythaemia vera (PV)*	Essential thrombocythaemia (ET)*	Primary myelofibrosis (PMF)*
Major criteria	1. Haemoglobin >16.5 g/dL (men) >16 g/dL (women) or Haematocrit >49% (men) >48% (women)	1. Platelet count ≥450 × 10^9/L	1. Megakaryocyte proliferation and atypia*** accompanied by either reticulin and/or collagen fibrosis or†
	2. BM trilineage myeloproliferation with pleomorphic megakaryocytes	2. Megakaryocyte proliferation with large and mature morphology	2. Not meeting WHO criteria for CML, PV, ET, MDS, or other myeloid neoplasm
	3. Presence of *JAK2* mutation	3. Not meeting WHO criteria for CML, PV, PMF, MDS, or other myeloid neoplasm	3. Presence of *JAK2*, *CALR*, or *MPL* mutation
		4. Presence of *JAK2*, *CALR*, or *MPL* mutation	

(*Continued*)

Table 6.1 *contd.*

	Polycythaemia vera (PV)*	Essential thrombocythaemia (ET)*	Primary myelofibrosis (PMF)*
Minor criteria	1. Subnormal serum erythropoietin level	1. Presence of a clonal marker (e.g. abnormal karyotype) **or** absence of evidence for reactive thrombocytosis	1. Presence of a clonal marker (e.g. abnormal karyotype) **or** absence of evidence for reactive bone marrow fibrosis
			2. Presence of anaemia **or** palpable splenomegaly
			3. Presence of leukoerythroblastosis†† **or** increased lactate dehydrogenase††

*PV diagnosis requires meeting either all three major criteria or the first two major criteria and one minor criterion.

*ET diagnosis requires meeting all four major criteria or first three major criteria and one minor criterion.

*PMF diagnosis requires meeting all three major criteria or the first two major criteria and all three minor criteria.

***Small to large megakaryocytes with aberrant nuclear/cytoplasmic ratio and hyperchromatic and irregularly folded nuclei and dense clustering.

†or In the absence of reticulin fibrosis, the megakaryocyte changes must be accompanied by increased marrow cellularity, granulocytic proliferation and often decreased erythropoiesis (i.e. prefibrotic PMF).

††degree of abnormality can be borderline or marked and institutional reference range should be used for lactate dehydrogenase level

Key: BM, bone marrow; WHO, World Health Organization; CML, chronic myelogenous leukaemia; MDS, myelodysplastic syndromes

Adapted from Arber DA, et al. The 2016 revision to the World Health Organization classification of myeloid neoplasms and acute leukemia. *Blood*. 127(20):2391–405. https://doi.org/10.1182/blood-2016-03-643544. Reprinted with permission from the American Society of Hematology.

- About 5% and 10% of patients with *JAK2* wild-type ET or PMF, respectively, harbour point mutations located at codon 515 of *MPL*, the gene encoding for the thrombopoietin receptor; occasional patients with somatically acquired S505N mutation, most commonly associated with familial thrombocytosis, have also been reported. The tryptophan residue located at position 515 is part of a short aminoacidic stretch (K/RWQFP), located in the intramembrane, juxta cytoplasmic portion of the protein, whose integrity is mandatory to prevent the constitutive, ligand independent, activation of the receptor; any aminoacid change at this level (the most frequent being L, K, A) induces instability of the receptor and its activation. Retroviral expression of *MPL*W515L in a mouse model resulted in an aggressive MPN-like disease with extreme thrombocytosis, rapid development of bone marrow fibrosis, splenomegaly, and shortened survival. Patients with ET and PMF harbouring any of the *MPL*W515 substitutions present more extensive thrombocytosis when compared with *JAK2*V617F mutated, lower levels of haemoglobin and, in case of PMF, are more at risk of being transfusion dependent.

The discovery of mutations in the calreticulin gene (*CALR*) in 2013, by Green, Kralovics, and colleagues, impacts on the diagnostic criteria of MPN. Mutations in *CALR* are present in 60–88% of patients with ET and PMF, who are negative for the *JAK2* and *MPL* mutations. *CALR* mutations are represented by insertions or deletions restricted to exon 9; more than 80% of cases present two alternative mutations, either a 52-bp deletion (type 1; 45–53% of all cases) or a 5-bp insertion (type 2; 32–41%). However, more than 50 variants, divided broadly into type 1-like and type 2-like, have now been reported. All known mutations cause a +1nt frameshift with the resulting production of a novel C-terminal peptide. Theoretically, this represents a new antigen potentially suitable for labelling and targeting. Vannucchi and colleagues have reported that a rabbit antibody selectively labelled mutated calreticulin preferentially expressed in cells of megakaryocytic lineage in *CALR* mutated subjects, an observation which may impact diagnosis. The frequency of the diverse mutations observed in patients with MPN is depicted in Figure 6.1.

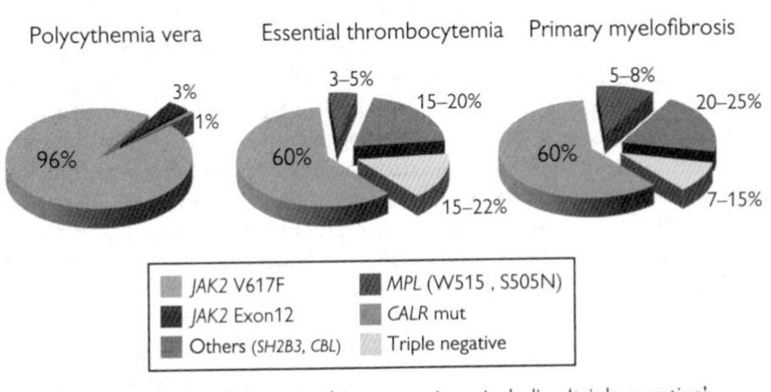

Figure 6.1 Frequency of the main driver mutations, including 'triple negative' patients with MPN.

*JAK2*V617F mutated patients may express the mutation in a heterozygous or homozygous status, meaning that the proportion of mutated allele is lower (heterozygous) or higher (homozygous) than 50% when assayed in whole blood nucleated cells or preferably purified granulocytes that are a heterogeneous cell population. Therefore, although commonly used as such, this terminology is not strictly appropriate since the concept of hetero- or homozygosity points to the single cell rather than to a heterogeneous cell population where the proportion of clonal *JAK2*V617F mutated cells and polyclonal normal cells is variable. Homozygosity is acquired through a process of mitotic recombination. Levels of *JAK2*V617F allele burden in blood cells greater than 50% are definitely more common in PV than in ET; in PMF, and even more in myelofibrosis developed from previous PV (PPV-MF) or ET (PET-MF), the large majority of patients have allele burden over 50%, but one-quarter of the patients may present levels lower than 20%. Therefore, quantifying *JAK2*V617F allele burden is not useful for making differential diagnosis among the different MPN, although a diagnosis of ET with a high levels of *JAK2*V617F mutated allele should prompt the clinician to re-analyse data to definitely confirm such diagnosis, since homozygosity in ET patients involved only 4% in a large series. Homozygosity in PV has been shown to result from the selective expansion of a founder homozygous clone that takes over the others, while in some ET patients the few emerging homozygous clones are restrained in their growth and do not amplify.

The level of *JAK2*V617F allele remains substantially stable over time in many patients and is not obviously modified by cytotoxic drugs, although some decline with long-term busulfan has been reported. Therefore, it is not informative, nor has any clinical implications, to obtain serial measurements of *JAK2*V617F allele during an uneventful disease as well as in patients receiving conventional treatment. With prolonged observation, some patients show progressive increase in the amount of mutated allele, and accumulation of V617F allele has been associated with progression to post-PV or post-ET MF. In case of *MPL* mutation, the mutant allele burden ranged from 1% to 95% among 62 mutated patients, being significantly higher in PMF or PET-MF than in ET. Homozygosity for *MPL* mutation was due to acquired copy-neutral loss of heterozygosity at 1p. Levels of *MPL*-mutated allele burden greater than 50% were associated with occurrence of marrow fibrosis, overall suggesting a pathogenetic role of accumulation of *MPL*-mutated alleles in the development of fibrosis. However, the current criteria for the diagnosis of post-PV/post-ET MF, as outlined by the International Working Group for Myeloproliferative Neoplasms Research and Treatment (IWG-MRT), are based on a set of clinical, haematological, and histopathological variables that do not include the levels of *JAK2*V617F or *MPL* allele. Therefore, in the clinical practice, outside a clinical trial, it is not informative to have MPN patients sequentially evaluated for their *JAK2*V617F or *MPL*W515L/K/A allele burden.

Using pegylated interferon (IFN)-alpha2a in PV patients, reduction of *JAK2*V617F allele burden from a baseline of 45% and 64% to 5% and 12% after therapy was respectively reported in two studies, while in another study that used either pegylated interferon alpha 2b or 2a no such degree of reduction was observed. Notably, decrease of *JAK2*V617F allele burden was not overtly correlated with clinical and haematological responses, and no clear explanation for the observed differences among different types of IFN can be anticipated. Furthermore, in two patients with *CALR* mutated ET, peg-IFN alpha therapy resulted in sustained complete haematologic responses that were associated with progressive reductions in allele burden. Therefore, in patients who have been in continuous treatment with pegIFN for at least 1 year, a time around which the first evidences of mutated allele reduction may occur, it may be reasonable to assess variations in the mutated allele burden; furthermore, a sustained complete molecular remission might prompt the physician to consider stopping treatment. Varying degree of reduction of the *JAK2*V617F allele burden in patients with MF and PV receiving the JAK1 and JAK2 inhibitor ruxolitinib have been described, but complete molecular remission may occur only occasionally in patients after long period of treatment. Some patients who maintained such molecular response even after treatment discontinuation have been anecdotally reported, but it remains to be demonstrated prospectively whether the attainment of molecular remission represents a criterion for managing therapy, and what is the final significance of the disappearance of measurable *JAK2*V617F allele for disease progression. In such instances of complete molecular remissions obtained with drugs (IFNα, type I JAK2 inhibitor), one must consider the availability of diagnostic assays that should be able to reproducibly measure levels of *JAK2*V617F allele burden with at least 10^{-4} performance. This is of particular relevance in the settings of haematopoietic stem cell transplantation (HSCT), where careful monitoring of the *JAK2*V617F allele burden may contribute to the optimized management of patients by providing information about the disappearance of the mutated clone and the identification of subjects that are at increased risk of relapse. The use of *JAK2*V617F allele monitoring for timely and successful delivery of donor lymphocyte infusions has been reported. Similarly, patients with MPL and *CALR* mutations may be evaluated for outcome after HSCT, but until now the reliability and sensitivity of available tests for these mutations remain to be fully ascertained.

The discovery of *CALR* mutations deserved a major impact on the diagnostic approach to suspected MPN targeting that 40% of PMF and ET cases that were *JAK2* and *MPL* unmutated. *CALR* mutations were found very infrequently in a few cases of atypical chronic myeloid leukaemia, chronic myelomonocytic leukaemia or chronic neutrophilic leukaemia and in occasional patients with myelodysplastic syndromes (MDS), particularly with refractory anaemia with ring sideroblasts, therefore mutated *CALR* is considered a highly specific marker of *JAK2* and *MPL* wild-type MPN. However, analysis of *CALR* mutated patients quite unexpectedly revealed to be extremely useful in the process of prognostic assessment for ET and particularly PMF patients. In the era of '*JAK2*V617 or *MPL* mutation-only', no clear-cut impact of those mutations, as well as the respective allele burden on disease outcome was realized. In patients with PMF, *JAK2*V617F homozygosity was associated in some studies to shorter survival and greater risk of transformation to leukaemia, while others reported that a low *JAK2*V617F allele burden was prognostically adverse. In ET, patients who are *JAK2*V617F mutated had a 2-fold higher rate of thrombosis compared with the wild-type ones, and a mutated allele burden in excess of 50% and

75% was associated with increased risk of thrombosis in ET and PV, respectively. However, additional confirmatory work is required prior to the systematic use of mutation asset for prognostication except in the case of ET. The International Prognostic Score of thrombosis includes the presence of *JAK2V617F* positivity as one risk variable for accurate prediction of thrombosis in patients with ET (Table 6.2). Conversely, ET patients who express the *CALR* mutation are at significantly lower risk of thrombosis when compared with *JAK2V617F* and *MPL*-mutated ones, with a relative risk very close to the 'triple negative'. The positive impact of *CALR* mutation in ET may be particularly pronounced among the youngest patients; no measurable differences in outcome according to the type (1 vs. 2) mutation. The addition of *CALR* mutation to the variables already listed in the IPSET-thrombosis score did not affect its performance, owing the strong impact of the *JAK2V617* mutation as prognostically adverse variable. However, it is particularly in PMF that the impact of CALR mutation has been striking. In the largest study, which included over 800 patients with PMF, *CALR* mutation was associated with significant better overall survival (17.7 years) compared with *JAK2V617F* (9.2 years) and *MPL* (9.1 years) mutated patients. However, perhaps the most relevant findings is that triple negative patients are at very high risk of early death (overall survival 3.2 years) that was associated with lower cumulative incidence of anaemia (Hb <10 g/dL), leukocytosis (>25 × 10^9/L) and thrombocytopenia (<100 × 10^9/L) (Figure 6.2). Concurrent presence of *CALR* mutation with abnormalities in *ASXL1* partially mitigated the adverse impact of the latter. More subtle effects may also be dependent on the unique molecular lesion in *CALR*, with type 1 mutation being reported to account for better prognosis than type 2.

Table 6.2 The IPSET score for prediction of thrombosis in ET

Risk factor	HR
Age >60 y	1.50
Cardiovascular risk factors	1.56
Previous thrombosis	1.93
JAK2V617F mutation	2.04
Risk categories	**Score**
Low risk	0–1
Intermediate risk	2
High risk	≥3

Adapted from Barbui T, et al. (2012). Development and validation of an International Prognostic Score of thrombosis in World Health Organization–essential thrombocythemia (IPSET-thrombosis). *Blood*. 120(26):5128–33. DOI: 10.1182/blood-2012-07-444067. Reprinted with permission from the American Society of Hematology.

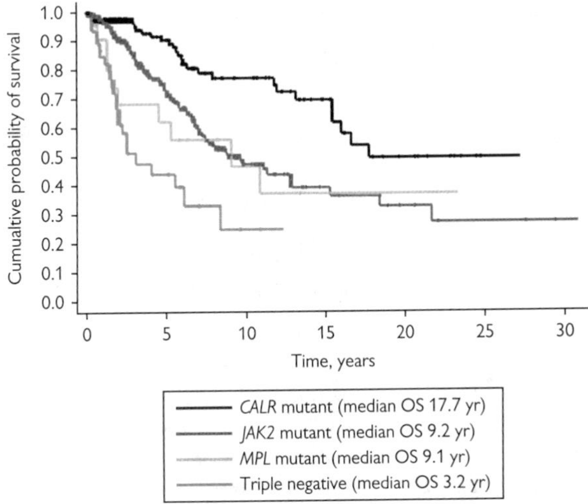

Figure 6.2 Kaplan–Meier analysis of the impact of phenotypic driver mutations (*JAK2*V617F, *MPL*W5151, and *CALR* mutations), and the condition of 'triple negativity', on overall survival in patients with PMF (also see plate section).

Adapted from Rumi E, et al. Clinical effect of driver mutations of JAK2, CALR or MPL in primary myelofibrosis. *Blood*. 124(7):1062–9. DOI: 10.1182/blood-2014-05-578435. Reprinted with permission from the American Society of Hematology.

Subclonal mutations: Less common, more complex, but prognostically meaningful

The molecular landscape of patients with MN is much more complex than originally believed. This is supported by evidence from several studies showing that many different mutations other than the phenotypic drivers, mainly falling in the functional categories of epigenetic regulators, genes of the spliceosome and oncogenes, may occur in a proportion of the patients. The most recurrent abnormalities reported to date are listed in Table 6.3. Generally speaking, these are definitely more frequent in PMF as compared to PV and ET, while others, in particular mutations of *TP53*, tend to accumulate at the time of leukaemic transformation. These same abnormalities occur with similar or even higher frequency in MDS and acute leukaemias, therefore they have no specific utility for the diagnosis of MPN a part for rare instances of unusual clinical presentation and absence of the phenotypic driver mutations where finding any one of these subclonal mutations might help to assess the existence of a clonal myeloid disorder. However,

Table 6.3 List of subclonal mutations reported in patients with MPN

	Localization	Function	Type of abnormalities
SIGNALLING			
JAK2ex14	9p24	Tyrosine kinase, signalling	Gain of function
JAK2ex12	9p24	Tyrosine kinase, signalling	Gain of function
MPL	1p34	Receptor, signalling	Gain of function
CALR	19p13	ER-associated multifunction protein	Unknown
SH2B3(LNK)	12q24	Adaptor, signalling	Loss of function
CBL	11q23	Adaptor, E3 ubiquitin ligase, signalling	Dominant negative
SOCS1	16p13.2	E3 ubiquitin ligase, signalling	Methylation
SOCS2	12q22	E3 ubiquitin ligase, signalling	Methylation
SOCS3	17q25.3	E3 ubiquitin ligase, signalling	Methylation, mutation
EPIGENETIC			
TET2	4q24	DNA hydroxymethylation	Loss of function
ASXL1	20q11.21	Chromatin modifications	Loss of function
EZH2	7q35	Chromatin methylation	Loss of function
JARID	6p24	Chromatin methylation	Loss of function
SUZ12	17q11.2	Chromatin methylation	Loss of function
EED		Chromatin methylation	Loss of function
SPLICING			
SRSF2	17q25.1	Spliceosome	Loss of function
SF3B1	2q33.1	Spliceosome	Loss of function
LEUKAEMIA PROGRESSION			
IDH1	2q33.3	Metabolism	Neomorphic enzyme
IDH2	15q26.1	Metabolism	Neomorphic enzyme
TP53	17p13.1	Cell cycle, apoptosis	Loss of function
SMD4	1q32	TP53 regulator	Amplification
DNMT3A	2p23	Chromatin modifications	Loss of function
RB	13q14	Cell cycle, apoptosis	Deletion
IKZF1	7p12	Transcription factor	Deletion
RUNX1	21q22.3	Transcription factor	Loss of function
NRAS	1p13.2	GTPase, signalling	Gain of function

Source: data from Vainchenker W, et al. (2011). New mutations and pathogenesis of myeloproliferative neoplasms. *Blood*. 118(7):1723–35. DOI: 10.1182/blood-2011-02-292102; and Guglielmelli P, et al. (2018). MIPSS70: Mutation-Enhanced International Prognostic Score System for Transplantation-Age Patients with Primary Myelofibrosis. *J Clin Oncol*. 36(4):310–18. DOI: 10.1200/JCO.2017.76.4886.

recent reports indicating that mutations within some of these genes may be found in normal elderly individual advocates caution in interpreting the results. On the other hand, mutations of these genes in the settings of an otherwise well characterized MPN patient deserve prognostic relevance.

In an international study involving 897 patients with PMF, of which 483 constituted a learning cohort and were evaluated at the time of diagnosis, and 396 a validation cohort including patients at any time after diagnosis, over a panel of 11 genes we found that the most frequently mutated were *ASXL1*, *TET2*, *SRSF2*, *EZH2*, while *IDH1* and *IDH2* mutations were the less frequent (Table 6.4). Mutations in *ASXL1*, *EZH2*, *SRSF2*, and *IDH1/2* individually, and in an IPSS or DIPSS-plus independent manner, correlated with reduced survival and increased rate of leukaemia. *ASXL1*, *SRSF2*, and *EZH2* mutations were significantly enriched in the IPSS high-risk group with mutational frequencies of 42%, 25%, and 12%, respectively, and the DIPSS-plus high-risk category (45%, p <0.0002 and 22%, p <0.004, respectively). In terms of overall survival, in a multivariable analysis all three mutations resulted independently correlated with reduced survival with HR of 1.91 (95% CI: 1.1–3.36) for *EZH2*, 2.21 (95% CI: 1.57–3.11) for *ASXL1* and 2.6 (95% CI: 1.63–41.6) for *SRSF2*. As to the risk of leukaemia, the corresponding HR figures were 2.5 for *ASXL1* (95% CI: 1.5–4.1), 2.73 for *SRSF2* (95% CI: 1.34–5.55) and 2.66 for *IDH1* or *IDH2* (95%CI: 1.10–6.47), while mutations of *EZH2* were not significant (HR: 1.98, 95% CI: 0.88–4.46). We thereby defined as being at 'high molecular risk' (HMR) those patients who presented any one mutation in anyone of the aforementioned four genes, and multivariable analysis confirmed their statistically significant association with shorter survival, again IPSS and adverse cytogenetic independently. Furthermore, the cumulative risk of leukaemia using competitive risk analysis resulted significantly increased (HR: 2.96; 95% CI: 1.85–4.76) versus low molecular risk (LMR) patients (Figure 6.3). These observations, made in patients analysed within 1 year from diagnosis, were independently confirmed in patients included in the validation series against the DIPSS-plus scoring system. A direct comparison discovered that the rate of occurrence of those mutations was superimposable in patients evaluated at diagnosis (the IPSS series) or during the disease course (DIPSS-plus series); this suggests that most mutations are already present at diagnosis and that a mutational assessment at that time may be well predictive of outcome (Table 6.4). In addition, when the individual genes were evaluated for their prognostic impact, mutations in *ASXL1* turned out to be the most significant. As a matter of fact, a subsequent study showed that in patients coexpressing mutated *CALR* and *ASXL1*, the prognostic advantage driven by the *CALR* mutation was limited to *ASXL1* unmutated subjects, with the prognostically worse category being comprised of *ASXL1* mutated/*CALR* unmutated patients. Others have shown that splice factor gene mutations are less frequently associated with *CALR* mutation, possibly contributing to the better outcome of CALR mutated PMF patients also in the settings of stem cell transplantation. The relevance of a HMR status definition for the management of PMF patients is supported by the findings that 22% of subjects considered as being at low and intermediate-1 risk according to the IPSS score are actually harbouring prognostically adverse mutations, therefore their apparent good outcome may be overestimated. It remains to be established

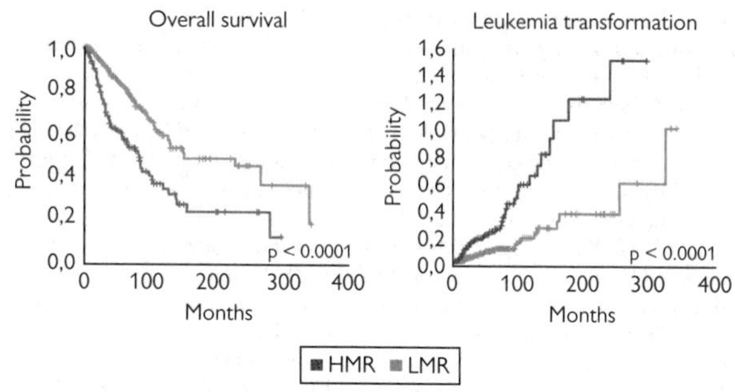

Figure 6.3 Kaplan–Meier analysis of the impact of a high molecular risk (HMR) versus low molecular risk (LMR) status on overall survival and leukaemia transformation in patients with PMF.

Adapted with permission from Vannucchi AM, et al. (2013). Mutations and prognosis in primary myelofibrosis. *Leukemia*. 27(9):1861–9. DOI: 10.1038/leu.2013.119.

Table 6.4 HMR mutations occurrence in a cohort of 863 patients with PMF

	IPSS n = 490	DIPSS n = 315
ASXL1 (%)	23.1	35.9
SRSF2 (%)	6.9	13.3
EZH2 (%)	6.3	3.7
IDH1/2 (%)	2.7	4.4

Source: data Guglielmelli P, et al. (2018). MIPSS70: Mutation-Enhanced International Prognostic Score System for Transplantation-Age Patients with Primary Myelofibrosis. *J Clin Oncol*. 36(4):310–18. DOI: 10.1200/JCO.2017.76.4886.

in prospective studies whether the use of more aggressive therapies, including stem cell transplantation, in this subgroup of patients might result in improved survival. Of interest, an analysis of MF patients treated with ruxolitinib in the context of the prospective, phase 3 COMFORT-2 study confirmed the adverse prognosis of the HMR status and demonstrated that the clinical efficacy in terms of enlarged spleen volume reduction and symptomatic improvement were similar in HMR and LMR groups. Furthermore, ruxolitinib provided a trend for improved survival in both molecularly characterized categories as well. In subsequent studies, it was also provided evidence that differences in outcome (survival and leukaemia transformation) exist within the HMR group when patients are categorized according to the number of HMR mutations they harbour (i.e. only one versus two or more mutations). Similar data were generated in an extended analysis of recurrent mutations.

Conclusions

The understanding of the mutation landscape of MPN has witnessed significant advances in the last few years with the discovery of phenotypic driver mutations that have revolutionized the diagnostic approach and paved the way for novel treatments with drugs targeting the key JAK/STAT signalling pathway. Patients lacking the three phenotypic driver mutations are very likely harbouring novel genetic abnormalities, the objective of intensive efforts from several groups. In addition, findings of recurrent subclonal mutations have added further insights into a previously unforeseen molecular complexity, and much still remains to be learned. On this basis, emergent data support the use of some genetic abnormalities for more accurate prognostication of MPN patients, particularly with PMF, and if substantiated in prospective studies might turn out the management of MPN patients.

Further reading

Arber DA, Orazi At, Hasserjian R, et al. The 2016 revision to the World Health Organization (WHO) classification of myeloid neoplasms and acute leukemia. *Blood*. 2016;127(20):2391–405.

Barbui T, Finazzi G, Carobbio A, et al. Development and validation of an International Prognostic Score of thrombosis in World Health Organization–essential thrombocythemia (IPSET-thrombosis). *Blood*. 2012;120(26):5128–33.

Barosi G, Bergamaschi G, Marchetti M, et al. JAK2 V617F mutational status predicts progression to large splenomegaly and leukemic transformation in primary myelofibrosis. *Blood*. 2007;110(12):4030–6.

Baxter EJ, Scott LM, Campbell PJ, et al. Acquired mutation of the tyrosine kinase JAK2 in human myeloproliferative disorders. *Lancet*. 2005;365(9464):1054–61.

Dusa A, Mouton C, Pecquet C, Herman M, Constantinescu SN. JAK2 V617F constitutive activation requires JH2 residue F595: a pseudokinase domain target for specific inhibitors. *PLoS One*. 2010;5(6):e11157.

Finazzi G, Carobbio A, Guglielmelli P, et al. Calreticulin mutation does not modify the IPSET score for predicting the risk of thrombosis among 1150 patients with essential thrombocythemia. *Blood*. 2014;124(16):2611–12.

Guglielmelli P, Barosi G, Specchia G, et al. Identification of patients with poorer survival in primary myelofibrosis based on the burden of JAK2V617F mutated allele. *Blood*. 2009;114(8):1477–83.

Guglielmelli P, Biamonte F, Rotunno G, et al. Impact of mutational status on outcomes in myelofibrosis patients treated with ruxolitinib in the COMFORT-II Study. *Blood*. 2014;123(10):2157–60.

Guglielmelli P, Lasho TL, Rotunno G, et al. The number of prognostically detrimental mutations and prognosis in primary myelofibrosis: an international study of 797 patients. *Leukemia*. 2014;28(9):1804–10.

Guglielmelli P, Nangalia J, Green AR, Vannucchi AM. CALR mutations in myeloproliferative neoplasms: hidden behind the reticulum. *Am J Hematol*. 2014;89(5):453–6.

James C, Ugo V, Le Couedic JP, et al. A unique clonal JAK2 mutation leading to constitutive signalling causes polycythaemia vera. *Nature*. 2005;434(7037):1144–8.

Klampfl T, Gisslinger H, Harutyunyan AS, et al. Somatic mutations of calreticulin in myeloproliferative neoplasms. *N Engl J Med*. 2013;369(25):2379–90.

Kralovics R, Passamonti F, Buser AS, et al. A gain-of-function mutation of JAK2 in myeloproliferative disorders. *N Engl J Med*. 2005;352(17):1779–90.

Levine RL, Wadleigh M, Cools J, et al. Activating mutation in the tyrosine kinase JAK2 in polycythemia vera, essential thrombocythemia, and myeloid metaplasia with myelofibrosis. *Cancer Cell*. 2005;7(4):387–97.

Nangalia J, Massie CE, Baxter EJ, et al. Somatic CALR mutations in myeloproliferative neoplasms with nonmutated JAK2. *New Engl J Med*. 2013;369(25):2391–405.

Passamonti F, Elena C, Schnittger S, et al. Molecular and clinical features of the myeloproliferative neoplasm associated with JAK2 exon 12 mutations. *Blood*. 2011;117(10):2813–16.

Pikman Y, Lee BH, Mercher T, et al. MPLW515L is a novel somatic activating mutation in myelofibrosis with myeloid metaplasia. *PLoS Med*. 2006;3(7):e270.

Rotunno G, Mannarelli C, Guglielmelli P, Pacilli A, Pancrazzi A, Pieri L, et al. Impact of calreticulin mutations on clinical and hematological phenotype and outcome in essential thrombocythemia. *Blood*. 2014;123(10):1552–5.

Rumi E, Pietra D, Guglielmelli P, et al. Acquired copy-neutral loss of heterozygosity of chromosome 1p as a molecular event associated with marrow fibrosis in MPL-mutated myeloproliferative neoplasms. *Blood*. 2013;121(21):4388–95.

Rumi E, Pietra D, Pascutto C, et al. Clinical effect of driver mutations of JAK2, CALR or MPL in primary myelofibrosis. *Blood*. 2014;124(7):1062–9.

Scott LM, Tong W, Levine RL, et al. JAK2 exon 12 mutations in polycythemia vera and idiopathic erythrocytosis. *N Engl J Med*. 2007;356(5):459–68.

Tefferi A, Thiele J, Vannucchi AM, Barbui T. An overview on CALR and CSF3R mutations and a proposal for revision of WHO diagnostic criteria for myeloproliferative neoplasms. *Leukemia*. 2014;28:1407–13.

Tefferi A, Wassie EA, Guglielmelli P, et al. Type 1 vs Type 2 calreticulin mutations in essential thrombocythemia: a collaborative study of 1027 patients. *Am J Hematol*. 2014;28:1568–70.

Vainchenker W, Delhommeau F, Constantinescu SN, Bernard OA. New mutations and pathogenesis of myeloproliferative neoplasms. *Blood*. 2011;118(7):1723–35.

Vannucchi AM, Antonioli E, Guglielmelli P, et al. Prospective identification of high-risk polycythemia vera patients based on JAK2(V617F) allele burden. *Leukemia*. 2007;21(9):1952–9.

Vannucchi AM, Antonioli E, Guglielmelli P, et al. Characteristics and clinical correlates of MPL 515W>L/K mutation in essential thrombocythemia. *Blood*. 2008;112:844–7.

Vannucchi AM, Antonioli E, Guglielmelli P, et al. Clinical profile of homozygous JAK2V617F mutation in patients with polycythemia vera or essential thrombocythemia. *Blood*. 2007;110(3):840–6.

Vannucchi AM, Antonioli E, Guglielmelli P, Pardanani A, Tefferi A. Clinical correlates of JAK2V617F presence or allele burden in myeloproliferative neoplasms: a critical reappraisal. *Leukemia*. 2008;22(7):1299–307.

Vannucchi AM, Lasho TL, Guglielmelli P, et al. Mutations and prognosis in primary myelofibrosis. *Leukemia*. 2013;27(9):1861–9.

Vannucchi AM, Rotunno G, Bartalucci N, et al. Calreticulin mutation-specific immunostaining in myeloproliferative neoplasms: pathogenetic insight and diagnostic value. *Leukemia*. 2014;28(9):1811–18.

Chapter 7

Chronic myeloid leukaemia

Tariq I. Mughal

Introduction *94*
Epidemiology *95*
Aetiology *95*
Natural history *95*
Clinical features and diagnosis *96*
Cytogenetics *96*
Molecular biology *98*
Prognostic factors *100*
Management *101*
First-generation TKI *102*
Second-generation TKIs *105*
Third-generation TKI *106*
Adverse effects associated with *ABL1* TKIs *107*
Investigational approaches *108*
Allogeneic stem cell transplantation *109*
Discontinuing *ABL1*-TKI treatment *110*
Treatment of patients with CML in blast transformation *110*
Future prospects *111*

Introduction

The term chronic myeloid leukaemia (CML), historically used interchangeably with the terms chronic myelogenous leukaemia, chronic myelocytic, or chronic granulocytic leukaemia, describes a subtype of clonal chronic myeloproliferative neoplasms (MPN) in which every leukaemic progeny of the CML stem cell harbours the *BCR-ABL1* founder driver gene. This gene encodes an oncoprotein, $p210^{BCR\text{-}ABL1}$, with a constitutive active ABL tyrosine kinase activity that is generally thought to be the principal initiating event leading to the chronic phase (CP) of CML. Efforts, over the past three decades, to inhibit this abnormal kinase activity have, arguably, proven to be one of the most successful in adult cancer medicine. Today, following oral therapy with one of the several licensed ABL tyrosine kinase inhibitors (TKI), most adult patients who are able to achieve substantial reduction of the CML cells, defined as a major molecular remission (MMR), can anticipate a normal overall life expectancy, even though the TKIs might not completely eradicate the *BCR-ABL1*-positive CML cells from the body (Figure 7.1). A current challenge now is how to be able to discontinue TKI therapy successfully in patients who have achieved deeper molecular remission (DMR), and also improve outcomes for children diagnosed with CML, which remains an unmet clinical need. Resistance to TKIs can also emerge and in some cases allogeneic stem cell transplantation (allo-SCT) may be useful. Allo-SCT currently remains the only therapy that can reliably produce long-term (10 years or more) DMR [also referred to as complete molecular remissions (CMR), variably defined as 4 or more log reduction of the *BCR-ABL1* ($MR^{4.0}$, $MR^{4.5}$ or $MR^{5.0}$) transcripts from the baseline and in many cases cured.

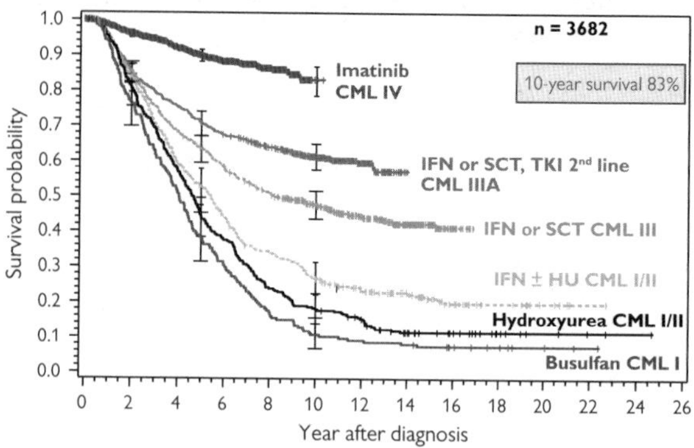

Figure 7.1 Survival with CML over time (1993–2013): the German CML-Study Group experience (also see plate section).

Reproduced with courtesy of Rüdiger Hehlmann, German CML Study Group, Germany.

Epidemiology

The worldwide incidence of CML, with the possible exception of India and China, appears to be about 1.0 to 1.5 per 100 000 of the adult population per annum in all countries where cancer registries are adequately maintained. The median age of CP onset is about 55 years, with males affected slightly more often than females; it is possible that the age of onset in India is considerably lower, but this requires confirmation. Childhood CML appears very rare, accounting for less than 5% of all leukaemias. Though CML is a rare disease, the prevalence rate has recently increased by use of TKIs treatment and survival near age-adjusted population rates, and an estimated current CML-related mortality of 2%.

Aetiology

The only currently known risk of developing CML appears to be exposure to high doses of ionizing radiation, as occurred in survivors of the atomic bombs exploded in Hiroshima and Nagasaki (Japan) in 1945. There appears to be no familial predisposition, nor any definite association with human leukocyte antigen (HLA) genotypes or any infectious diseases. The risk of CML is probably increased with age.

Natural history

In the absence of treatment CML is a remarkably heterogenous disease, characterized by two or three well-defined phases. Most patients present in the CP, which in the pre-TKI era lasted about 4 to 6 years, and was often followed by an accelerated phase (AP), lasting about 6–9 months, and thereafter a blast crisis (BC), also known as blast phase, with an overall historical survival of less than 6 months. About a one-third to one-half of patients in CP have a biphasic disease, and transform directly to BC, without a clear-cut AP. TKIs have clearly impacted the natural history, with the CP being significantly longer in most, if not all, patients (Box 7.1).

Box 7.1 World Health Organization 2016 criteria for accelerated phase of CML

- Persistent or increasing WBC (>10 × 10^9/L), unresponsive to therapy.
- Persistent or increasing splenomegaly, unresponsive to therapy.
- Persistent thrombocytosis (>1000 × 10^9/L), unresponsive to therapy.
- Persistent thrombocytopenia (<100 × 10^9/L) unrelated to therapy.
- 20% or more basophils in the peripheral blood.
- 10–19% blasts in the peripheral blood and/or bone marrow.
- Additional clonal chromosomal abnormalities in Ph-positive cells at diagnosis that include 'major route' abnormalities (second Ph, trisomy 8, isochromosome 17q, trisomy 19), complex karyotype, or abnormalities of 3q26.2.
- Any new clonal chromosomal abnormality in Ph-positive cells that occurs during therapy.

Source: data from Arber DA, et al. (2016). The 2016 revision to the World Health Organization classification of myeloid neo-plasms and acute leukemia. *Blood.* 127(20):2391–405. https://doi.org/10.1182/blood-2016-03-643544.

Clinical features and diagnosis

Currently, about 50% of patients who are diagnosed with CML in CP tend to be asymptomatic, and the diagnosis is made following a blood test for unrelated reasons; the remainder present with symptoms such as fatigue, bleeding, weight loss, sweating, and abdominal discomfort due to splenomegaly. Less common symptoms include priapism, bone pain, gout, or skin infiltration.

Laboratory findings include marked leukocytosis, anaemia, and thrombocytosis. The peripheral blood smear typically shows leukocytosis with a fairly normal differentiation; occasionally basophilia or eosinophilia may be present, and can herald the transformation to AP. The bone marrow aspirate typically tends to be hypercellular with an increased myeloid: erythroid ratio and a blast cell count of 5–10% of cells (Figure 7.2).

Although the haematological findings from the blood test are helpful, cytogenetic and molecular genetic tests are required to confirm the diagnosis by demonstrating the presence of the Philadelphia (Ph) chromosome and the *BCR-ABL1* fusion gene (Figure 7.3a). The Ph chromosome analysis is best performed on a bone marrow aspirate sample, and *BCR-ABL1* gene should be detected by fluorescence *in situ* hybridization (FISH), and best by using reverse transcriptase quantitative polymerase chain reaction (PCR) on a peripheral blood or bone marrow aspirate sample using standardized protocols (Figure 7.3b). Indeed, standard practice today dictates the use of PCR for *BCR-ABL1* to be conducted at diagnosis and used thereafter to monitor patients on therapy, in accordance to established international treatment monitoring guidelines (see next).

Cytogenetics

Over 95% of all patients diagnosed with CML have the hallmark cytogenetic abnormality, the Ph chromosome (22q-), and the founder *BCR-ABL1* gene in every CML cell. The origins of the Ph chromosome, an acquired abnormality that is formed by a balanced translocation between chromosome 9 and 22 [t(9;22)(q34;q11)] that results in the *BCR-ABL1* fusion gene, is

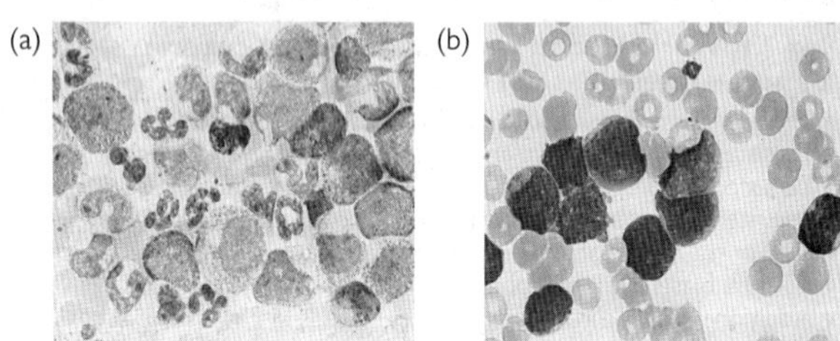

Figure 7.2 Peripheral blood appearances of a patient with CML at diagnosis. Note the increased number of leucocytes including immature granulocytes and occasional blast cells (also see plate section).

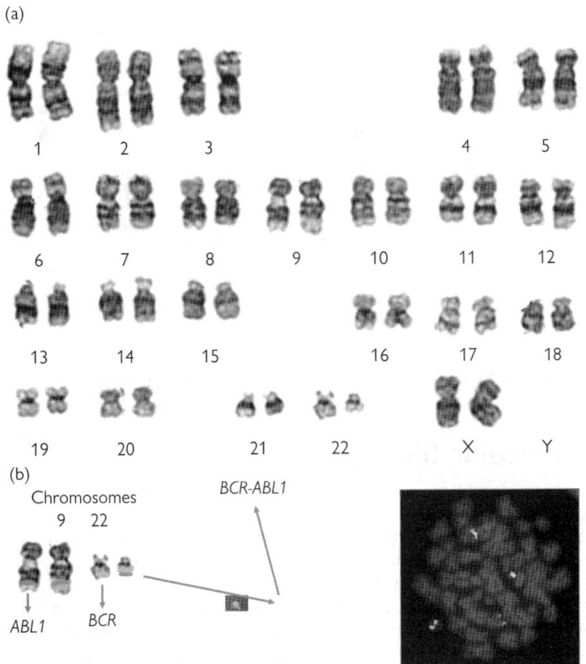

Figure 7.3 (a) Ph chromosome by conventional cytogenetics; (b) BCR-ABL1 by fluorescence in situ hybridization (FISH) (also see plate section).

Reproduced with permission from Mughal TI, et al. (2016) Chronic Myeloid Leukemia: Reminiscences and Dreams. *Haematologica*. 101(5):541–58. DOI:10.3324/haematol.2015.139337. Copyright © 2016 Ferrata Storti Foundation.

unknown (Figure 7.4). It is of some interest that the *BCR-ABL1* gene on the Ph chromosome is expressed in all CML patients, but the *ABL1-BCR* gene on the 9q+ derivative is expressed in about 70% of patients, and its precise role remains speculative with some observations suggesting prognostic implication. In patients who do not harbour the 'classical', Ph chromosome, a number of variant cytogenetic translocations involving chromosome 22 and an alternative partner chromosome have been described; a very small minority have mutations in the *RAS* or *SETBP1* genes. Recent observations suggest a number of non-random additional cytogenetic abnormalities, such as +8, +19, +Ph, and other complex abnormalities, which appear to be associated with inferior outcomes to TKIs and a shorter time to transforming to AP and BC. Other CML-associated genes with the emergence of advanced disease have also been described, which is discussed next.

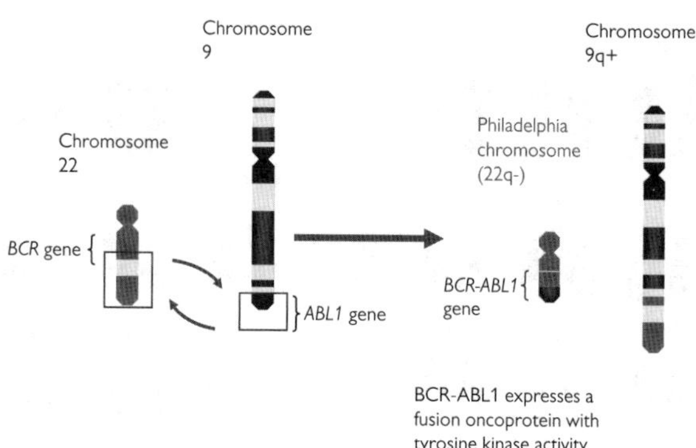

Figure 7.4 A schematic representation of the 'origin' of the Philadelphia (Ph) chromosome.

Molecular biology

The generation of the chimeric *BCR-ABL1* gene in a pluripotential haematopoietic stem cell appears to result in the CP of CML by an uncontrolled expansion and proliferation of the granulocytic lineage, though the precise mechanism(s) remain an enigma. It is quite clear, however, that three diverse oncoproteins, designated $p210^{BCR\text{-}ABL1}$, $p190^{BCR\text{-}ABL1}$ and $p230^{BCR\text{-}ABL1}$, are produced by the expression of the *BCR-ABL1* gene dependent on the precise breakpoints involved, and these, in turn, have distinct leukaemogenic activity. Murine models confirm the role of these oncoproteins in inducing a CML-like disease, though the precise pathogenetic details remain scanty. During the formation of the *BCR-ABL1* gene, a 5' part of BCR and 3' part of ABL, created by break between exons 13 and e14 in the major breakpoint cluster region of the BCR gene and in the upstream portion of exon a2 in the ABL1 gene occurs (Figure 7.5). This results in a BCR-ABL1 gene which contains either an e13a2 or e14a2 junction, which probably function similarly, though there are some suggestions that this might not be the case. Regardless of this, the mRNA molecules transcribe into $p210^{BCR\text{-}ABL1}$, the principal oncoprotein found in CML. The other two BCR-ABL1-oncoproteins, both of which are exceedingly rare in CML, $P190^{BCR\text{-}ABL1}$ and $P230^{BCR\text{-}ABL1}$, are produced by variant breakpoints, e1a2 mRNA junction, and e19a2 mRNA junction, respectively in CML; $P190^{BCR\text{-}ABL1}$ is associated with Ph-positive acute lymphoblastic leukaemia (ALL), and $p230^{BCR\text{-}ABL1}$ with a rare form of Ph-positive chronic neutrophilic leukaemia. Figure 7.6 depicts a simplified representation of molecular signalling pathways activated in CML cells and the BCR-ABL1 domain structure. The unfolding genetic and epigenetic landscape of CML in BC suggests novel abnormalities, such as mutations in *TP53*, *RB*, and *CDKN2A*, or overexpression of *EV1* and *MYC*, being acquired, probably in tandem with additional cytogenetic

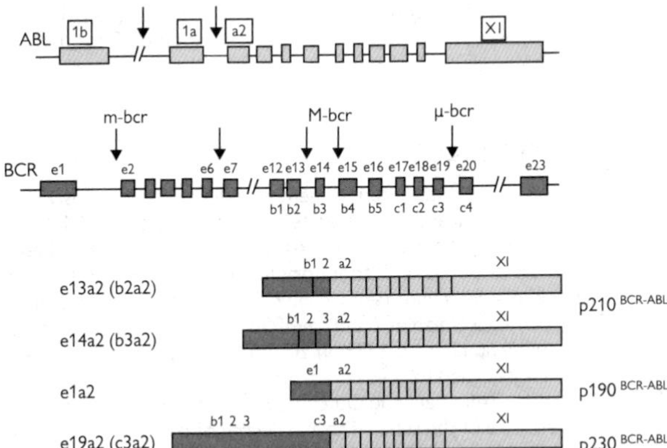

Figure 7.5 A schematic representation of the various breakpoints in the *ABL* and *BCR* genes and the proteins encoded in *BCR-ABL* positive leukaemias

Reproduced with permission from Mughal TI, et al. (2016) Chronic Myeloid Leukemia: Reminiscences and Dreams. *Haematologica*. 101(5):541–58. DOI:10.3324/haematol.2015.139337. Copyright © 2016 Ferrata Storti Foundation.

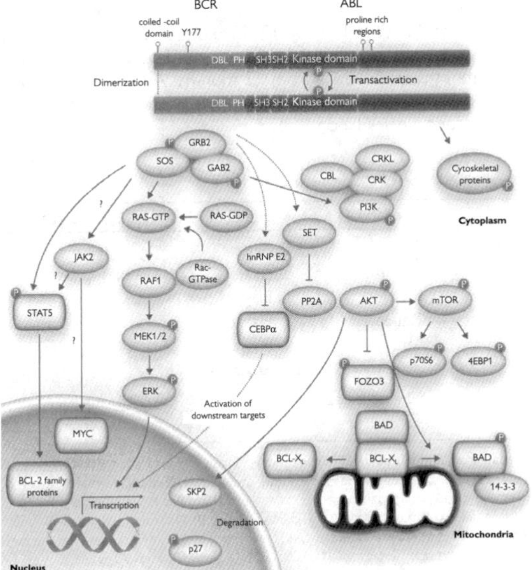

Figure 7.6 *BCR-ABL1* domain structure and simplified representation of molecular signalling pathways activated in CML cells.

abnormalities, such as t(3;12)(q26;q22), t(8;12)(q22;q22), t(7;11)(p15;p15) and inv(16)(p13;q22), which result in the transformation of CP to BC, either directly or via a transient AP.

Prognostic factors

The first important risk stratification method definable at diagnosis, was that introduced by Sokal and colleagues, termed *Sokal Score*, in 1984. It calculated an individual patient's risk of progressing from CP to BC, based on several validated clinical and laboratory features: age, blast cell count, spleen size, and platelet count (see Chapter 5) This was modified slightly, by the European LeukemiaNet (ELN) in 1998, by the inclusion of basophil and eosinophil numbers in 1998. In 2011, ELN proposed a prognostic score specifically designed to predict outcome to the original TKI, imatinib, EUTOS (European Treatment and Outcome Study), and was dependent on two parameters: size of the spleen size and degree of basophilia in the peripheral blood (Table 7.1). More recently, early response to TKI treatment has been recognized as a major prognostic factor, and suitable guidelines based on the *BCR-ABL1* transcript levels at 3, 6, or 12 months following the initiation of TKI treatment have been produced by the ELN (Table 7.2). It is, however, of interest that MMR, a significant therapeutic milestone, is not part of this ELN criteria for the definition of failure. Current efforts suggest that optimal clinical outcomes, patients receiving TKIs should achieve a complete cytogenetic responses (CCyR) (equivalent to $MR^{2.0}$) by 12 months, and MMR ($MR^{3.0}$) by 12–18 months. Optimal molecular responses are now defined as *BCR-ABL1* transcript levels <10% at 3 months, <1% at 6 months, and <0.1% from 12 months. Another prognostic parameter, telomere length of circulating CML cells, has been proposed but requires prospective validation.

Table 7.1 Prediction of prognosis in CML

	Sokal 1984	EURO 1998	EUTOS 2011
Parameters	Age Spleen Blasts Platelets	Age Spleen Blasts Platelets Eosinophils Basophils	Spleen basophils
Treatment	Chemotherapy	IFNα	Imatinib
Endpoint	survival	survival	CCyR

Source: data from Sokal JE, et al. (1984). Prognostic discrimination in 'good-risk' chronic granulocytic leukemia. *Blood.* 63(4):789–99; Hasford J, et al. (2011). Predicting complete cytogenetic response and subsequent progression-free survival in 20160 patients with CML on imatinib treatment: the EUTOS score. *Blood.* 118(3):686–92. DOI: 10.1182/blood-2010-12-319038; and Hoffman VS, et al. (2017). Treatment and outcome of 2904 CML patients from the EUTOS population-based registry. *Leukemia.* 31(3):593–601. DOI: 10.1038/leu.2016.246.

Table 7.2 European LeukemiaNet 2020 Milestones for treating CML

	Optimal	Warning	Failure
Baseline	NA	High-risk ACA*, high-risk ELTS** score	Not applicable
3 months	*BCR-ABL1* ≤10%	*BCR-ABL1*>10%	*BCR-ABL1* >10% if confirmed within 1-3 months
6 months	*BCR-ABL1* <1%	*BCR-ABL1*>1-10%	*BCR-ABL1*>10%
12 months	*BCR-ABL1* ≤0.1%	*BCR-ABL1* >0.1–1%	*BCR-ABL1* >1%
Any time	*BCR-ABL1* ≤0.1%	*BCR-ABL1* >0.1–1%	*BCR-ABL1*>1%, resistance mutations, high-risk ACA

*ACA, additional chromosome abnorm alities in Ph-positive cells; **ELTS, EUTOS long term survival score.

Adapted under a Creative Commons Attribution 4.0 International License from Hochhaus A, et al. (2020). European LeukemiaNet 2020 recommendations for treating chronic myeloid leukemia. *Leukemia*. 34:966–984. https://doi.org/10.1038/s41375-020-0776-2.

Management

The remarkable success in the therapeutic use of TKIs for newly diagnosed adults and most, if not all, children with CML in CP have resulted in a major contribution and resulted in complete paradigm shift. Current treatment guidelines recommend commencing patients on the original TKI, imatinib, or one of the several licensed second-generation (2G-) TKIs, and monitoring response stringently by testing the *BCR-ABL1* transcript levels using standardized protocols and the international scale for reporting. This minimizes variability among laboratories, and reduces the risk of misinterpretation of results (Box 7.2). Responding patients first demonstrate normalization of blood count, second elimination of the Ph chromosome

Box 7.2 Monitoring patients with CML who are on TKI therapy

- Haematologic: At diagnosis, then every 2 weeks or, more frequently, in the event of haematologic toxicity, until complete haematologic response (CHR), then every 3 months for 2 years, then 3–6 monthly.
- Cytogenetic (bone marrow) and molecular (peripheral blood): At diagnosis to exclude other clonal abnormalities, and then at 3 months, and thereafter every 6 months until CCyR confirmed. Increasingly, most patients and clinicians now prefer to monitor molecularly with reverse transcriptase quantitative polymerase chain reaction (RQ-PCR) on blood cells at least once every 3 months until MMR is confirmed, then every 6 months.
- Mutational analysis (peripheral blood), preferably by next-generation sequencing in patients who are not responding optimally or have failed TKIs treatment.

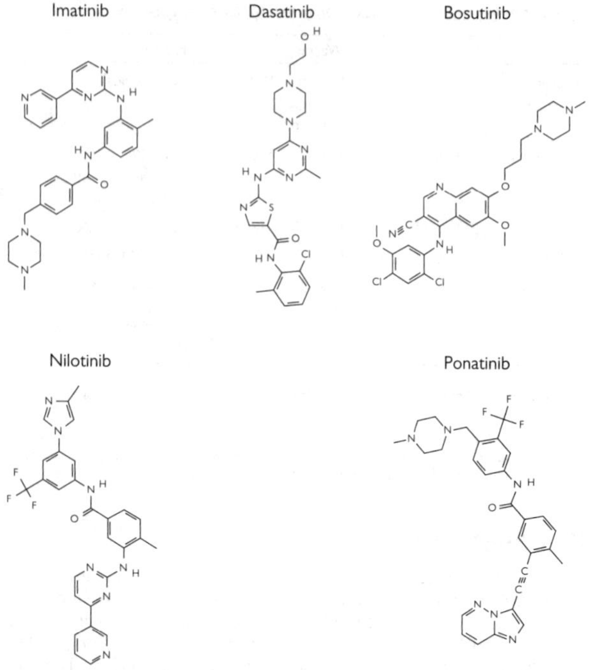

Imatinib Dasatinib Bosutinib

Nilotinib Ponatinib

Figure 7.7 Currently licensed TKIs for CML.

Reproduced with permission from Mughal TI, et al. (2016) Chronic Myeloid Leukemia: Reminiscences and Dreams. *Haematologica*. 101(5):541–58. DOI:10.3324/haematol.2015.139337. Copyright © 2016 Ferrata Storti Foundation.

(CCyR; equivalent to MR^{2}) and finally elimination of the *BCR-ABL1* transcripts (CMR; MR^{4} or MR$^{4.5}$ or MR^{5}). Figure 7.7 depicts some of the currently licensed TKIs for CML.

First-generation TKI

The original ABL1 TKI, now named imatinib, and previously known as imatinib mesylate (CPG57168 or STI-571), a 2-phenylaminopyrimidine, occupies the adenosine 5'-triphosphate (ATP)-binding pocket of the kinase component of the *BCR-ABL1* oncoprotein, and therefore blocks tyrosine phosphorylation by competing with ATP (Figure 7.8). It also works by binding to an adjacent part of the kinase domain in a manner than holds

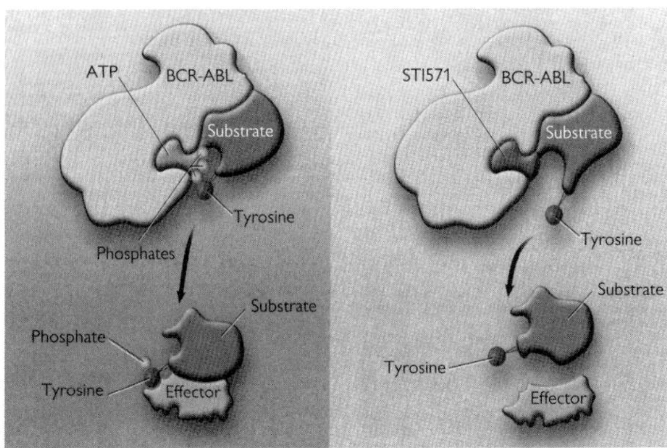

Figure 7.8 The presumed initial mechanism of action of imatinib (previously known as STI571).

the ABL–activation loop of the oncoprotein in an inactive configuration. The drug was known to be a potent *v-ABL* and *PDGFR* inhibitor in murine models and it entered the clinics in 1998, initially for treatment of interferon alpha-resistant or refractory CML in CP, and subsequently to treat newly diagnosed adult patients with CML in CP. In 2001, following the impressive results from the prospective randomized phase III study (*IRIS*), it was licensed for all newly diagnosed patients with CML in CP at a fixed dose of 400 mg/day. Almost two decades later we know that about 83% of patients achieve durable CCyR and the progression from CP to advanced phases was also significantly delayed (Figure 7.1). The safety analysis of the drug is also impressive, with very few potentially serious long-term side effects, which are discussed next. Higher doses of imatinib, up to 800 mg/day, have also been tested and found to result in a greater proportion of patients achieving CMR, but significant more side effects, in particular cytopenias and hepatotoxicity. Data from several other studies, such as the French SPIRIT and Australian TIDEL II studies, also suggest that higher dose imatinib (~600 mg) is as good as 2G TKIs in the first-line setting. The 10 years+ of follow-up of the *IRIS* study observes about 40% of the study cohort to have failed imatinib therapy, though non-compliance contributes to some of these failures. Imatinib resistance, both primary and secondary, accounts for the majority of these failures. Primary resistance is quite rare, and primary resistance to imatinib is largely associated with poor gastrointestinal absorption, potential interactions with other medications, and abnormal drug efflux and influx proteins, MDR1 and hOCT1, respectively. Acquired resistance arises largely from the emergence of mutants, both simple and complex, with the gatekeeper mutant, *T315I*, being particularly deleterious (Figure 7.9). Rarely acquired resistance can arise from *BCR-ABL1*

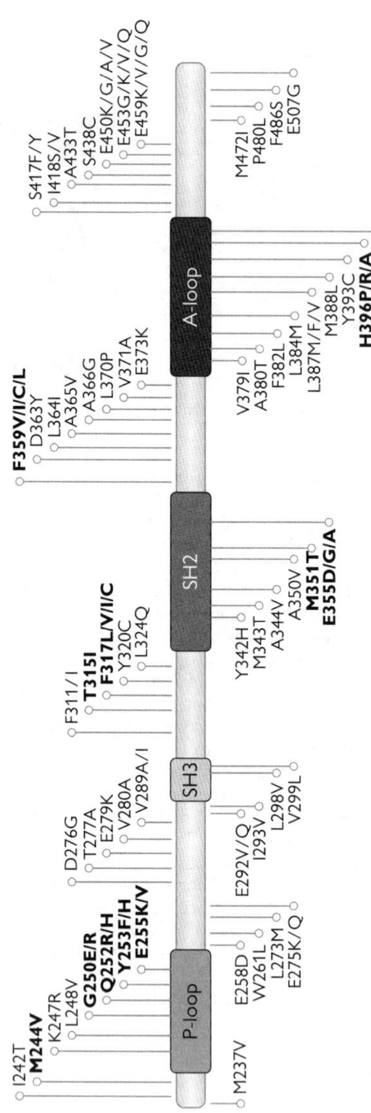

Figure 7.9 The ten most frequent mutations, accounting for ~70% of TKI-resistant CML patients are bold.

gene amplification. The treatment options for patients who fail imatinib at standard dose, but are still in CP include the use of higher doses of imatinib, 2G-TKIs, allo-SCT, or consideration for a clinical trial

Second-generation TKIs

The recognition, following a 3–4 years' follow-up of the *IRIS* study, that over 50% of patients might require alternative therapy, paved the way for the development of the oral 2G-TKIs (notably nilotinib, dasatinib and bosutinib) and inhibitors of the *T315I* mutant. Based on *in vitro* studies, all of the 2G-TKIs are more potent than imatinib. Nilotinib, a modified version of imatinib engineered to bind more tightly in the ATP pocket, is about 30 times more potent than imatinib, and dasatinib, a dual SRC-ABL kinase inhibitor, is about 300 times more potent than imatinib, and though it bears no structural resemblance works like imatinib. Bosutinib, a dual *SRC-ABL1* kinase inhibitor, is also more potent than imatinib and works by binding to the kinase domain of *BCR-ABL1* in an active or inactive confirmation. All three drugs were tested in patients with CML in CP who were imatinib resistant or refractory patients and found to be effective and with acceptable safety profiles. Notably none of these three drugs were sensitive to CML patients with mutant *T315I*.

In 2006 the drugs entered phase III randomized studies where they were tested against standard dose imatinib. Two doses of nilotinib, 300 mg/day or 400 mg/day, was tested in the *ENESTnd* study, dasatinib at 100 mg/day in the *DASISION* study, and bosutinib at 500 mg/day in the *BELA* study. All three studies demonstrated increased benefits compared with imatinib, in terms of achieving deeper and faster molecular responses, both MMR (MR^3) and CMR, in a higher proportion of patients, and a reduction in the risk of transformation to advanced phases, though the results with bosutinib showed superiority compared with imatinib at the 24 months follow-up. The discontinuation rate for all three drugs was about 30% for treatment failure for any cause or progression following a 2-year follow-up, rising up to about 36% at the 3-year follow-up milestone. In 2010, nilotinib and dasatinib, but not bosutinib, were licensed for first-line use in CML in CP. Bosutinib was the tested at a slightly reduced dose of 400 mg/day, due to side effects (discussed next) in the BFORE study, which confirmed the drug's efficacy and better safety, and the drug was licensed in 2017.

Table 7.3 depicts the results of both trials, following 4 years of follow-up. Currently none of these three drugs demonstrate an overall statistically significant survival benefit, compared to imatinib, though rates of progression to the advanced phases of CML have continued to be decreased. Dasatinib, but not nilotinib nor bosutinib, has also been tested in children and found to be effective and safe, but longer-term follow-up is recommended.

Table 7.3 Results from different studies comparing dasatinib or nilotinib to imatinib at 5 years.

	Dasatinib 100 mg qd n = 259	Imatinib 400 mg qd n = 260	Imatinib 400 mg qd n = 283	Nilotinib 300 mg bid n = 282	Nilotinib 400 mg bid n = 281
MMR at 5yr	76%	64%	60%	77%	77%
Overall progression to AP/BC	11 (4.6%)	18 (7.3%)	20 (7.5%)	10 (3.5%)	6 (2.1%)
Overall survival	91%	90%	91.6%	93.6%	96%
Progression-free-survival	85%	86%	95.3%	92%	91.1%

Reproduced with permission from Mughal TI, et al. (2016) Chronic Myeloid Leukemia: Reminiscences and Dreams. *Haematologica*. 101(5):541–58. DOI:10.3324/haematol.2015.139337. Copyright © 2016 Ferrata Storti Foundation.

Third-generation TKI

Ponatinib, previously known as AP24534, and now termed a third generation (3G-)TKI, is an oral multikinase inhibitor, with activity against *ABL1*, *SRC*, and several other tyrosine kinases including *KIT, PDGFRA, FGFR1*, and *FLT3*. It was developed as a consequence of novel chemical modification of a purine scaffold. The drug was rationally developed so that its central triple carbon-carbon bond, which extends from the purine scaffold allows it to take up a unique position with no steric hindrance attributable to the T315I mutation. The drug's credentials against the *T315I* mutated CML in CP were confirmed in a phase 1 study, and it then entered a phase 2 study (*PACE*) in patients with CML resistant to all the licensed TKIs (notably imatinib, dasatinib, nilotinib or bosutinib) at a dose of 45 mg/day. Results from this study suggested considerable activity in the study cohort, including some patients with compound mutations, and the drug was licensed in 2012 for second-line use in patients with CML resistant to imatinib, dasatinib or nilotinib, irrespective of the presence or absence of a T315I mutation. Thereafter a randomized phase 3 study (*EPIC*), testing ponatinib 45 mg/day against imatinib 400 mg/day in newly diagnosed patients with CML in CP was embarked upon. The study was closed by the Food and Drug Administration (FDA) in 2013 following the observation of an increased incidence of arterial thrombotic events, hypertension, and hepatitis in the longer-term follow-up of the *PACE* study. The EPIC study remains on hold and efforts are now assessing lower doses, based on the notion that the serious cardiovascular and other effects are dose-related, in the *OPTIC* post-marketing study. Recent observations confirm the emergence of resistance to ponatinib as a consequence of new mutations, such as *T315M* and *T315L*, as well as compound mutations.

Adverse effects associated with *ABL1* TKIs

Several studies have now shown that up 14% and 25% of all patients receiving first-line or second-line treatment, respectively, discontinue treatment due to side effects. This, in turn, impacts on treatment continuity, compliance, and adherence, resulting in poorer quality of life and clinical outcomes, particularly in patients with pre-existing medical conditions, such as diabetes and other metabolic disorders. The negative impact on survival has been observed in some studies incorporating the Charlson Comorbidity Index (CCI), such as the German CML IV study, as well as real-world examples. The majority of TKI-related side effects in general, in particular those associated with imatinib, tend to be mild and reversible. Indeed, the recent observations following almost 17 years of imatinib in the clinics for CML in CP confirms' the drug's safety profile. Imatinib associated side effects include nausea, rash, infraorbital oedema, and fluid retention; severe cytopenias and hepatitis occur less commonly and usually in the first 12 months of therapy (Table 7.4). The longer-term follow-up of the imatinib *IRIS* study, now 17 years, suggests no severe or late unexpected side effects, but do indicate chronic low-grade debilitating fatigue, particularly in younger female patients. Nilotinib has been associated with increased risk of peripheral arterial occlusive disease and potentially serious metabolic effects, such as hyperglycaemia, and rarely pancreatitis; importantly the FDA has issued a black box warning for QTc prolongation and cardiac death. Dasatinib has been associated with cytopenias, pleural effusions and, rarely, pulmonary hypertension and haemorrhagic colitis. Bosutinib is associated with diarrhoea, which appears to be dose-related, hepatotoxicity and very rarely anaphylactic shock (Table 7.4). Ponatinib is associated with dose-related serious arterial thrombotic effects in about 9% of patients, and this notably led to the *EPIC* trial being placed on hold. Other side effects associated with ponatinib include thrombocytopenia, rash, and platelet dysfunction.

The precise underlying pathogenesis for vascular toxicity, particularly associated with nilotinib and ponatinib, is an enigma. It is possible that age-related somatic mutations (ARCH) and clonal haematopoiesis of indeterminate potential (CHIP) may play a role in the cardiovascular and metabolic side effects. There is also emerging evidence suggestive of endothelial cell injury raising the prospect of proteomic profiling of TKI effects on human endothelial cells to predict vascular toxicity.

Table 7.4 Adverse events related to TKIs in patients with CML

	Imatinib	Dasatinib	Nilotinib	Bosutinib	Ponatinib
Peripheral oedemas	++				
Pulmonary hypertension		+			
Effusions		+++		+	
Diarrhoea	+			+++	++
Rash	+	+	++	+	
Nausea	+			+	++
Hyperglycaemia			++		
PAOD*			+++		++
Arterial thrombosis		+	++		+++
Venous thrombosis					++
Asthenia	++				
Skin fragility	++				
Muscle cramps	++				

*PAOD, Peripheral arterial occlusive disease.

Reproduced with permission from Mughal TI, et al. (2016) Chronic Myeloid Leukemia: Reminiscences and Dreams. *Haematologica.* 101(5):541–58. DOI:10.3324/haematol.2015.139337. Copyright © 2016 Ferrata Storti Foundation.

Investigational approaches

Although imatinib and the other TKIs have achieved much from a therapeutic perspective for patients with CML in CP, many important challenges remain. For example, it appears that none of the current TKIs are able to eradicate the CML stem cells completely. The current wave of the discontinuation trials suggests that about only 40% of patients are able to remain in sustained CMR on stopping the TKIs, and the remainder relapse and require further treatment. Clearly while BCR-ABL1 remains a seminal target in CML, it is also important to focus on other molecular pathogenesis mechanisms involved in this disease. Many studies are testing specific inhibitors in targeting signal transduction pathways that play a role in the survival and maintenance of CML stem cells. As illustration, such pathways involve the JAK/STAT, mTOR, PI3K/AKT, and autophagy signalling pathway, to mention a few (Figure 7.10). Many of these inhibitors are now in formal clinical studies. There is also considerable interest in the allosteric inhibitor, asciminib (ABL001; previously known as GNF-5), a novel BCR-ABL1 inhibitor that targets the myristoyl pocket, and maintains activity against currently known mutants that confer resistance to ATP-binding site, is currently being tested in a randomized phase 3 trial versus bosutinib. Earlier studies established the drug's candidacy and safety, leading to this study in patients with CML who have had at least two previous lines of therapy. There is

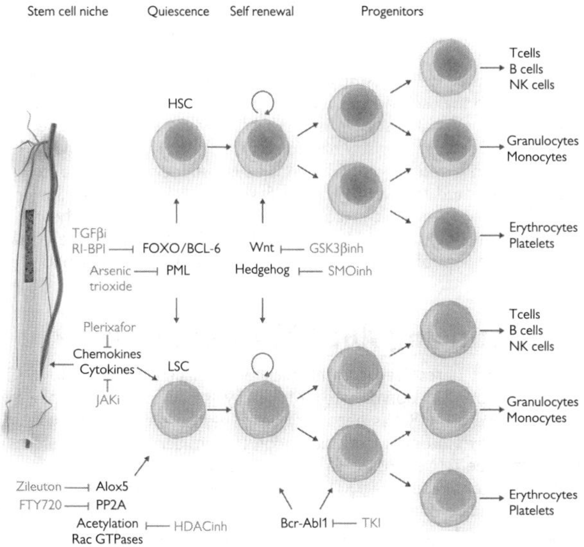

Figure 7.10 Investigational approaches for CML.

also interest in testing a second-generation ABL1 TKI, radotinib, which resembles nilotinib. This agent is actually licensed for first line use in CML in CP in South Korea. Another drug of interest is pioglitazone, a peroxisome proliferator-activated receptor gamma agonist, which was found to accord CMR in a small French study assessing patients with CML in CP who have had a suboptimal response to imatinib. In this regard, there is also renewed interest to assess the role of interferon alfa, in particular the pegylated form, or vaccines developed against *BCR-ABL1*-specific peptides in patients who fail to achieve deeper molecular responses with ABL1 TKI therapies.

Allogeneic stem cell transplantation

It is almost half a century since allo-SCT was tested in patients with CML, and subsequently became the only treatment to eradicate CML stem cells in selected patients and cure CML. Today it remains the only curative therapy, but still carries the risk of much morbidity and some mortality from graft versus host disease (GvHD) and opportunistic infections, even when the transplantation conditioning is substantially reduced. Novel strategies targeting antigens involved in the graft versus leukaemia (GvL) effects should help reduce some of the risks of serious complications. Clearly the definition of the various factors influencing survival, such as patient's age, disease phase at time of allo-SCT, duration of CML in CP, degree of donor-recipient histocompatibility, and patient/donor gender has had a significant positive impact. Current registry data, which is discussed in greater detail in Chapter 16, suggest that 5-year leukaemia-free survival of 80% are achieved with the use of conventional allo-SCT using an HLA-matched sibling donor; comparable survival is about 670% with a suitable matched unrelated donor. Recent registry data for an allograft performed in a low-risk transplant score patient with CML in CP suggest additional improvement, with an estimated survival of 85% at 5 years and a significantly lowered transplant-related mortality. At present most specialists debate whether to offer an adult patient with CML in CP an allo-SCT after they have failed two lines or three lines of TKI therapies, and a suitable donor is available.

Discontinuing *ABL1*-TKI treatment

An important unresolved current question in patients with CML in CP who are responding optimally to TKI therapy, is how long to continue this therapy once a DMR has been achieves. The therapeutic value of such therapy is beyond doubt, and the notion to consider a safe and effective treatment-free remissions (TFR) is attractive. TFR allows for the safe and effective discontinuation of TKI therapy, and its inclusion should enable additional personalization of the treatment algorithm and facilitate an improved focus on daily life and improving quality of life. It should reduce treatment-related risks, optimize treatment adherence, financial burdens, and better inform on the precise definition of treatment goals and milestones, treatment choice, and monitoring.

The concept appears particularly attractive when the more potent 2G-TKIs are utilized, since current studies suggest they accord speedier and deeper molecular remissions, compared with imatinib. Mahon and colleagues (Bordeaux, France) get considerable credit in introducing the TFR concept, which has now been testerd in numerous single-arm studies involving imatinib, dasationib and nilotinib, and found to be successful in about 40% of patients. In a small minority, a second TFR is possible following the failure of the first. Another important area being studied is the use of lower TKI doses once a DMR has been achieved. Collectively, it seems that many of the questions related to TFR successfully should be addressed within the next few years. This should then be a seminal milestone in the real-world treatment of patients with CML.

Treatment of patients with CML in blast transformation

This is discussed in Chapter 12.

Future prospects

It is remarkable how the translational science story of CML led to the successful development of an oral therapy which empowers the concepts of precision medicine and offers substantial survival benefits compatible with a normal lifespan for patients with this disease. A principal challenge now is to ensure long-term drug safety, and to discontinue therapy safely once a sustained molecular remission has been achieved. Current experience suggests that the 2G-TKIs accord durable CMRs earlier compared with imatinib, and better protection against progression, compared to imatinib. It, however, remains to be seen if these findings will translate to better survival rates. Furthermore, the risk of serious adverse events, in particular cardiovascular, with nilotinib and ponatinib, are significant. Currently, imatinib remains the most popular first-line drug, with the 2G-TKIs being used for suboptimal responders. Figure 7.11 depicts a possible treatment algorithm for patients who are considered to be imatinib failures, and this will undoubtedly to evolve as longer-term safety and efficacy data, becomes available. Resistance associated with the use of TKIs remains a problem, but a number of well-studied further treatments, including allo-SCT, are now available for eligible patients. Clearly although much has indeed been achieved for patients with CML, many issues either remain or need clarification. These include, the mechanisms that underlie the origin of the Ph chromosome, the dysregulation of many of the molecular pathways involved, the emergence of resistance, efforts to eradicate the CML stems without recourse to an allo-SCT, Some questions also remain in patients with CML who have antecedent CHIP prior to the acquisition of *BCR-ABL1* mutation. The renewed interest in immunotherapy, including pegylated interferons in TKI suboptimal responders, and improving allo-SCT procedure is also appealing.

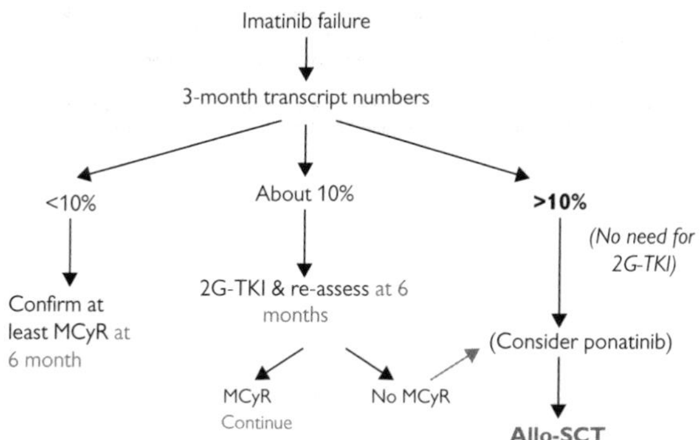

Figure 7.11 Suggested management of imatinib failure (if there is a possible transplant donor).

Further reading

Ben-Neriah Y, Daley GQ, Mes-Masson AM, et al. The chronic myelogenous leukemia-specific P210 protein is the product of the bcr/abl hybrid gene. *Science*. 1986;233:212–14.

Daley GQ, van Etten, Baltimore D. Induction of chronic myelogenous leukemia in mice by P210 BCR/ABL gene of the Philadelphia chromosome. *Science*. 1990;247:824–30.

Druker BJ, Guilhot F, O'Brien SG, et al. Five-year follow-up of patients receiving imatinib for chronic myeloid leukemia. *N Engl J Med*. 2006;355:2408–17.

Druker BJ, Tamura S, Buchdunger E, et al. Effects of a selective inhibitor of the Abl tyrosine kinase on the growth of Bcr-Abl positive cells. *Nat Med*. 1996;2:561–6.

Fialkow PJ, Garler SM, Yoshida A. Clonal origin of chronic myelocytic leukemia in man. *Proc Natl Acad Sci USA*. 1967;58:1468–71.

Groffen J, Stephenson JR, Heisterkamp N, de Klein A, Bartram CR, Grosveld G. Philadelphia chromosomal breakpoints are clustered within a limited region, bcr, on chromosome 22. *Cell*. 1984;36:93–9.

Hochhaus A, Larson RA, Guilhot F, et al. Long-term outcomes of imatinib treatment for chronic myeloid leukemia. *N Engl J Med*. 2017;376:917–27.

Hochhaus A, Baccarani M, Silver RT, et al. European LeukemiaNet 2020 recommendations for treating chronic myeloid leukemia. *Leukemia*. 2020; doi.org/10.1038/s41375-020-0776-2.

Issa GC, Kantarjian HM, Gonzalez GN, et al. Clonal chromosomal abnormalities appearing in Philadelphia chromosome-negative metaphases during CML treatment. *Blood*. 2017;130:2084–91.

Kantarjian H, Sawyers C, Hochhaus A, et al. Hematologic and cytogenetic responses to imatinib mesylate in chronic myelogenous leukemia. *N Engl J Med*. 2002;346(9):645–52.

Kantarjian H, Shah NP, Hochhaus A, et al. Dasatinib versus imatinib in newly diagnosed chronic-phase chronic myeloid leukemia. *N Engl J Med*. 2010;362:2260–70.

Mughal TI, Lion T, Abdel-Wahab, O, et al. Precision immunotherapy, mutational landscape, and emerging tools to optimize clinical outcomes in patients with classical myeloproliferative neoplasms. *Haematol Oncol*. 2018;36(5):740–8.

Mughal TI, Radich JP, Deininger MW, et al. Chronic myeloid leukemia: reminiscences and dreams. *Haematologica*. 2016;101:541–58.

Nowell PC, Hungerford DA. A minute chromosome in human granulocytic leukemia. *Science*. 1960;132:1497.

Radich JR. Chronic myeloid leukemia: global impact from a local laboratory. *Cancer*. 2017;123(14):2594–6.

Rea D, Nicolini FE, Tulliez M, et al. Discontinuing of dasatinib or nilotinib in chronic myeloid leukemia: interim analysis of the STOP 2G-TKI study. *Blood*. 2017;129:846–54.

Rowley JD. Letter: a new consistent chromosomal abnormality in chronic myelogenous leukaemia identified by quinacrine fluorescence and Giemsa staining. *Nature*. 1973;243:290–3.

Saglio G, Kim DW, Issaragrisil S, et al. Nilotinib versus imatinib for newly diagnosed chronic myeloid leukemia. *N Engl J Med*. 2010;362:2251–9.

Sauselle S, Hehlmann R, Fabarius A, et al. Defining therapy goals for major molecular remission in chronic myeloid leukemia: results of the randomized CML study IV. *Leukemia*. 2018;32(5):1222–8.

Chapter 8

Polycythaemia vera

Tiziano Barbui, Tariq I. Mughal, and Guido Finazzi

Introduction *114*
Epidemiology and aetiology *114*
Contemporary clinical features *114*
Diagnosis *116*
Management *117*

Introduction

Polycythaemia vera (PV) was probably the first form of erythrocytosis with overlapping features of leukaemia (maladie de Vaquez) to be recognized as a distinct entity towards the end of the nineteenth century. Modern views on its biology, and risk of leukaemic or fibrotic transformation, did not result until much later (see Chapter 1). In 1951, following the recognition of PV to share unique biological and clinical features with chronic myeloid leukaemia (CML), essential thrombocythaemia (ET) and primary myelofibrosis (PMF), the term 'myeloproliferative disorders' (MPD) was introduced, by Dameshek, to describe them. In 2008, a panel of the World Health Organization (WHO)-appointed experts replaced the term MPD with myeloproliferative neoplasm (MPN) in alignment with the first important clue to its molecular pathogenesis. PV is characterized by a clonal proliferation of haematopoietic stem cells that results in a progressive increase in the red cell mass (RCM), and the presence of mutually exclusive, though not always, *JAK2*, *CALR*, and *MPL* driver mutations. Current genetic analysis confirms the presence of a *JAK2*^{V617F} mutation in 97% and *JAK2* exon 12 or a variant in the remainder; *CALR* and *MPL* mutations are typically absent. The current 2016 WHO revised classification criteria includes seven subtypes of MPN, and the term 'classic' MPN is often used to refer to PV, ET, PMF, and CML. Here, we briefly summarize recent advances in our understanding of the disease biology and risk stratification, and indicate how these have important therapeutic implications.

Epidemiology and aetiology

PV is probably the second most common subtype of MPN, following ET. The annual incidence of PV is reported to be around 0.84 to 1.9 per 100 000 adults, a prevalence of 44 to 57 per 100 000 persons and a median age of about 60–70 years, with a slight male predominance. However, after 2016 WHO diagnostic criteria, it is very likely that PV will be diagnosed with a greater frequency as the haemoglobin (Hb) and haematocrit (Hct) threshold values have been lowered in comparison with pre-2016 diagnosis. There are no specific risk factors that have been associated with PV, though there are several well-characterized, but rare, pedigrees with autosomal dominant pattern of susceptibility in some families.

Contemporary clinical features

Systemic symptoms and signs

The central feature of PV is an expansion of the total RCM and a significant risk of thrombosis, which can be arterial, venous, or microvascular. The increased RCM manifests itself as a raised Hb)/Hct and packed cell volume (PCV). This is often, accompanied by leucocytosis, thrombocytosis; palpable splenomegaly is seen in about 40–50% of patients. Most patients present with substantial symptom-burden which includes fatigue, pruritis, night sweats, bone pain, and microcirculatory symptoms; rarely patients present with bleeding. The importance of symptom-burden was confirmed in a recent internet-based survey of 1179 MPN patients, including 405 with PV. The study observed the presence of fatigue in 85%, pruritus in 65%, night sweats in 49%, and bone pain in 43% of the cohort. Given the significant morbidity associated with these symptoms, specific assessment tools, such as the MPN-Symptom Assessment Form (MPN-SAF), were developed and validated to quantitatively assess the extent of disease burden. Notably, no correlation between PV clustered patients by MPN-SAF total symptom score (TSS) and PV risk category was found.

Incidence and type of thrombosis

The estimated rate of thrombosis at diagnosis for PV varies from 12% to 39%, and perhaps higher for patients with early and 'masked' disease (mPV), many of whom do not fulfil the current WHO diagnostic criteria (next) and exhibit thrombosis in unusual anatomic sites. Arterial thrombosis can present myocardial infarcts, ischaemic strokes, transient ischaemic attacks, mesenteric and limb ischaemia; microvascular occlusions can affect the extremities and lead to erythromelalgia. Venous thrombosis can lead to abdominal venous thrombosis (AVT), such as Budd–Chiari syndrome and obstruction of the portal, mesenteric, and splenic circulation, occurs in up to 35% of all patients with PV, but considerably fewer with other subtypes of MPN.

Several attempts have been made over the past two decades to establish the impact of thrombosis and the efficacy and safety of antithrombotic drugs in patients with PV. The first such large study was the prospective European Collaboration on Low-dose Aspirin in Polycythemia Vera Investigators (ECLAP) study which assessed the use of low-dose aspirin in 1638 patients diagnosed with PV using the Polycythemia Vera Study Group (PVSG) criteria that antedated the WHO criteria. Following a median follow-up period of 2.8 years, the cumulative rate of vascular events (cardiovascular deaths and non-fatal thrombotic events) was observed to be 5.5 events per 100 persons per year and the bleeding history was 2.9%. A second more recent study, the Cytoreductive Therapy in PV (CYTO-PV) study, examined the cardiovascular events and intensity of treatment in 365 adult patients with WHO-defined PV. The study observed significantly lower risk of cardiovascular deaths and major thrombosis (2.7% patients per year) following the reduction of Hct to less than 45% with conventional treatment. Similar findings were observed in another recent International Working Group for MPN Research (IWGMRT) retrospective study, which found major thrombosis rate of 2.6% patients per year, and overall incidence of arterial thrombosis in 17% and venous thrombosis in 12%. Both of these studies show figures lower than those described for the ECLAP study, which may have arisen as a consequence of different diagnostic criteria and potential treatment differences. Clearly the importance of an earlier diagnosis and treatment is therapeutically valuable for the improved thrombosis outcome in contemporary PV patients, though the precise contributions and goals might need additional clarity.

Natural history and risk factors for survival

The median survival of patients with PV is approximately 14 and 24 years, for patients older than 60 years or younger than 40 years of age, respectively. Though the disease is characterized by risk of transformation to myelofibrosis (MF) or acute myeloid leukaemia (AML), the principal cause of PV-related deaths remains cardiovascular mortality due to thrombotic complications. As illustration, the ECLAP study, demonstrated cardiovascular mortality to be almost twice that of the general Italian population, accounting for 41% of all PV-related deaths (1.5 deaths per 100 adults per year). In striking contrast to this, deaths due to transformation to MF or AML are considerably lower. The estimated rate of PV to transform to MF is about 12–20% and related to disease duration, JAK2 allelic burden >50%, age >60 years, leucocyte count > 13×10^9/L, thrombosis, and the presence of additional genetic, in particular ASXL1, SRSF2 and IDH2 mutations, or cytogenetic abnormalities. Interestingly, a recent study of 1500 strictly defined WHO-PV patients observed patients with two or three of these factors had a 10-year relative survival of 26%, compared with 59% and 84% in patients with one and no risk factors, respectively. The 10-year risk to transform to AML is about 15% and related to advanced age, leukocytosis, and abnormal cytogenetics. In the seminal ECLAP study, MF and AML transformations accounted for 13% of all PV-related deaths; notably, secondary solid tumours accounted for 20% of all PV deaths (20%).

Diagnosis

A diagnosis of PV requires both the presence of either three major criteria or two major and one minor criterion defined by the 2016 WHO revised diagnostic criteria and the exclusion of other causes of polycythaemia. The WHO diagnostic criteria are based on a composite assessment of clinical and laboratory features depicted in Box 8.1, and now validated by several independent efforts. It requires the presence of a JAK2 mutation and documentation of an increase in the level of Hb/Hct, >18.5 g/dL/ >55.5% in men, and >16.5 g/dL/ >49.5% in women. In addition, it is useful to assess the bone marrow (BM) morphology, which can help distinguish the JAK2-positive MPN subtypes, in particular distinguishing early stage PV and mPV, which do not fulfil the WHO Hb/Hct required levels, from ET, and other causes of increased Hct. Measurement of the serum erythropoietin (Epo) level, which is low in about 85% of patients with PV, can also be helpful. In the past RCM measurements, thought to be an accurate indicator of the blood red cell content, played an important diagnostic role, in particular in early stage and indeed have comprised a major criterion for the diagnosis of PV since 1967. The test is analytically well validated and standardized, but the practical clinical utility has now been challenged, with the availability of mutation screening, serum Epo level, and BM examination. RCM measurements remain useful in particular for patients with mPV and help optimize MPN classification. Parenthetically, the diagnostic Hb values required by the WHO guidelines have been considered surrogate of increased RCM.

Box 8.1 Revised (2016) World Health Organization criteria for polycythaemia vera

Diagnosis of PV requires meeting either all three major criteria, or the first two major criteria and the minor criterion**

Major criteria

1. Haemoglobin >16.5 g/dL in men
   Haemoglobin >16.0 g/dL in women
   or
   Haematocrit >49% in men
   Haematocrit >48% in women
   or
   Increased red cell mass (RCM)*
2. BM biopsy showing hypercellularity for age with trilineage growth (panmyelosis) including prominent erythroid, granulocytic, and megakaryocytic proliferation with pleomorphic, mature megakaryocytes (differences in size)
3. Presence of JAK2V617F or JAK2 exon 12 mutation

Minor criterion

- Subnormal serum erythropoietin level
- Diagnosis of PV requires meeting either all three major criteria, or the first two major criteria and the minor criterion**

* > 25% above mean normal predicted value.

** criterion number 2 (BM biopsy) may not be required in cases with sustained absolute erythrocytosis: haemoglobin levels >18.5 g/dL in men (haematocrit 55.5%) or >16.5 g/dL in women (haematocrit 49.5%) if major criterion 3 and the minor criterion are present. However, initial myelofibrosis (present in up to 20% of patients) can only be detected by performing BM biopsy; this finding may predict a more rapid progression to overt myelofibrosis (post-PV MF).

Reproduced from Arber DA, et al. (2016). The 2016 revision to the World Health Organization classification of myeloid neoplasms and acute leukemia. *Blood.* 127(20):2391–405. https://doi.org/10.1182/blood-2016-03-643544.

Management

In contrast to most myeloid malignancies, patients with PV appear to have a remarkable long natural history, and many patients have a survival that is similar to that of the general population. PV is generally assumed to be incurable and is treated palliatively with several current treatment modalities, whose safety and effectiveness has been well validated. Since thrombosis is the most common serious and potentially life-threatening complication of PV, the principal goal of any form of treatment is to prevent thrombotic complications and their dire consequences. Thrombosis is a multifactorial process and its pathogenesis results from an interplay of various disease-related and other factors, such as cardiovascular risks. Consequently, the identification and appropriate management of disease-independent risk factors, in particular tobacco smoking, and the promotion of a healthy lifestyle, is pivotal.

It is important to stratify the risk of all PV patients carefully in order to avoid unnecessary treatment and treatment-related side effects. For the time being, the treatment should employ phlebotomy (venesection) to keep Hct<45% and low-dose (81 mg) ASA (aspirin) in the absence of contraindications. Cytoreductive therapy, most commonly hydroxyurea (hydroxycarbamide), can be considered for patients unable to have phlebotomy and those with high-risk disease. Clearly the identification of the JAK2V617F mutation generated much interest in the development of therapeutic JAK2 inhibitors for patients with MPN, including high-risk PV. Indeed, one such drug, ruxolitinib, a JAK1 and type II JAK2 inhibitor with a short half-life, is currently licensed as second-line therapy for patients with PV who are intolerant or have an inadequate response to hydroxyurea.

Risk stratification according to thrombotic and other risks

The clinical relevance and therapeutic importance of thrombosis risk stratification in PV has been determined in several studies conducted over the past two decades using slightly different diagnostic criteria for PV. The PVSG 01 clinical trial and the ECLAP study, assessing PVSG-criteria patients with PV, and the subsequent WHO criteria PV patients, it is generally accepted that older patients with history of arterial or venous vascular events, remain at a significant risk for recurrent thrombotic events. Therefore, both age and a past history of thrombosis need to be considered when assessing 'thrombotic risk'. This is high when the age is >60-years or thrombosis history, and low in the absence of both risk factors (Table 8.1).

In addition, the risk may be enhanced in the presence of the most known cardiovascular disease risk factors as in the general population. In particular, it should be noted that among these factors, arterial hypertension is prevalent likely due to the increased blood volume that characterizes PV disease. The risk associated with gender and the presence of thrombophilia do not seem to enhance significantly the risk in men, in contrast to ET.

Treatment of patients with a low thrombotic risk

The mainstay of treatment of patients with a low thrombotic risk is regular phlebotomy, provided the patients can tolerate it and low-dose aspirin. This treatment works by inducing iron deficiency which can help lower the Hct. The European LeukemiaNet (ELN) and the National Comprehensive Cancer Network (NCCN) treatment guidelines recommends a target Hct of 45%, based on the established proportional increase of thrombotic risk with higher Hct. This recommendation is based on the results of Cyto-PV trial, in which, 365 adult patients with PV were randomly allocated to achieve a target Hct <45% or 45 to 50% following regular phlebotomies. After a median follow-up of 31 months, the primary endpoint of

Table 8.1 Risk stratification in polycythaemia vera based on thrombotic risk

Risk category	Risk variables
Low	Age <60 years old; and no thrombosis history
High	Age ≥60 years old; and/or thrombosis history

thrombotic events or deaths from cardiovascular causes was recorded in 2.7% of the low-Hct cohort, in contrast to 9.8% of the high-Hct patients ($p = 0.007$), leading confirmatory support to the current treatment guidelines. There remains some uncertainty with regards to the precise frequency of phlebotomies required for optimal risk reduction and the need to additional therapies, either aspirin or cytoreductive therapy. A single study suggests that patients requiring more than three phlebotomies annually may have higher risk to develop a thrombotic event, but this finding should not be attributed to phlebotomies *per se*, but rather be related to the fact that patients requiring more phlebotomies are those who have an inadequate control of the Hct.

The addition of low-dose (100 mg/d) aspirin to regular phlebotomies has been tested in a double-blind, placebo-controlled, randomized clinical trial, ECLAP, and found to reduce thrombotic complications in low thrombotic risk PV patients without contraindication to the drug. Notably, the relative risk of bleeding associated with aspirin was not significantly increased in this study. There is now emerging evidence that some patients, in particular those with high-risk disease, might benefit from higher doses of aspirin, for example, 100 mg twice daily. This may possibly be related to better thromboxane A2 suppression and procoagulant changes in platelets. Clearly there are a number of poorly understood factors involved, which collectively conspire to worsen the thrombotic risk, and further studies are required.

Treatment of patients with a high thrombotic risk

Hydroxyurea (hydroxycarbamide)

Patients with high-risk PV should have regular phlebotomy to maintain Hct below 45%, low-dose aspirin, and a cytoreductive drug, most commonly hydroxyurea. Hydroxyurea, an antimetabolite that prevents DNA synthesis, has been in clinical use of patients with PV for over five decades and on the WHO's current list of essential medicines, having been found to be effective and safe for diverse medical indications. The drug is administered orally, typically at a dose of 500 mg to 2 grams daily, and reduces the Hct, and the platelet and leucocyte count. In general, it is very well tolerated, with leucopoenia and thrombocytopenia being the most common side effects.

Hydroxyurea was first tested in patients with PV by the PVSG in a small non-randomized study, which demonstrated the drug's efficacy and safety. At a median follow-up of 8.6 years, treatment with hydroxyurea resulted in a reduction in thrombotic events, compared to phlebotomy alone (6.6% vs. 14% at 2 years). These results were thereafter confirmed in several other studies, some of which suggested that the drug may increase the inherent leukaemogenic risk associated with the disease. Notably, these studies included patients who had received alkylating agents or P32 (hazard ratio 7.58). In the ECLAP study, the risk of AML was significantly increased by exposure to P32, busulfan, or pipobroman (hazard ratio 5.46), but not hydroxyurea alone. A French PV randomized study compared hydroxyurea to pipobroman in 292 PV patients, and found pipobroman to be associated with a shorter survival and increased leukaemic risk, compared with hydroxyurea. The general consensus at present is that there is no convincing evidence to show that hydroxyurea, when used as a single cytoreductive therapy, significantly increases the risk of AML, although one cannot be absolutely certain due to the inherent leukaemic risk of the disease.

Rarely, hydroxyurea can cause painful leg ulcers, gastrointestinal side effects, and photosensitivity in susceptible patients. A large multicentre retrospective study of 3411 patients with MPN, including PV, estimated the frequency and the clinical relevance of drug-related fever, pneumonitis, and cutaneous or mucosal lesions. This study demonstrated that clinically relevant hydroxyurea-related side effects in accordance with the criteria of 'intolerance' established by the ELN consensus conference, occur in 5% of patients even after long exposure time. Of note, the long-term exposure to this drug has been associated with a significant increase of non-melanoma skin cancer.

Interferon alpha

Another drug of considerable interest for patients with high-risk is interferon alpha (IFNα). The drug was first introduced in 1982 for the initial therapy of CML, and following successful experience, has been tested in patients with PV over the past three decades. IFNα, in particular the pegylated form (peg-IFNα), has now been found to be effective and safe, with unprecedented high rates of clinical, haematological, molecular, and BM histological remissions. However, treatment-related toxicity, in particular flu-like symptoms and chronic fatigue, has been a principal limitation to its broader use. Efforts to improve the drug's tolerability have led to the introduction of several alternative long-acting forms, such as ropeginterferon alfa-2b, a peg-proline IFNα-2b. It has now been tested in two randomized phase 3 trials, the *PROUD-PV* and *CONTINUATION-PV*, comparing it to hydroxyurea (hydroxycarbamide), and the recent results confirm ropeg IFN-α-2b's safety and efficacy. Although the study results demonstrated similar efficacy and safety after 12 months, superiority of ropeg IFNα-2b over hydroxyurea was significant in terms of haematological and molecular responses, at the 2- and 3-year milestones. This study led to the licensing of IFNα in MPN. In addition, sustained clinical, molecular, and morphological responses, including measurable residual disease (MRD), after ropeg IFNα-2b discontinuation supports the drug's ability to eradicate the PV clone in selected patients. In contrast, in the MPD-Consortium randomized clinical trial comparing Peg-IFN to HU, no difference in haematological response between the two arms was found at 12 and 24 months. Meaningful differences in response and toxicity between these two agents over time were not observed and both agents appear to be effective therapies for treatment naïve PV patients. Importantly since the drug is considered to pose no teratogenic effects, it can potentially be used safely in patients with PV who are pregnant

Ruxolitinib

Following the impressive success of imatinib for patients with CML, there was considerable optimism as the JAK2 inhibitors entered clinical trials. But the results, for the most part, suggest a qualified success with significant symptomatic benefit for MF and, to a lesser extent, high-risk PV patients but no major change in the natural history nor an impact on the $JAK2^{V617F}$ allelic burden.

Ruxolitinib, the first-in-class JAK1/2 inhibitor, is currently licensed as second-line therapy for patients with PV who are intolerant, resistant, or have an inadequate response to hydroxyurea (Table 8.2). The approval was based on the results of a randomized phase 3 (RESPONSE) trial, which compared ruxolitinib to best available therapy in PV patients resistant or intolerant to hydroxyurea. By week 32, 72% and 24% of ruxolitinib-treated patients had a decrease in spleen size and complete haematological remission from baseline compared with 33% and 9% in the control arm, respectively; even though fewer thrombotic events were observed in the ruxolitinib-treated cohort the number of events are very limited to allow a conclusion on this regard. Ruxolitinib was also superior to the control arm in improving PV-related symptoms, as assessed by the MPN-SAF criteria. A currently ongoing study (RELIEF) is assessing the symptom-burdens in these patients further.

Other investigational agents

Inhibition of histone deacetylases (HDAC) has proven to be clinically valuable in diverse malignancies including MPN. In patients with PV, an Italian study assessed the efficacy and safety of a potent HDAC inhibitor,

Table 8.2 Criteria of clinical resistance and intolerance to hydroxyurea in polycythaemia vera based on the European LeukemiaNet consensus

Type	Criteria
Resistance	
1	Need for phlebotomy to keep Hct <45% after 3 months of ≥2 g/day of hydroxyurea, OR
2	Uncontrolled myeloproliferation, i.e. platelet count >400 × 10^9/L AND white blood cell count >10 × 10^9/L after 3 months of ≥2 g/day of hydroxyurea, OR
3	Failure to reduce massive* splenomegaly by more than 50% as measured by palpation, OR failure to completely relieve symptoms related to splenomegaly after 3 months of ≥2 g/day of hydroxyurea, OR
Intolerance	
4	Absolute neutrophil count <1.0 × 10^9/L OR platelet count <100 × 10^9/L or Hb <100 g/L at the lowest dose of hydroxyurea required to achieve a complete or partial clinico-haematological response†, OR
5	Presence of leg ulcers or other unacceptable hydroxyurea-related non-haematological toxicities, such as mucocutaneous manifestations, gastrointestinal symptoms, pneumonitis, or fever at any dose of hydroxyurea

* Organ extending by >10 cm from the LCM.

† Complete response was defined as Hct <45% without phlebotomy, platelet count ≤400 × 10^9/L, white blood cell count ≤10 × 10^9/L, and no disease-related symptoms. Partial response was defined as: Hct <45% without phlebotomy, or response in three or more of the other criteria (European LeukemiaNet criteria).

Reproduced with permission from Barbui T, et al. (2018). Philadelphia-chromosome-negative classical myeloproliferative neoplasms: Revised management recommendations from the European LeukemiaNet. *Leukemia*. 32(5):1057–69. DOI: 10.1038/s41375-018-0077-1.

givinostat, in two phase 2 trials. The first assessed patients with PV and other MPN who were either intolerant or refractory to hydroxyurea, and the second evaluated potential to combine givinostat with hydroxyurea in patients who appeared refractory to conventional doses of hydroxyurea. Both studies observed modest efficacy in terms of reducing Hct and according symptom relief, and further studies are desirable. Another HDAC inhibitor, vorinostat, has also been evaluated in newly diagnosed and intolerant/relapsed/refractory PV patents and found to be able to accord haematological responses and also reduce pruritus and splenomegaly. The drug, however, was associated with substantial toxicity and further development discontinued.

Summary of recommendations

Since the majority of patients diagnosed with PV can be anticipated to have an excellent prognosis, with overall survival that is not dissimilar to that of the general population, it is critical to develop a risk-based treatment algorithm which ensures an emphasis on a healthy lifestyle to minimize cardiovascular risk factors, and minimize potential treatment-related side effects. PV currently remains incurable and the main objective of specific therapy is to prevent serious and potentially life-threatening thrombotic complications. PV patients with a low risk of thrombosis (age <60 years and no previous history of thrombosis) are managed with regular phlebotomy to keep Hct <45%, and low-dose aspirin to reduce the thrombotic risks. In high-risk patients, hydroxyurea, the efficacy, and safety of which has been established

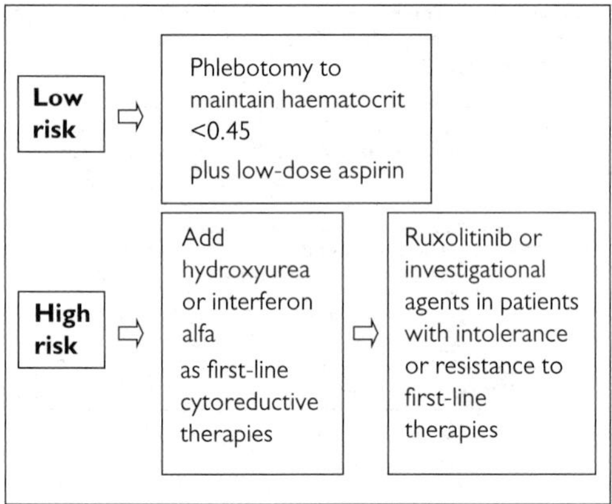

Figure 8.1 Flow-chart of recommended risk-adapted treatment for patients with polycythaemia vera.

Reproduced with permission from Barbui T, et al. (2013). Myeloproliferative neoplasms and thrombosis. *Blood*. 122(13):2176–84. DOI: 10.1182/blood-2013-03-460154. Copyright © 2013 by The American Society of Hematology.

over five decades, or IFNα are generally considered the most useful drugs. In patients resistant or intolerant to such first-line treatment, ruxolitinib, or participation in prospective clinical trials should be considered. Current recommendations for management of patients with PV are summarized in Figure 8.1. Specific recommendations for unique scenarios, such as the optimal management of venous thrombosis in unusual sites, and the management of the pregnant PV patient, are summarized in Box 8.2 and Box 8.3, respectively.

Box 8.2 Management of thrombosis in unusual sites

Cerebral vein thrombosis

- Common presenting symptoms
  - Severe headache (>90% of cases)
  - Paresis, aphasia
  - Seizures, mental status disorder
- Recommended diagnostic procedures
  - Magnetic resonance imaging
  - Angiography
- Treatment
  - Anticoagulant therapy (long-life?)

Abdominal vein thrombosis (hepatic, portal, mesenteric)

- Common presenting symptoms
  - Abdominal pain
  - Hepatomegaly and ascites (in hepatic thrombosis)
- Recommended diagnostic procedures
  - CT scan
  - Hepatic ultrasonography (in hepatic thrombosis)
  - Angiography
- Treatment
  - Long-life anticoagulant therapy*
  - Invasive procedures if needed (in hepatic thrombosis)

* Anticoagulant therapy: full heparinization followed by oral anticoagulation with PT INR range 2.0–3.0.

Source: data from Barbui T, et al. (2011). Philadelphia-negative classical myeloproliferative neoplasms: Critical concepts and management recommendations from European LeukemiaNet. *J Clin Oncol.* 29(6):761–70. DOI: 10.1200/JCO.2010.31.8436.

Box 8.3 Recommendations for management of pregnancy in polycythaemia vera

1. Risk stratification
   - At least one of the following defines high-risk pregnancy:
     - previous major thrombotic or bleeding complication
     - previous severe pregnancy complications*
2. Therapy
   - Low-risk pregnancy
     - Target haematocrit should be kept below 45%
     - Aspirin 100 mg/day
     - LMWH 4000 U/day after delivery until 6 weeks postpartum
   - High-risk pregnancy. As above, plus
     - If previous major thrombosis or severe pregnancy complications: LMWH 4000 U/day throughout pregnancy (stop aspirin if bleeding complications)
     - If myelosuppression is required:** consider IFN-α

* Severe pregnancy complications: >3 first-trimester or >1 second or third-trimester losses, birth weight <5th centile of gestation, pre-eclampsia, intrauterine death, or stillbirth.

** disease-related prior reason for cytoxic therapy or uncontrolled haematocrit or progressive myeloproliferation (leukocytosis, thrombocytosis, splenomegaly)

Reproduced with permission from Barbui T, et al. (2018). Philadelphia-chromosome-negative classical myeloproliferative neoplasms: Revised management recommendations from the European LeukemiaNet. *Leukemia*. 32(5):1057–69. DOI: 10.1038/s41375-018-0077-1.

Further reading

Barbui T, Barosi G, Birgegard G, et al. Philadelphia-negative classical myeloproliferative neoplasms: critical concepts and management recommendations from European Leukemia Net. *J Clin Oncol*. 2011;29:761–70.

Barbui T, Carobbio A, Rumi E, et al. In contemporary patients with polycythemia vera, rates of thrombosis and risk factors delineate a new clinical epidemiology. *Blood*. 2014;124;3021–3.

Barbui T, Finazzi G, Falanga A. Myeloproliferative neoplasms and thrombosis. *Blood*. 2013;122:2176–84.

Barbui T, Tefferi A, Vannucchi AM, et al. Philadelphia chromosome-negative classical myeloproliferative neoplasms: revised management recommendations from European Leukemia Net. *Leukemia*. 2018;32:1057–69.

Barbui T, Thiele J, Gisslinger H, et al. The 2016 WHO Classification and Diagnostic Criteria for Myeloproliferative Neoplasms: document summary and in-depth discussion. *Blood Cancer J*. 2018;8:15.

Barbui T, Thiele J, Vannucchi AM, Tefferi A. Rethinking the diagnostic criteria of polycythemia vera. *Leukemia*. 2014;28:1191–5.

Barosi G, Birgegard G, Finazzi G, et al. A unified definition of clinical resistance and intolerance to hydroxycarbamide in polycythaemia vera and primary myelofibrosis: results of a European LeukemiaNet (ELN) consensus process. *Br J Haematol*. 2010;148:961–3.

De Stefano V, Ruggeri M, Cervantes F, et al. High rate of recurrent venous thromboembolism in patients with myeloproliferative neoplasms and effect of prophylaxis with vitamin K antagonists. *Blood Cancer J*. 2016;6:e493.

Finazzi G, Caruso V, Marchioli R, et al. Acute leukemia in polycythemia vera. An analysis of 1,638 patients enrolled in a prospective observational study. *Blood*. 2005;105:2664–70.

Finazzi G, Vannucchi AM, Martinelli V, et al. A phase II study of Givinostat in combination with hydroxycarbamide in patients with polycythaemia vera unresponsive to hydroxycarbamide monotherapy. *Br J Haematol*. 2013;161:688–94.

Geyer HL, Mesa RA. Therapy for myeloproliferative neoplasms: when, which agent, and how? *Blood*. 2014;124:3529–37.

Geyer HL, Scherber RM, Dueck AC, et al. Distinct clustering of symptomatic burden among myeloproliferative neoplasm patients: retrospective assessment in 1470 patients. *Blood*. 2014;123:3803–10.

Kiladijan JJ, Mesa RA, Hoffman R. The renaissance of interferon therapy for the treatment of myeloid malignancies. *Blood*. 2011;117:4706–15.

Landolfi R, Marchioli R, Kutti J, et al. Efficacy and safety of low-dose aspirin in polycythemia vera. *N Engl J Med*. 2004;350:114–24.

Marchioli R, Finazzi G, Landolfi R, et al. Vascular and neoplastic risk in a large cohort of patients with polycythemia vera. *J Clin Oncol*. 2005;23:2224–32.

Marchioli R, Finazzi G, Specchia G, et al. Cardiovascular events and intensity of treatment in polycythemia vera. *N Engl J Med*. 2013;368:22–33.

Tefferi A, Barbui T. Polycythemia vera and essential thrombocythemia: 2019 update on diagnosis, risk-stratification and management. *Am J Hematol*. 2019;94:133–43.

Tefferi A, Rumi E, Finazzi G, et al. Survival and prognosis among 1545 patients with contemporary polycythemia vera: an international study. *Leukemia*. 2013;27:1874–81.

Tefferi A, Thiele J, Orazi A, et al. Proposals and rationale for revision of the World Health Organization diagnostic criteria for polycythemia vera, essential thrombocythemia, and primary myelofibrosis: recommendations from an ad hoc international expert panel. *Blood*. 2007;110:1092–7.

Vannucchi AM. How I treat polycythemia vera. *Blood*. 2014;124:3212–20.

Verstovsek S, Komrokji RTS. Novel and emerging therapies for the treatment of polycythemia vera. *Expert Rev Hematol*. 2014;8(1):101–13.

Verstovsek S, Passamonti F, Rambaldi A, et al. A phase 2 study of ruxolitinib, an oral JAK1 and JAK2 Inhibitor, in patients with advanced polycythemia vera who are refractory or intolerant to hydroxyurea. *Cancer*. 2014;120:513–20.

Chapter 9

Myelofibrosis

Claire Harrison, Yan Beauverd, and Donal McLorran

Introduction to myelofibrosis *127*
Epidemiology *127*
Pathophysiology *127*
Clinical and biological features *130*
Complications and evolution *132*
Diagnosis *133*
Risk stratification and prognostic factors *137*
Management, treatment, and response to treatment *139*

Introduction to myelofibrosis

Myeloproliferative neoplasms include chronic myelogenous leukaemia, *BCR-ABL1*–positive (CML) and BC *BCR-ABL1*-negative diseases: polycythaemia vera (PV), essential thrombocythaemia (ET), primary myelofibrosis (PMF), chronic neutrophilic leukaemia (CNL), chronic eosinophilic leukaemia, not otherwise specified (CEL-NOS), mast cell disease (MCD), and myeloproliferative neoplasm (MPN) unclassifiable. In the BCL-ABL negative myeloproliferative neoplasms, PV, ET, and PMF are the most frequent and share similarity in term of pathogenesis. PMF is a 'proper' primary disease in its own right but myelofibrosis can also be secondary to PV and ET which are formerly named post-PV myelofibrosis and post-ET myelofibrosis. PMF, post-PV myelofibrosis, and post-ET myelofibrosis have a similar pathogenesis, clinical presentation, evolution, and treatment. With regard to these similarities, they are often indifferently included in ongoing therapeutic trials. In this chapter except where otherwise stated we shall refer to them together as myelofibrosis (MF) this is distinct from myelofibrosis due to other condition usually reactive but an important condition to discriminate is myelodysplasia with fibrosis.

The current WHO classification published in 2016 revised previous diagnostic criteria published in 2008. PMF has been known by a number of sometimes confusing terms: chronic idiopathic myelofibrosis, agnogenic myeloid metaplasia, myelosclerosis with myeloid metaplasia, or chronic granulocytic-megakaryocytic myelosis. Most current epidemiological knowledge of PMF is based on retrospective cohorts using previous diagnostic criteria and classifications.

Epidemiology

PMF is the least frequent myeloproliferative neoplasm with an incidence of 0.22 to 1.5 per 100 000 per year, and without sex predominance. Diagnosis occurs most frequently in the seventh decade (median age of 67 years old). Less than 5% are less than 40 years old at the time of diagnosis and it is a very rare condition in childhood. The rate of transformation to MF from PV is around 12–21% and 9–10% from ET, this risk increases over time. No specific epidemiological risk factor is associated with most cases of PMF. Some rare cases are associated with benzene and toluene exposure or ionizing radiations (people exposed to atomic bomb at Hiroshima or thorium-based radiographic contrast product). Factors associated with transformation from PV and ET are also not clear but have been reported to be different according to the underlying genetic mutation *CALR* vs. *JAK2* V617F, greater risk with higher *JAK2* V617F allele burden in PV, may differ with different therapies, and becomes more likely over time.

Pathophysiology

PMF is a clonal disease of the myeloid lineage. It is a multiple step disease starting with clonal proliferation followed by increase of what have

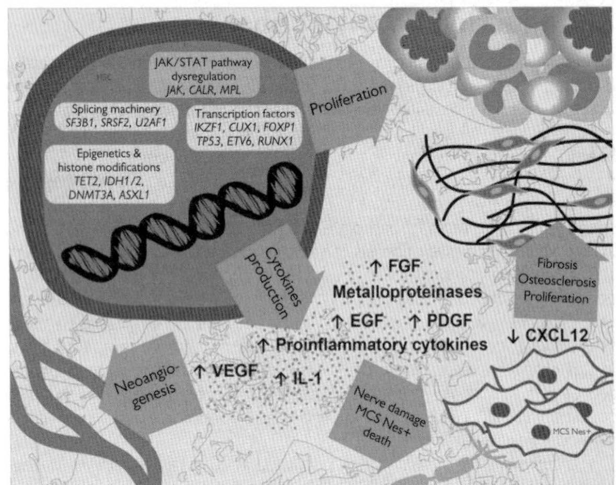

Figure 9.1 Schematic representation of HSC mutations and relations with the bone marrow niche.

traditionally been believed to be non-clonal fibroblast and mesenchymal cell proliferation and collagen deposition secondary to cytokine stimulation. In PMF, circulating red cells, myeloid cells, and thrombocytes are all clonal cells. Myeloblasts (CD34+) are increased compared to controls or others myeloproliferative neoplasms as ET or PV. Recent data have shown that the *JAK2* V617F mutation may not only be present on haemopoietic stem cells but also in endothelial progenitor cells in some patients with specific phenotypes. A schematic representation of factors implicated in the pathogenesis of MF is shown in Figure 9.1.

JAK/STAT pathway and genes mutations involved in genes regulation

Constitutional activation of the JAK/STAT pathway is the hallmark of *BCR-ABL1* negative myeloproliferative neoplasms where different mutations are described and discussed in detail in Chapters 2 and 3. The most frequent are *JAK2* V617F mutation (present in ~60% of patients) and *MPL* exon 10 mutation (mutations W515L and W515K), present in ~5% of patients and encoding for the thrombopoietin receptor. These mutations confer a gain-of-function and permanently activate the JAK/STAT pathway. In 2013, several mutations affecting exon 9 of the Calreticulin gene (*CALR*) were described. *CALR* mutation is almost exclusive (virtually never associated with *JAK2* or *MPL* mutation) and present in ~30% of PMF. Only few patients do not present a *JAK2*, *MPL* or *CALR* mutation (~5%) these are known as 'triple negative'. Similar to *JAK2* or *MPL* mutations, *CALR* mutation also seem to activate the JAK/STAT pathway.

The JAK/STAT pathway targets genes encoding for cell proliferation and survival, it is currently believed to be responsible for proliferative characteristics (hypercellular bone marrow, leucocytosis, and thrombocytosis). JAK/STAT also targets genes involved in production of inflammatory cytokines that are also likely to be responsible for some of the constitutional symptoms associated with myelofibrosis (night sweats, fever, or fatigue).

In addition to the constitutive activation of the JAK/STAT pathway, numerous other mutations have been observed in MF. Epigenetics and histones acetylation are an important component of gene expression and their modification can cause dysregulation in gene expression. In MF, different genes involved in epigenetics or histone component have shown mutations, as *TET2, IDH1/2, DNMT3A, ASXL1*. Moreover, regulation of transcription factors and mutations in genes coding them (*IKZF1, FOXP1, ETV6, CUX1, TP53*, or *RUNX1*) were also described. These mutations could participate in the dysregulation of the cell cycle or DNA damage response. Finally, mutations of the genes *SF3B1, SRSF2*, or *U2AF1* were reported in MF and involve the splicing machinery.

The bone marrow niche

The term 'haematopoietic niche' refers to a concept of strong interactions and cross talk between haematopoietic stem cell and stromal cells involved in stem cell regulation, quiescence, proliferation, or differentiation. Major components of the haemopoietic niche which have shown an impact of haematopoietic stem cell (HSC) maintenance are multipotent stromal cell expressing nestin (MSC Nes+), endothelial cell, and the non-myelinated Schwann cell. Viability of MSC Nes+ is dependent of its innervation by sympathetic nerves which requires integrity of Schwann cell. MSC Nes+ produce the cytokine CXCl12 which is involved in regulation, migration, and quiescence of HSC and participate to maintain a normal haemopoiesis, as well as regulate production and proliferation of fibroblasts. Some evidence for this comes from a JAK2 mutant mice model expressing excess interleukin IL-1b which caused Schwann cell death, there was neuroglial damage and subsequently reduction of the number of MCS NES+. Diminution of MCS NES+ reduces production of CXCl12 and promotes HSC proliferation and migration and impairs normal haemopoiesis, as well as triggering fibrosis and new bone formation.

In addition, some MPN patients with the *JAK2V617F* mutation have detectable clonal endothelial progenitor cells (cEPC) which exhibit the same mutation, and furthermore the presence of cEPC seems to confer a higher risk of thrombosis in such patients. This observation points in the direction of a common haematopoietic and endothelial progenitor being implicated in the pathogenesis of MPN. Both these models suggest that in responses in the microenvironment, vascular endothelium may not merely be reactive and may present future therapeutic targets.

Cytokines and their implication in the aetiology of fibrosis

Transforming growth factor-beta (TGF-β) is thought to be a cornerstone cytokine involved in the development of fibrosis and is produced in excess in patients with MF. Moreover, a dysregulated balance between matrix metalloproteinases (MMP) and tissue inhibitors of MMPs is probably also implicated in the abnormal deposition of fibrosis. Other cytokines are also increased, such as epidermal growth factor (EGF), basic fibroblast growth factor (FGF), platelet derived growth factor (PDGF), vascular endothelial growth factor (VEGF) and are potentially important in the fibrosis as well as in increase of microvascularization. A schematic presentation of MF pathogenesis is summarized in Figure 9.1.

In conclusion, in addition to gene mutations involved in the JAK/STAT pathway, numerous other genes mutations in the splicing machinery, in epigenetics or histone modifications as well as in transcription factors seem to play a role in the MF pathogenesis. Moreover, dysregulation in the HSC niche in now well established and is of first importance.

Clinical and biological features

Myelofibrosis is a progressive disease, as discussed it also often evolves from a precursor disease state without any clinical symptoms and only few laboratory anomalies—often only thrombocytosis (sometimes mimicking ET) -, to more symptomatic disease with numerous clinical findings and laboratory anomalies. As the disease progresses clinically often but not always concordant progression is evident histologically, with a so-called prefibrotic stage usually related to less symptomatic disease progressing to densely fibrotic and then a burnt out osteomyelofibrotic phase usually related to more symptomatic features.

Symptoms

Constitutional symptoms are prevalent with around 15% of patients are reported to be asymptomatic at diagnosis. Fatigue is the most common symptom reported in 47–70% of patients and thought to be associated with a hypercatabolic state secondary to cytokine overproduction. Other symptoms related to this hypercatabolic state are involuntary loss of weight and night sweats, low grade fever, as well as bone pain splenomegaly-related symptoms (abdominal discomfort or pain due to spleen enlargement or splenic infarct, early satiety, or dyspepsia) are observed in 25–50% of patients. Pruritus is also frequent and sometimes very debilitating. Other symptoms may of course relate to abnormal blood cell production (e.g. bleeding and the presence of extramedullary haemopoiesis).

Signs

Splenomegaly is one of the cardinal characteristics of MF (present in more than 90% of patients at diagnosis), often massive (23% of patients have splenomegaly >23 cm below the costal margin) and easily palpable on examination. Hepatomegaly is also very frequent (39% of patients). Splenomegaly is caused by extramedullary haemopoiesis and can be worsened by portal hypertension secondary to hepatomegaly. Causes of hepatomegaly are multiple: such as extramedullary haemopoiesis and/or due to increase of splanchnic blood flow following spleen enlargement. Portal hypertension can develop (secondary to hepatomegaly or portal or hepatic vein thrombosis), resulting in ascites, oesophageal and gastric varices, and increasing risk of gastrointestinal bleeding.

The hallmark of the disease is the ineffective haemopoiesis secondary to fibrosis this often leads to extramedullary haemopoiesis. The main organs involved in extramedullary haematopoiesis are spleen and liver but occasionally the vertebral column, lymph nodes, retroperitoneum, lungs or pleura, genitourinary system, or skin. These deposits may then cause specific signs for example those related to pulmonary hypertension.

Laboratory anomalies

Anaemia is frequently found in myelofibrosis and 50% of patients have a haemoglobin level less than 100 g/L at diagnosis. Anaemia results from a decrease of erythropoiesis in fibrotic bone marrow and an ineffective extramedullary erythropoiesis. Defective red cell production can be worsened by splenic sequestration due to enlarged spleen or bleeding promoted by portal hypertension, gastric and oesophageal varices, and thrombocytopaenia, autoimmune haemolysis may also occur. Over time with disease progression, anaemia generally progress, and some patients require red blood cell transfusion. Blood film appearances include anisopoikilocytosis, with teardrop cells (dacrocytes) and nucleated red cells typically were observed. An example of typical blood film is shown in Figure 9.2.

White blood cells are typically increased and myeloid series is usually left-shifted. Increased leucocyte count (13% of patients have >25x10 at diagnosis time) can be marked and some myeloblasts (37–45% of patients have ≥1% blasts present at diagnosis time) can be seen on blood film. Leucopenia may also occur. The platelet count is variable for example, 37% have a low platelet count and 13% a high platelet count at diagnosis. With

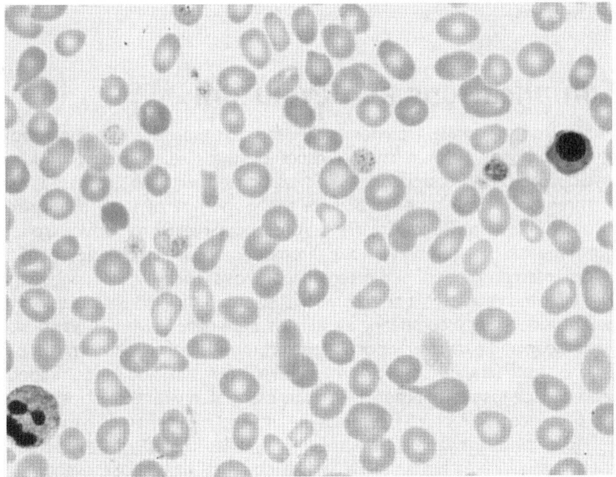

Figure 9.2 Blood film with typical teardrop cell and nucleated red cell (also see plate section).

progression of disease, the platelet count tends to go down, likely as a consequence of splenic sequestration with progressive splenomegaly, increasingly ineffective haemopoiesis, and perhaps immune phenomena. Platelet morphology can be altered with anisocytosis, abnormalities of granulation, and some fragmented megakaryocytes can also be seen. With ineffective haemopoiesis and increase of cell turnover, markers of cell lysis as lactate dehydrogenase and uric acid are often elevated. Liver enzymes can also be increased secondary to liver infiltration with extramedullary haemopoiesis.

Bone marrow anomalies

The bone marrow is often difficult to aspirate due to fibrosis so-called dry tap. In all cases an aspirate is not sufficient to confirm diagnosis and a trephine biopsy is always required to determine fibrosis grading and to evaluate megakaryocytes morphology and their distribution in the bone marrow. When available, aspirates could show an increased number of megakaryocytes with some abnormal features. At diagnosis, more than 70% of patients were at fibrotic stage. At this stage, bone marrow biopsy demonstrates usually normo- or hypocellularity with an important increase of collagen or reticulin fibrosis. The hallmark is the presence of clusters of atypical megakaryocytes, usually increased in number, and the presence of vascular proliferation and dilatation of marrow sinuses with intraluminal haemopoiesis. Osteosclerosis (new bone formation) can be seen at this stage. Around 25% of patients are in a so-called prefibrotic stage at diagnosis characterized by absence or limited fibrosis and hypercellular bone marrow. Typical anomalies involve megakaryocyte lineage (increased in number and always atypical). These features are discussed in more detail in Chapter 4.

Complications and evolution

Apart from anaemia, splenomegaly, and extramedullary haematopoiesis (which are intrinsic characteristics of the disease), as with other myeloproliferative neoplasms MF is associated with an increased risk of thrombosis. In a large multicentre study, the rate of fatal (pulmonary thromboembolism, Budd–Chiari syndrome, portal vein thrombosis, stroke), and non-fatal thrombosis (venous thromboembolism, stroke, acute myocardial infarction, peripheral arterial thrombosis) was 1.7% patient-years. The adjusted rate of major thrombotic events (non-cardiovascular death was considered as a competing event) was 2.2% patient-years. Atypical site thrombosis and particularly portal vein thrombosis are well-known complications of MF (and other myeloproliferative neoplasms) and can sometimes precede diagnosis. Significant risk factors associated with thrombosis were the presence of *JAK2* V617F mutation and age older than 60 years. The frequency of major vascular events in MF is similar to ET (1–3% per patient-year) but overall is higher in PV where non-fatal thrombotic events and cardiovascular death was reported as 5.5% patient-years.

Evolution to leukaemia is a major complication associated with MF. By definition, acute leukaemia in this circumstance is diagnosed in the presence of ≥20% blasts in peripheral blood and/or bone marrow (while a blast count of 10–19% indicates an accelerated phase). Most transformations evolve towards acute myeloid leukaemia, but some transformations are phenotypically lymphoblastic, megakaryocytic, or mixed. In previous studies, the 10-year risk of leukaemic transformation was estimated at between 8% and 23%. Different risk factors associated with increased risk of leukaemic evolution were described as >3% peripheral blasts or platelet count <100 000/L at diagnosis. In the same way, presence of one or two of: bone marrow blasts >10% or high-risk karyotype (defined as del17p, −5, −7, and/or complex) increases the risk for 1-year leukaemia transformation from 2% to 13%. The mutational profile of MPN-related acute myeloid leukaemia is also different than *de novo* acute myeloid leukaemia. Mutation of *TET2, ALX1, TP53*, and *IDH1/2* is more often muted in MPN-related acute myeloid leukaemia (AML) while in the novo AML mutation of *FLT3, DNMT3A*, and *WT1* is more frequent. Unfortunately, the outcome of MPN-related AML is poor, with a 2-year overall survival of 15%.

Diagnosis

Diagnosis of PMF is often suspected following abnormalities in full blood count, detecting splenomegaly or the presence of constitutional symptoms. For patients already diagnosed with PV or ET, changes in clinical symptoms (hypercatabolic features, symptoms secondary to splenomegaly) or biological features (anaemia, thrombocytopenia, leukoerythroblastosis) may raise the suspicion of transformation to MF.

In 2016, WHO proposed a revision of diagnostic criteria for PMF. Diagnostic criteria include biological and clinical features as well as bone marrow histology findings, abnormal blood film and full blood count, molecular abnormalities, or splenomegaly as well as exclusion of other myeloid neoplasm. Presence of specific gene mutations (as *JAK2* V617F, *cMPL*, or *CALR*) demonstrates the clonal feature of the disease. Diagnosis requires meeting three major criteria and two minor criteria. Inclusion of recently discovered calreticulin mutation will probably be included in next diagnosis criteria revision. Diagnostic criteria are summarized in Box 9.1.

Post-PV and post-ET myelofibrosis criteria were defined by the International Working Group for Myelofibrosis Research and Treatment (IWG-MRT) in 2016 as shown in Table 9.1. In Table 9.2, we summarized the most important exams to perform at diagnosis time, as well as frequent associated anomalies.

It is important to realize that the presence of fibrosis in the bone marrow is not pathognomonic of MF and can be seen in others haematological neoplasms (MDS, AML, Hairy-cell leukaemia, etc.) as well as non-haematological conditions (immunologic disease, pulmonary hypertension, metastasis, etc.). A practical flowchart for diagnosis of MF is proposed in Figure 9.3.

Box 9.1 PMF diagnostic criteria according WHO 2016

Major criteria

- Presence of megakaryocyte proliferation and atypia, usually accompanied by either reticulin and/or collagen fibrosis, or, in the absence of significant reticulin fibrosis, the megakaryocyte changes must be accompanied by an increased bone marrow cellularity characterized by granulocytic proliferation and often decreased erythropoiesis (i.e. prefibrotic cellular-phase disease)
- Not meeting WHO criteria for PV, CML, MDS, or other myeloid neoplasm
- Demonstration of *JAK2* 617V>F or other clonal marker (e.g. *MPL* 515W>L/K), or in the absence of a clonal marker, no evidence of bone marrow fibrosis due to underlying inflammatory or other neoplastic diseases

Minor criteria

- Leukoerythroblastosis
- Increase in serum lactate dehydrogenase level
- Anaemia
- Palpable splenomegaly

Adapted from Arber DA, et al. (2016). The 2016 revision to the World Health Organization classification of myeloid neoplasms and acute leukemia. *Blood*. 127(20):2391–405. https://doi.org/10.1182/blood-2016-03-643544. Reprinted with permission from the American Society of Hematology.

Table 9.1 Post-PV and post-ET MF diagnostic criteria according to IWG-MRT

	Post-PV myelofibrosis diagnostic criteria according to IWG-MRT	Post-ET myelofibrosis diagnostic criteria according to IWG-MRT
Required criteria	• Documentation of a previous diagnosis of PV as defined by the WHO criteria. • Bone marrow fibrosis grade 2–3 (on 0–3 scale) or grade 3–4 (on 0–4 scale).	• Documentation of a previous diagnosis of ET as defined by the WHO criteria. • Bone marrow fibrosis grade 2–3 (on 0–3 scale) or grade 3–4 (on 0–4 scale).
Additional criteria (two are required)	• Anaemia or sustained loss of requirement of either phlebotomy (in the absence of cytoreductive therapy) or cytoreductive treatment for erythrocytosis. • A leukoerythroblastic peripheral blood picture. • Increasing splenomegaly defined as either an increase in palpable splenomegaly of greater than or equal to 5 cm (distance of the tip of the spleen from the left costal margin) or the appearance of a newly palpable splenomegaly.	• Anaemia and a greater than or equal to 2 mg mL-1 decrease from baseline haemoglobin level. • A leukoerythroblastic peripheral blood picture. • Increasing splenomegaly defined as either an increase in palpable splenomegaly of greater than or equal to 5 cm (distance of the tip of the spleen from the left costal margin) or the appearance of a newly palpable splenomegaly.

Table 9.1 *contd.*

	Post-PV myelofibrosis diagnostic criteria according to IWG-MRT	Post-ET myelofibrosis diagnostic criteria according to IWG-MRT
	• Development of greater than or equal to1 of three constitutional symptoms: >10% weight loss in 6 months, night sweats, unexplained fever (>37.5°C).	• Increased lactic acid dehydrogenase (LDH) (above reference level). • Development of greater than or equal to1 of three constitutional symptoms: >10% weight loss in 6 months, night sweats, unexplained fever (>37.5°C).

Source: data from Cervantes F, et al. (2009). New prognostic scoring system for primary myelofibrosis based on a study of the International Working Group for Myelofibrosis Research and Treatment. *Blood.* 113(13):2895–901. DOI: 10.1182/blood-2008-07-170449; and Thiele J, et al. (2005). Bone marrow histopathology in myeloproliferative disorders—current diagnostic approach. *Semin Hematol.* 42(4):184–95. https://doi.org/10.1053/j.seminhematol.2005.05.020.

Table 9.2 Screening tests for MF diagnosis

Exams	Frequent abnormalities
Blood analysis	
Full blood count	Anaemia, leucocytosis, or leukopenia, thrombocytosis, or thrombocytopenia.
Blood film	Teardrop cell, nucleated red cell, blast cell %.
LDH	Often increased (ineffective erythropoiesis and haemolysis). Not specific for MF.
EPO	If reduced, is a marker of response to EPO treatment.
Urate	Often increased (ineffective erythropoiesis and haemolysis) may not require therapy.
JAK2V617F, MPL, CALR	Frequent mutations associated with myelofibrosis.
BCR-ABL	To exclude CML.
Bone marrow analysis	
Aspirate	Often dry, but can show abnormal megakaryocytes.
Trephine	Prefibrotic stage: usually hypercellular with abnormal megakaryocytes. Fibrotic stage: increase of fibrosis, atypical megakaryocytes, dilatation of marrow sinuses with intraluminal haemopoiesis.
Karyotype	Needed to assess the disease risk (DIPSS-plus). If the aspirate is dry, peripheral blood can be analysed.
Other exams	
Abdominal ultrasound	Looking for splenomegaly, if not palpable on examination.

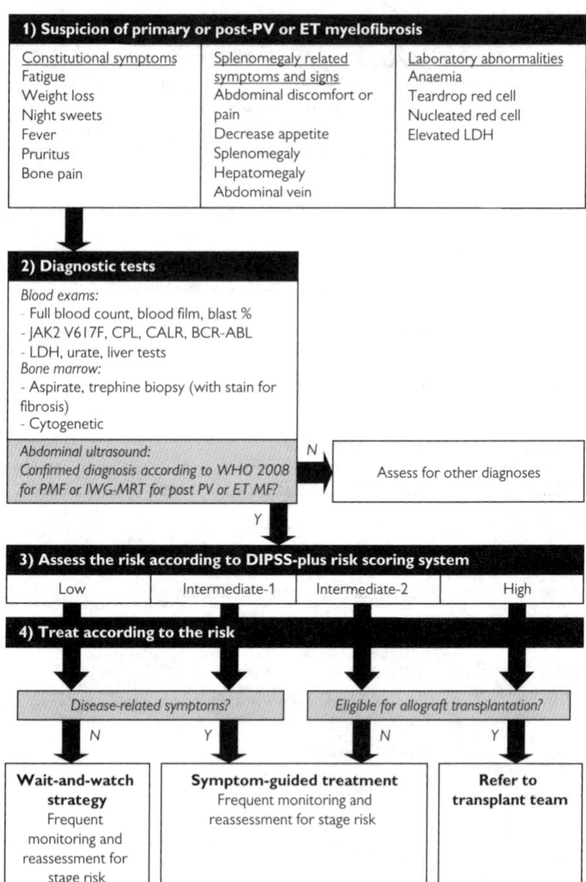

Figure 9.3 Diagnosis and management for primary and post-PV and ET MF.

Risk stratification and prognostic factors

Risk stratification is important to determine treatment options, specifically stem cell transplantation. In contrast to PV and ET where risk stratification is built around thrombosis, risk in MF this is tailored to prognosis. In 2009, the International Prognostic Scoring System (IPSS) was developed which delineates five predictive factors of survival; age >65 years, haemoglobin <100 g/L, leukocyte count >25 × 10^9/L, circulating blasts ≥1%, and presence of specific constitutional symptoms (weight loss, night sweats, and fever). According to the number of positive factor (0, 1, 2, ≥3), four-risk groups were highlighted with significant difference in term of overall survival. More recently, the dynamic IPSS (DIPSS) has been developed. This score can be applied at any time of the disease course and thus will demonstrate evolution. It includes the same variables as IPSS but the weight of anaemia changes: 2 points for haemoglobin <100 g/L. The last score developed was DIPSS-plus which integrates other prognostic factors, unfavourable cytogenetic (defined as sole or two abnormalities including +8, −7/7q−, i(17q), inv(3), −5/5q−, 12p−, or 11q23 rearrangement, or complex karyotype), red cell transfusion need, and platelet count <100 × 10^9/L. This eight-item risk score also results in four prognostic risk groups. All these scores are summarized in Table 9.3.

Currently, it is recommended to use DIPSS-plus to risk stratify patients with PMF. While none of these scores where validated for post-PV and post-ET myelofibrosis, they are frequently used in this context. One recent study has shown that IPSS do not accurately discriminate risk groups in post-ET and post-PV patients and DIPSS and DIPSS-plus were currently not evaluated for these patients.

Moreover, other prognostic markers were described. Recent data in the literature have shown that some molecular abnormalities could be independent prognosis factor. Overall survival was reduced in patients with *EZH2* mutation and low allele *JAK* V617F burden. In the same way, 'triple negative' patients (negative for *JAK2* V617F, *MPL*, and *CALR* mutations) seem to have a lower overall survival than patients with *JAK2* V617F, while *CALR* patients showed a better survival. Similarly, patients with *CALR* mutation are usually younger, with higher platelet count, and have lower DIPSS-plus scores and require less transfusion. The mutational status of the genes *CALR* and *ASXL1* has also been proposed as an independent prognostic factor, with a median overall survival of 20 years for *CALR+/ASXL1–*, 9 years for *CALR+/ASXL+* and *CALR–/ASXL1–* and 4 years for *CALR–/ASXL1+*. Furthermore, mutations on *SRFS2* gene is mutated in 17% of patients with PMF and is associated with shorten overall survival. Isocitrate dehydrogenase (IDH) mutations are found in 4% of patients and are also associated with shorter overall survival. Both of these overall survival markers are independent from the DIPSS-plus scoring system.

A new prognostic score integrating gene mutational status, the Mutation-Enhanced International Prognostic Scoring System (MIPSS) was been proposed in 2014 (see Chapter 6). This scoring system determines eight predictive factors of survival with different weight (age >60 year old: 1.5 point; haemoglobin <100 g/L: 0.5 point; presence of constitutional symptoms: 0.5 point; platelets <200x10e9/l: 1 point; triple negative mutational

Table 9.3 Prognostic scores for MF

Number of points for risk factor, according to risk score				
Risk factors	IPSS	DIPSS	DIPSS-plus	MIPSS
Age >65 years	1	1	1	1.5§
Haemoglobin <100 g/L	1	2	1	0.5
Leukocyte count >25 × 10^9/L	1	1	1	NA
Circulating blasts ≥1%	1	1	1	NA
Presence of constitutional symptoms*	1	1	1	0.5
Unfavourable cytogenetics#	NA	NA	1	NA
Red cell transfusion need	NA	NA	1	NA
Platelet count <100 × 10^9/L	NA	NA	1	NA
Platelet count <200 × 10^9/L	NA	NA	NA	1
Triple negativity	NA	NA	NA	1.5
JAK2 / *MPL* mutation	NA	NA	NA	0.5
ASXL1 mutation	NA	NA	NA	0.5
SRSF2 mutation	NA	NA	NA	0.5

Risk categorization and median survival according to point value for each score								
Risk	IPSS	Median survival	DIPSS	Median survival	DIPSS-plus	Median survival	MIPSS	Median survival
Low	0	11.3	0	NR	0	15.4	0–0.5	26.4
Int-1	1	7.9	1–2	14.2	1	6.5	1–1.5	9.7
Int-2	2	4	3–4	4	2–3	2.9	2–3.5	6.4
High	≥3	2.3	5–6	1.5	≥4	1.3	≥4	1.9

*: fever, nights sweet, weight loss >10% from baseline

#: +8, -7/7q-, i(17q), -5/5q-, 12p-, inv(3), 11q23 rearrangement

§: Age >60 years for MIPSS

Int-1: intermediate-1; Int-2: intermediate-2; NR: not reach

Source: data from Barosi G, et al. (2007). A unified definition of clinical resistance/intolerance to hydroxyurea in essential thrombocythemia: results of a consensus process by an international working group. *Leukemia*. 21(2):277–80. https://doi.org/10.1038/sj.leu.2404473.

status (*JAK2 V617F, MPL, CALR*): 1.5 point; *JAK* V617F or *MPL* mutation: 0.5 point; *ASXL1* mutation: 0.5 point; *SRSF2* mutation: 0.5 point). A four-risk group was derived (low for 0–0.5 point, intermediate-1 for 1–1.5 points, intermediate-2 for 2–3.5 points and high for ≥4 points) which is prognostic for median survival (26.4, 9.7, 6.4, and 1.9 years, respectively). This score is summarized in the Table 9.3. Moreover, this new score can identify subgroups of IPSS patient with poorer prognostic trajectory when compared with the former score and well as the lower risk patients have a much better median survival. However, this score was not yet been evaluated dynamically (during the disease evolution) and its impact in terms of treatment strategy is not established.

Cytokines levels have also been evaluated in the context of prognosis. In untreated patients, increased level of IL-8, IL-2R, IL-12, and IL-15 were independent prognostic factors for lower survival.

Management, treatment, and response to treatment

Current therapy for MF is mainly palliative and management of patient with MF depends upon a combination of the prognostic risk categorization and for most patients more specifically the most prominent and concerning (to both patient and clinician disease features). The range of management for such palliative care is wide, from a wait-and-see strategy (for low-risk and asymptomatic patients) to treatment targeted to features such as symptoms.

The only potentially curative treatment is allogeneic stem cell transplantation but is associated with an elevated risk of transplantation-related mortality and is currently only proposed for intermediate-2 and high-risk patients. Furthermore, as median diagnosis of myelofibrosis is in the seventh decade, most of patients are not eligible for allogeneic stem cell transplantation. Allogeneic stem cell transplantation will be specifically discussed in detail in Chapter 15.

Low-risk and asymptomatic patients

These patients are non-symptomatic and have a median of survival more than 10 years. Indeed, using the MIPSS score this may exceed 24 years. In this situation the most reasonable management is a wait-and-see approach, as the current medication does not change disease course. It is however necessary to regularly follow these patients, checking for the appearance of constitutional or other disease-related symptoms, changing in their blood count (apparition of anaemia, leucocytosis, or thrombocytopenia) or circulating blasts which would change the risk stratification and management. We find the MPN 10 or MF-SAF score helpful to continuously monitor for symptoms, Figure 9.4.

Low-risk symptomatic patients and intermediate-1 patients

As discussed earlier the symptoms of myelofibrosis are heterogeneous. In these patients, treatment should be directed initially by the specific symptoms, as it does not modify the disease course. Naturally it is also always

Fatigue

Absent	0	1	2	3	4	1	6	7	8	9	10	Worst imaginable

Filling up quickly when you eat (early satiety)

Absent	0	1	2	3	4	1	6	7	8	9	10	Worst imaginable

Abdominal discomfort

Absent	0	1	2	3	4	1	6	7	8	9	10	Worst imaginable

Inactivity

Absent	0	1	2	3	4	1	6	7	8	9	10	Worst imaginable

Problems with concentration – compared to before my diagnosis

Absent	0	1	2	3	4	1	6	7	8	9	10	Worst imaginable

Night sweats

Absent	0	1	2	3	4	1	6	7	8	9	10	Worst imaginable

Itching (pruritus)

Absent	0	1	2	3	4	1	6	7	8	9	10	Worst imaginable

Bone pain (diffuse, not join pain or arthritis) Fever (>37.8°C or 100°F)

Absent	0	1	2	3	4	1	6	7	8	9	10	Worst imaginable

Unintentional weight loss last 6 months

Absent	0	1	2	3	4	1	6	7	8	9	10	Worst imaginable

Figure 9.4 Example of Myeloproliferative Neoplasm Symptom Assessment Form Total Symptom Score (MPN-SAF TSS), otherwise known as MPN 10.

important to be aware that other conditions independent of MF may underlie these symptoms and require specific management

Anaemia

Different strategies can be employed for anaemia. Before introducing treatment, reversible and frequent causes such as iron or vitamin deficiency (cyanocobalamin, folate, etc.) should be ruled out and treated if present. Choice of starting a treatment should be guided by symptoms and comorbidities (e.g. ischaemic heart disease, renal impairment, etc.).

Androgen therapy is one of the treatments of choice for anaemia in myelofibrosis. Danazol is the most frequently used with a response rate of 37%. It is usually well tolerated, and most side effects are headaches, tiredness, muscle cramps, skin reactions, or mild increase of liver enzymes. The effect of danazol is not immediate with a median time to response of 5 months. It is recommended that patients should be treated for a minimum of six months. Others androgen drugs which have demonstrated to be efficient for anaemia are oxymetholone and fluoxymesterone (response rate of ~30%).

Erythropoiesis-stimulating agents (ESA) are another option and efficiency are probably better for patients with low erythropoietin (EPO) level (<125 mU/mL). However, ESA should be carefully considered in patients with prominent or troublesome splenomegaly due to the reported risk of drug-induced increase of spleen size.

Immunomodulating drugs as thalidomide and lenalidomide have shown some benefit in treating anaemia. However, their side effects cause frequent discontinuation hampering their benefit. Some side effects may be managed with small doses of corticosteroids which can be added concomitantly. Finally, pomalidomide alone or in combination with prednisone have shown only a slight benefice in term of anaemia with a response rate of 17–22%. However, a recent study which compared pomalidomide vs. placebo have showed no significant difference in term of rate or duration of red blood cell transfusion-independence response.

In drug refractory anaemic patients with troublesome splenomegaly, splenectomy can be discussed and reportedly can offer durable remission of transfusion-dependent anaemia in ~23% of patients. However, mortality (~9%) and postoperative morbidity (~31%, mostly thrombosis, bleeding, and infection) are important. In the other hand, splenectomy may precipitate hepatomegaly (increased liver sizes were observed in 16%) and can be implicated in hepatic failure due to extramedullary haemopoiesis. If a splenectomy is envisaged, patient must be educated about infection risk and vaccinated for encapsulated bacteria (Pneumococcal, Meningococcal and Haemophilus) following standard protocols.

Many patients unfortunately do not benefit from anaemia-directed treatments or experience side effects and require recurrent transfusion. Due to risk of iron overload, iron chelation can be introduced for patients with long life expectancy and may be particularly important in potential candidates for allogeneic stem cell transplantation. However, the benefit of iron chelation in the majority of MF patients has yet to be established.

Splenomegaly and constitutional symptoms

A wait-and-see approach has been considered reasonable until symptoms appear. Symptoms are generally size-related and include abdominal symptoms such as discomfort or pain, but also symptoms of portal hypertension (ascites, varices with risk of gastrointestinal bleeding) and cytopenias related to hypersplenism. This situation may change in the future.

JAK inhibitors

Following a better understanding of pathogenesis of myelofibrosis, drugs targeting JAK2 activation were investigated and developed. Currently, ruxolitinib (JAK1/2 inhibitor) is the only one of these agents approved for myelofibrosis. The two most pivotal trials (COMFORT-I and COMFORT-II), compared oral ruxolitinib versus placebo or best available therapy respectively. The COMFORT-I study[79] showed a dramatic improvement in spleen size (spleen volume reduction of at least 35%) in more than 40% of patients at 24 weeks and additionally 45% experienced a reduction of disease-related symptoms as determined by a 50% reduction in total symptom score using a bespoke MF-symptom assessment form (MF-SAF or MPN 10 (Figure 9.4)). Similar results were observed in the COMFORT-II trial, 28% of patients achieving the target spleen reduction at 48 weeks in the ruxolitinib arm vs. 0% in the control arm (which included standard care therapies such as hydroxycarbamide) and a better reduction in symptoms associated with myelofibrosis compared with control. In addition, ruxolitinib therapy resulted in a demonstrable improvement in quality-of-life measures. The MRI presented in the Figure 9.5 shows the reduction in spleen size of a patient treated with ruxolitinib.

This treatment is usually well tolerated and main haematological side effects are anaemia and thrombocytopenia which are dose dependent and sometimes requiring reducing or rarely discontinuing the treatment. It is currently recommended to adapt dosage based upon initial platelet count, but some studies are currently ongoing to determine safety in thrombocytopenic patients. Ruxolitinib therapy is not recommended in patients with platelet counts below 50×10^9/L, this can be a limitation of this therapy. Anaemia as discussed is a direct consequence of ruxolitinib therapy but dose modifications are not recommended. In practice we individualize therapy in the presence of anaemia. Main non-haematological side effects are headaches and dizziness. Deregulation of immune response was described and some case reports of infection reactivations such as tuberculosis and B hepatitis or opportunistic infections as *Cryptococcus* and *Pneumocystis jirovecii pneumonitis* were described. Patients should be advised about the potential risk of infection and screening for hepatitis B and tuberculosis could be proposed. Finally, a rapid reduction or discontinuation of ruxolitinib can produce a rebound of cytokines production and disease-related symptoms as fever, night sweat, and rapid increase spleen size. Some case of tragic evolution (acute respiratory distress syndrome, disseminated intravascular coagulation-like syndrome or lysis syndromes) were described and it is advisable to slowly taper ruxolitinib dose, closely monitor the patient for recurrent splenomegaly and consider the use of corticosteroids to ameliorate a withdrawal syndrome. An additional 12 weeks of follow up of COMFORT-I and longer-term analysis of COMFORT-II have

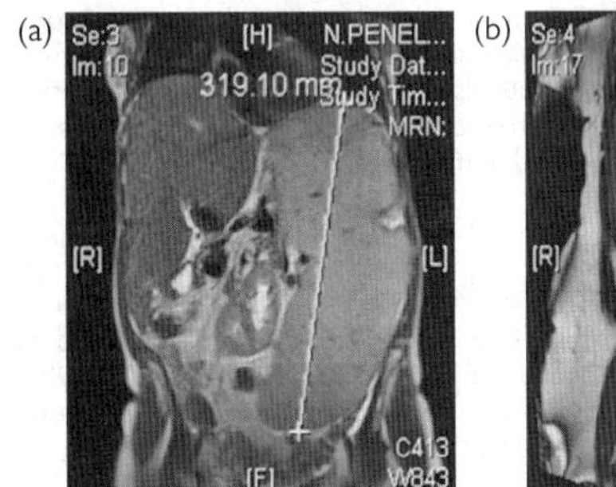

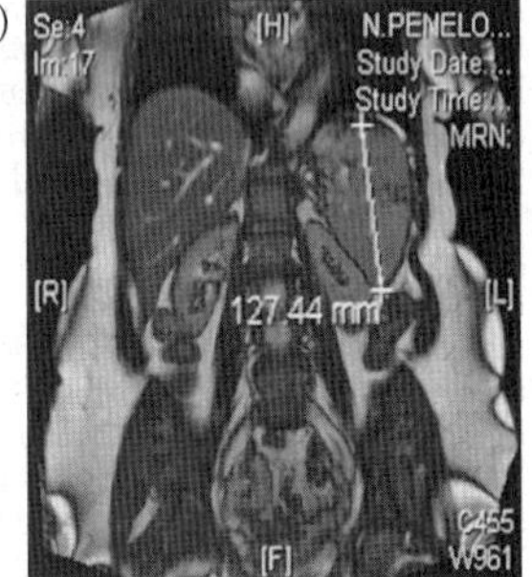

Figure 9.5 MRI from a patient before and 72 weeks after ruxolitinib therapy.

Reproduced courtesy of Claire Harrison, Professor and Clinical Director, Guy's and St Thomas' NHS Foundation Trust, London, UK.

been reported to show a longer overall survival for patients treated with ruxolitinib. These data should be interpreted with caution, the design of the trials particularly cross-over has led to much discussion. Nonetheless the trial data along with retrospective comparisons and reports of major biological improvements in isolated patients are all concordant with this theme.

The decision whether or not to continue ruxolitinib should be based upon a complex interplay balance between efficiency and toxicities. Ruxolitinib should be continued for a patient with good response in term of general symptoms and splenomegaly and in absence of any toxicity. In the opposite scenario, ruxolitinib should be discontinued for a patient without efficiency and presenting toxicities. Between both extremities, treatment continuation should be discussed from case to case bearing in mind the availability of therapeutic alternatives. One proposed algorithm is shown in Figure 9.6.

Other treatments

Cytoreductive drugs as hydroxycarbamide were the cornerstone of the treatment of MF for many years before ruxolitinib era. They have modest efficiency in reducing splenomegaly, disease-related symptoms, and other features such as leucocytosis and thrombocytosis associated with myelofibrosis. However, these benefits have not been analysed robustly and at least in the COMFORT-II cohort were lower in magnitude than with ruxolitinib. A main non-haematological drug-related side effect are ulcers (mouth or leg) which often necessitate discontinuing treatment and are associated with high dose and long-term use. Previous treatment-related ulcers often recur on rechallenge with hydroxycarbamide. In the case of cytopenia or intolerance to hydroxycarbamide, thalidomide or lenalidomide

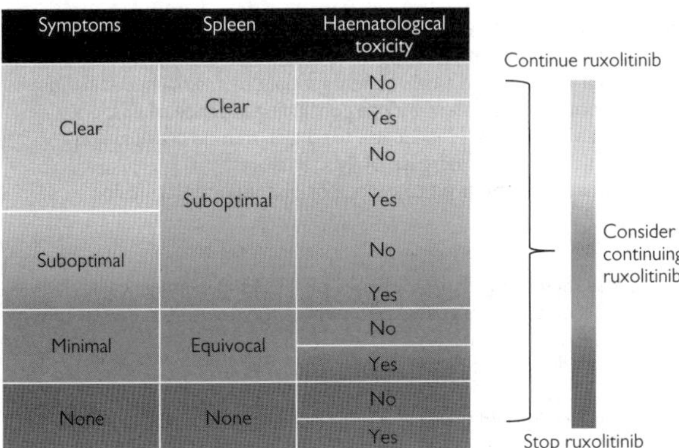

Figure 9.6 Considerations in the decision to continue or discontinue ruxolitinib therapy (also see plate section).

Reproduced with permission from Reilly JT, et al. (2014). Use of JAK inhibitors in the management of myelofibrosis: a revision of the British Committee for Standards in Haematology Guidelines for Investigation and Management of Myelofibrosis 2012. *Br J Haematol.* 167(3):418–20. DOI: 10.1111/bjh.12985.

could be an alternative. In the past, alkylating agents were used as oral melphalan or busulfan were used with some response in term of anaemia, leucocytosis, and splenomegaly. However, due to the haematological toxicity and the potential long-term risk of leukemogenicity, these treatments are not frequently used in routine clinical practice. As discussed earlier a surgical approach to splenomegaly should be reserved for drug-intolerant or ineligible patients, principally because of the high rate of morbidity and peri-operative mortality. Radiotherapy for splenomegaly-related symptoms should be reserved for such patients, and usually those not suitable for splenectomy. Our practical approach and recommendations for palliative management is summarized in the Box 9.2.

Intermediate-2 and high-risk patients

Much of our prior discussion concerning anaemia and splenomegaly is appropriate for these patients but we specifically want to emphasize that due

Box 9.2 Palliative management of MF-related symptoms

Practical management of symptomatic anaemia

First line

- Red cell packed transfusion.
- Frequency should be adapted according to symptoms and haemoglobin level.
- Iron chelation should be considered for patient with long-term red cell transfusion and potentially eligible for allograft.

And/or

- Danazol
  - **Dose**: Starting with 200 mg once a day, then slightly increase to 200 mg three-time a day. Patients should be maintained minimum 6 month on treatment before concluding absence of efficiency.
  - **Main side effects**: Headaches, tiredness, muscle cramps, skin reactions, or mild increase of liver enzymes.
  - **Remarks**: can be tried to reduce or discontinue transfusion.

And/or

- EPO
  - **Dose**: Starting with 10 000 units of rEPO three times weekly or darbepoetin 150 μg weekly. Doubling the dose after 1–2 months in absence of response.
  - **Main side effects**: Hypertension, headaches, increases risk of thrombosis.
  - **Remarks**: Should be reserved for patients with low EPO level (<125 mU/mL)

Second line

- Thalidomide + low-dose prednisolone.
  - **Dose**: Thalidomide 50 mg once a day + prednisone 0.5 mg/kg/d.
  - **Main side effects**: peripheral neuropathy, headaches, nausea, constipation, muscle cramps.

- Lenalidomide + low-dose prednisone (generally only for those with 5q cytogenetic abnormality).
  - **Dose**: lenalidomide 10 mg once a day.
  - **Main side effects**: neutropenia, thrombocytopenia, increase risk of thrombosis, muscle cramps, rash, diarrhoea, constipation, headaches.

Practical management of constitutional symptoms

First line

- Ruxolitinib
  - **Dose**: The recommended starting dose is 5 mg twice daily if platelets are less than 50 000/mm^3; 15 mg twice daily where platelet count is between 100 000/mm^3 and 200 000/mm^3, and 20 mg twice daily where platelet count is more than 200 000/mm.
  - **Main side effects**: Anaemia, thrombocytopenia, dizziness, headaches, increased risk of infection, AST, and alanine transaminase (ALT) elevation.
  - **Remarks**: Full blood count should be assessed frequently, and dose adapted according to haematological toxicities.

Second line

- Hydroxyurea/hydroxycarbamide
  - **Dose**: Starting dose could be 500 mg once a day. Increasing dose should be guided by response of constitutional symptoms and haematological toxicities.
  - **Main side effects**: Anaemia, thrombocytopenia, neutropenia. Stomatitis, nausea, diarrhoea. Mucocutaneous ulceration, squamous cell lesions. Possible increased risk of malignancy and leukaemic transformation.

Third line

- Busulfan
  - **Dose**: Variable strategies used, including stat pulses, courses, or 1–2 weeks, or daily dosing with careful monitoring.
  - **Main side effects**: haematopoietic toxicity, nausea, increased risk of leukaemic transformation.
- Melphalan
  - **Dose**: 2.5 mg three times a week, every 3 to 6 months.
  - **Main side effects**: haematopoietic toxicity, nausea, increased risk of leukaemic transformation.
- Splenectomy
  - **Remarks**: should be reserved for transfusion-dependent anaemia, rarely successful for thrombocytopenia may be indicated for symptoms of splenomegaly not controlled with other treatment.
  - High perisurgery morbidity and mortality.
- Splenic irradiation
  - **Remark**: may be used to reduce symptoms related to spleen enlargement.
  - Effects are often transient and may be associated with pancytopenia.

to the poor median of survival of these patients and the absence of curative treatment, they should be screened for suitability for allogeneic stem cell transplantation and referred for discussion if appropriate to transplant team. In patients non-eligible for allograft, a palliative approach using treatments previously discussed should be preferred. A possible treatment algorithm is presented in the Figure 9.3.

Personalized treatment approach to myelofibrosis

Our current treatment approaches to MF are principally based on disease risk groups as determined by IPSS, DIPSS, or DIPSS-plus scoring system. The relative few risk factors for each of them make them easy to use but has the potential to mask some subpopulations of patients with different outcomes. As shown with the proposed MIPSS scoring system, it is likely that some subgroups of patients with specific characteristics (e.g. different mutational status) have distinct outcomes which can currently undergo under- or overtreatment, or may fare better with specific targeted therapies. A further example of this is the use of lenalidomide for MF associated with the 5q-cytogenetic abnormality. In the future, investigation of more risk factors or biological features will lead to more personal treatment approach.

Investigational drug-therapies or strategies

Current investigational drugs target the specific dysregulations associated with myelofibrosis and particularly the JAK/STAT pathway.

Pacritinib is a novel oral JAK2/FLT3 inhibitor that has demonstrated antitumor activity in mouse models of human malignancies and showed evidence of efficacy in phase II trials, with limited haematologic toxicity. It was being investigated in phase III studies results, but all studies where put on a preliminary hold by the Food and Drug Administration (FDA) in January 2016 in view of potential excessive toxicity. Momelotinib is a JAK1/2 inhibitor. When evaluated in phase 1/2 trials, it was associated with improvement of anaemia, reduction of spleen size, and improvement of constitutional symptoms and is also currently being evaluated in phase 3 trials.

If development of novel therapeutic agents for MF is an option, drug combination is another strategy. In Table 9.4, we present the most recent data on new drugs and drug combinations for MF.

Currently, most of patients eligible for haematopoietic stem cell transplantation (HSCT) are also treated with ruxolitinib. Data available for HSCT and ruxolitinib use is currently weak and the need to continue or not ruxolitinib prior to HSCT is not clear. Continuation of ruxolitinib could be useful to maintain a better performance status which has shown a relationship with better survival. In the same way, reduction of spleen size could be associated with a faster haematological recovery. Finally, ruxolitinib seems to reduce graft versus host disease (GVHD) which is one of the main causes of morbidity following HSCT. However, ruxolitinib increase the risk of infections which could be theoretically deleterious for immunocompromised HSCT patients. Impairing natural killer (NK) cell function, ruxolitinib could also reduce the graft-versus-leukaemia (GVL) effect and increase the risk of relapse. Finally, some harmful side effects as cardiogenic shocks and tumour

Table 9.4 Novel agents and drugs associations

Drug	Results	References
Ruxolitinib + Panobinostat (JAK1/2 inhibitor + pan-deacetylase inhibitor)	Phase 2 study: 48% of patients achieved ≥35% of spleen volume at 24 weeks MSE: anaemia, thrombocytopenia, diarrhoea, asthenia	Kiladjian JJ, et al. (2014). Efficacy, safety, and confirmation of the recommended phase 2 dose of ruxolitinib plus panobinostat in patients with intermediate or high-risk myelofibrosis: Abstract#711. Available from http://www.primeoncology.org/app/uploads/prime_activities/8764/ASH2014_Kiladjian_Abs711_AS.pdf
Ruxolitinib + sonidegib (JAK1/2 inhibitor + Hedgehog signalling pathway inhibitor)	Phase 1 study: 65% of patients achieved ≥50% reduction of spleen volume MSE: Fatigue, anaemia, abdominal pain, dysgeusia, alopecia	Gupta V, et al. (2014). Phase 1b dose-escalation study of sonidegib (LDE225) in combination with ruxolitinib (INC424) in patients with myelofibrosis. *Blood*. 124(21):712. https://doi.org/10.1182/blood.V124.21.712.712.
INCB039110 (JAK1 inhibitor)	Phase 2 study: Improvement in MF-related symptoms at 24 weeks (~47% of patients) MSE: anaemia, thrombocytopenia, fatigue, nausea	Mascarenhas et al. (2014). Primary analysis results from an open-label phase II study of INCB039110, a selective JAK1 inhibitor, in patients with myelofibrosis. *Haematologica*. 102(2):327–335. DOI: 10.3324/haematol.2016.151126.
PRM-151 (recombinant form of pentraxin-2)	Phase 2 study: 35% achieved ORR (symptoms, spleen size, and/or decrease in BM fibrosis)	Verstovsek et al. (2014). Phase 2 trial of PRM-151, an antifibrotic agent, in patients with myelofibrosis: stage 1 results. *J Clin Oncol*. 32(15 suppl):7114–7114. DOI: 10.1200/jco.2014.32.15_suppl.7114
Imetelstat (telomerase inhibitor)	Pilot study: 44% achieved ORR, 22% experienced reversal of BM fibrosis. Some patients experience complete molecular response MSE: thrombocytopenia, anaemia, neutropenia	Tefferi A, et al. (2013). Imetelstat, a telomerase inhibitor, induces morphologic and molecular remissions in myelofibrosis and reversal of bone marrow fibrosis. *Blood*. 122(21):622. https://doi.org/10.1182/blood.V122.21.662.662.
Ruxolitinib + buparlisib (JAK1/2 inhibitor + pan PIK3 inhibitor)	Phase 1b study: For naïve JAK inhibitors and non-naïve patients, 70% and 54% respectively achieved ≥50% reduction of spleen volume	Durrant S, et al. (2015). HARMONY: An open-label, multicenter, 2-arm, dose-finding, phase 1b study of the combination of ruxolitinib and buparlisib (BKM120) in patients with myelofibrosis (MF). *Blood*. 124(21):710. https://doi.org/10.1182/blood.V124.21.710.710.

BM, bone marrow; MSE, main side effects; ORR, overall response rate.

lysis syndromes were described during conditioning in patients previously treated with ruxolitinib.

Monitoring and response criteria

A reproducible evaluation of treatment response is important, particularly for trials. Evaluation of myelofibrosis-related symptoms is of first importance. One of the tools to determine this is The Myeloproliferative Neoplasm Symptom Assessment Form Total Symptom Score: (MPN-SAF TSS), also known as MPN10, is a simple and reproducible tool including ten items focusing on disease-related symptoms developed and validates for that. It can be used in clinical practice to help physician for treatment adaptation and modification or for trial. An example of this scoring system is shown in Figure 9.4.

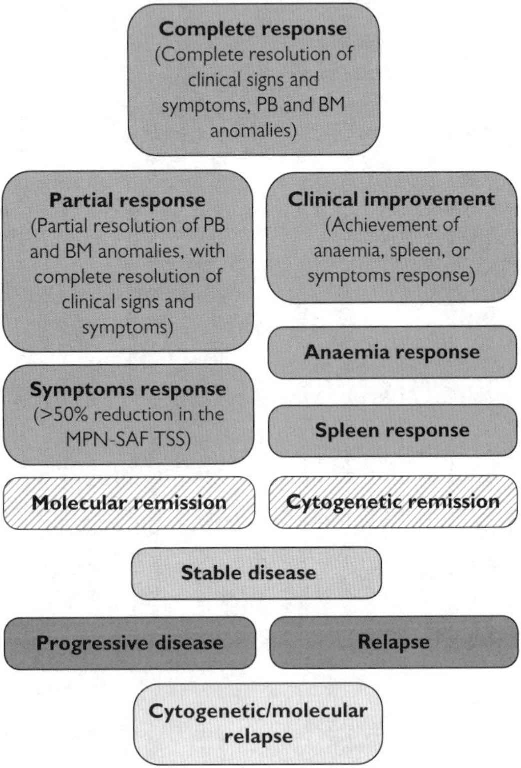

Complete response (Complete resolution of clinical signs and symptoms, PB and BM anomalies)

Partial response (Partial resolution of PB and BM anomalies, with complete resolution of clinical signs and symptoms)

Clinical improvement (Achievement of anaemia, spleen, or symptoms response)

Anaemia response

Symptoms response (>50% reduction in the MPN-SAF TSS)

Spleen response

Molecular remission

Cytogenetic remission

Stable disease

Progressive disease

Relapse

Cytogenetic/molecular relapse

Figure 9.7 Schematic representation of response criteria for MF.

In 2013, The European LeukemiaNet (ELN) and the International Working Group-Myeloproliferative neoplasms Research and Treatment (IWG-MRT) have published a consensus on response criteria for myelofibrosis. Response criteria include biological (bone marrow and peripheral blood) and clinical variables (spleen and liver size, extramedullary haemopoiesis). These response criteria for MF are shown in Figure 9.7; they are complex and not intended for routine clinical practice. However, there are no formal criteria for clinical purposes, so our management tends to be tailored to individual factors and preidentified targets.

The future of MF therapy

MF remains a complex disease the past decade has seen major advances in our understanding of the pathogenesis of this condition, which are beginning to be translated into clinical practice. The therapeutic landscape for MF has therefore changed dramatically and patients have benefitted considerably. Nonetheless there are significant ongoing challenges to address in the coming years areas of particular interest are factors implicated in the transition of ET and PV to MF, how to best risk stratify patients, when to apply higher risk therapies such as transplant and best combine this modality with agents such as ruxolitinib. In testing novel therapies and therapeutic combinations surrogate markers of response are clearly required.

Further reading

Barbui T, Carobbio A, Cervantes F, et al. Thrombosis in primary myelofibrosis: incidence and risk factors. *Blood*. 2010;115:7

Baxter EJ, Scott LM, Campbell PJ, et al. Acquired mutation of the tyrosine kinase JAK2 in human myeloproliferative disorders. *Lancet*. 2005;365:1054–61.

Brecqueville M, Rey J, Bertucci F, et al. Mutation analysis of ASXL1, CBL, DNMT3A, IDH1, IDH2, JAK2, MPL, NF1, SF3B1, SUZ12, and TET2 in myeloproliferative neoplasms. *Genes Chromosomes Cancer*. 2012;51:743–55.

Cervantes F, Dupriez B, Pereira A, et al. New prognostic scoring system for primary myelofibrosis based on a study of the International Working Group for Myelofibrosis Research and Treatment. *Blood*. 2009;113:2895–901.

Cervantes F, Tassies D, Salgado C, Rovira M, Pereira A, Rozman C. Acute transformation in nonleukemic chronic myeloproliferative disorders: actuarial probability and main characteristics in a series of 218 patients. *Acta Haematologica*. 1991;85:124–7.

Gangat N, Caramazza D, Vaidya R, et al. DIPSS plus: a refined Dynamic International Prognostic Scoring System for primary myelofibrosis that incorporates prognostic information from karyotype, platelet count, and transfusion status. *J Clin Oncol*. 2011;29:392–7.

Harrison C, Kiladjian JJ, Al-Ali HK, et al. JAK inhibition with ruxolitinib versus best available therapy for myelofibrosis. *N Engl J Med*. 2012;366:787–98.

Harrison CN, Campbell PJ, Buck G, et al. Hydroxyurea compared with anagrelide in high-risk essential thrombocythemia. *N Engl J Med*. 2005;353:33–45.

Harrison CN, Mesa RA, Kiladjian JJ, et al. Health-related quality of life and symptoms in patients with myelofibrosis treated with ruxolitinib versus best available therapy. *Br J Haematol*. 2013;162:229–39.

Hernandez-Boluda JC, Pereira A, Gomez M, et al. The International Prognostic Scoring System does not accurately discriminate different risk categories in patients with post-essential thrombocythemia and post-polycythemia vera myelofibrosis. *Haematologica*. 2014;99:e55–7.

James C, Ugo V, Le Couedic JP, et al. A unique clonal JAK2 mutation leading to constitutive signalling causes polycythaemia vera. *Nature*. 2005;434:1144–8.

Kiladjian J-J, Heidel FH, Vannucchi AM, et al. Efficacy, safety, and confirmation of the recommended phase 2 dose of ruxolitinib plus panobinostat in patients with intermediate or high-risk myelofibrosis; 2014. Available at: https://www.primeoncology.org/app/uploads/prime_activities/8764/ASH2014_Kiladjian_Abs711_AS.pdf

Klampfl T, Gisslinger H, Harutyunyan AS, et al. Somatic mutations of calreticulin in myeloproliferative neoplasms. *N Engl J Med*. 2013;369:2379–90.

Kralovics R, Passamonti F, Buser AS, et al. A gain-of-function mutation of JAK2 in myeloproliferative disorders. *N Engl J Med*. 2005;352:1779–90.

Levine RL, Wadleigh M, Cools J, et al. Activating mutation in the tyrosine kinase JAK2 in polycythemia vera, essential thrombocythemia, and myeloid metaplasia with myelofibrosis. *Cancer Cell*. 2005;7:387–97.

Nangalia J, Massie CE, Baxter EJ, et al. Somatic CALR mutations in myeloproliferative neoplasms with nonmutated JAK2. *N Engl J Med*. 2013;369:2391–405.

Passamonti F, Cervantes F, Vannucchi AM, et al. A dynamic prognostic model to predict survival in primary myelofibrosis: a study by the IWG-MRT (International Working Group for Myeloproliferative Neoplasms Research and Treatment). *Blood*. 2010;115:1703–8.

Passamonti F, Maffioli M, Cervantes F, et al. Impact of ruxolitinib on the natural history of primary myelofibrosis: a comparison of the DIPSS and the COMFORT-2 cohorts. *Blood*. 2014;123:1833–5.

Passamonti F, Rumi E, Arcaini L, et al. Prognostic factors for thrombosis, myelofibrosis, and leukemia in essential thrombocythemia: a study of 605 patients. *Haematologica*. 2008;93:1645–51.

Passamonti F, Rumi E, Pietra D, et al. A prospective study of 338 patients with polycythemia vera: the impact of JAK2 (V617F) allele burden and leukocytosis on fibrotic or leukemic disease transformation and vascular complications. *Leukemia*. 2010;24:1574–9.

Reilly JT, McMullin MF, Beer PA, et al. Guideline for the diagnosis and management of myelofibrosis. *Br J Haematol*. 2012;158:453–71.

Reilly JT, McMullin MF, Beer PA, et al. Use of JAK inhibitors in the management of myelofibrosis: a revision of the British Committee for Standards in Haematology Guidelines for Investigation and Management of Myelofibrosis 2012. *Br J Haematol*. 2014;167:418–20.

Rumi E, Pietra D, Ferretti V, et al. JAK2 or CALR mutation status defines subtypes of essential thrombocythemia with substantially different clinical course and outcomes. *Blood*. 2014;123:1544–51.

Tefferi A, Cervantes F, Mesa R, et al. Revised response criteria for myelofibrosis: International Working Group-Myeloproliferative Neoplasms Research and Treatment (IWG-MRT) and European LeukemiaNet (ELN) consensus report. *Blood*. 2013;122:1395–8.

Tefferi A, Guglielmelli P, Larson DR, et al. Long-term survival and blast transformation in molecularly annotated essential thrombocythemia, polycythemia vera, and myelofibrosis. *Blood*. 2014;124:2507–13.

Tefferi A, Lasho TL, Jimma T, et al. One thousand patients with primary myelofibrosis: the mayo clinic experience. *Mayo Clinic Proc*. 2012;87:25–33.

Tefferi A. Myelofibrosis with myeloid metaplasia. *N Engl J Med*. 2000;342:1255–65.

Verstovsek S, Mesa RA, Gotlib J, et al. A double-blind, placebo-controlled trial of ruxolitinib for myelofibrosis. *N Engl J Med*. 2012;366:799–807.

Zhang SJ, Rampal R, Manshouri T, et al. Genetic analysis of patients with leukemic transformation of myeloproliferative neoplasms shows recurrent SRSF2 mutations that are associated with adverse outcome. *Blood*. 2012;119:4480–5.

Chapter 10

Essential thrombocythaemia

Carlos Besses, Beatriz Bellosillo, Alberto Alvarez-Larrán, and Tariq I. Mughal

Introduction to essential thrombocythaemia *152*
Pathophysiology and molecular biology *152*
Clinical features *153*
Clinical and laboratory features at diagnosis *153*
Diagnosis *156*
Clinical management *159*
Summary *166*

Introduction to essential thrombocythaemia

The revised 2016 edition of the World Health Organization (WHO) myeloid and lymphoid diseases classification recognizes myeloproliferative neoplasms (MPN) to comprise of classic, as a reference to the original description of myeloproliferative disorders (MPDs) by Dameshek (Chapter 1), and non-classic (atypical) categories. In this chapter we discuss essential thrombocythaemia (ET) which is a subtype of the classic *BCR-ABL1*-negative MPN, and also include polycythaemia vera (PV), primary myelofibrosis (PMF), and patients who transform to myelofibrosis (MF) from PV (post-PV MF) or ET (post-ET MF). Collectively they are a group of clonal haematological malignancies that are characterized by excessive accumulation of one or more myeloid cell lineages and an inherent ability to transform to acute myeloid leukaemia (AML). ET is the most common of these disorders and associated with an excellent prognosis. Morphology and clinical laboratory analysis remain important, the unfolding genomic landscape enables better diagnostic work-up and help distinguish ET from secondary/reactive thrombocytosis in challenging cases

Though patients have an increased tendency to experience thrombotic and bleeding tendencies, most have survival approaching that of the general population. At present there are no therapies which impact the ET malignant clone and the principal objective of treating patients is to prevent thrombotic/bleeding events and reduce the risk of transformation to MF and AML. In this regard, the European LeukemiaNet (ELN) and other national/international expert groups have developed clinical management guidelines, though many controversies, in particular on the use of antiplatelet and cytotoxic therapies persist. The refinement in the design of accurate and individualized prognostic systems of thrombosis and the incorporation of drugs able to modify the increasingly complex genetic abnormalities and abnormal histology are the future steps in the therapeutic landscape.

Pathophysiology and molecular biology

Biology

- ET is a clonal stem cell haematopoietic disorder as was demonstrated in studies using the X-chromosome linked glucose-6-phosphate dehydrogenase locus. The presence of a single G6PD isoenzyme type in platelets, granulocytes, and red cells of ET patients established the common stem cell origin of the disease.
- An important landmark in the study of ET was the discovery of the *JAK2*V617F, a pivotal phenotypic driver of most *BCR-ABL1*-negative MPN, the thrombopoietin receptor (*MPL*) gene at exon 10, and the calreticulin (*CALR*) gene at exon 9, between 2005 and 2013. Current data suggest the presence of mutations in the *JAK2*, *CALR*, and *MPL* genes, in about 60%, 20%, and 5%, respectively, of all ET patients.

These mutations comprise the 2016 WHO diagnostic criteria, and tend to be mutually exclusive, though not always.

- About 15% of ET patients are considered negative for these driver mutations and labelled 'triple negative' ET. About one-third of triple-negative ET patients present with atypical or variant mutations in the *MPL* and *JAK2* genes.
- Somatic mutations in several other genes, such as the epigenetic genes (*ASXL1, TET2, EZH2, IDH1, IDH2, DNMT3A*), RNA splicing genes (*SRSF2, U2AF1, U2AF2, SF3B1*), or transcription regulatory genes (*TP53, IKZF1, NF-E2, CUX1*) can be found in about a third of patients, and may have a prognostic and therapeutic relevance.
- The order of mutation acquisition appears to influence the biology and clinical features in ET and other subtypes of MPN. As an illustration, if *JAK2*V617F is acquired before *TET2, DNMT3A*, or acquired uniparental disomy (aUPD) of chromosome 14q, the individual is more likely to develop PV than ET compared to patients in whom *JAK2*V617F is acquired late.
- The search for the *JAK2*V617F mutation must be the first-line genetic test in the investigation of a patient with thrombocytosis and clinical suspicion of MPN. In case of negativity, the second recommended step is to check for the existence of *CALR* mutations. If both are negative, the next procedure is to search for *MPL* mutations (W515K/L, S505N).
- Approximately, 80–85% of *CALR*-mutated ET patients present somatic 52-bp deletions (type 1 mutation) or recurrent 5-bp insertions (type 2 mutation), being the remaining mutation variants. ET patients with *CALR* mutations show male predominance, younger age, lower haemoglobin, and leucocyte counts, higher platelet counts, and lower risk of thrombotic complications than *JAK2*-mutated ET patients.

Clinical features

Epidemiology

- In a 2014 meta-analysis, ET was the most common subtype of classic MPN with an annual incidence ranging from 0.21 to 2.27 per 100 000 people and prevalence rate between 11 and 43 per 100 000 people.
- Median age at diagnosis is around 60 years, with 15–20% of all patients <40 years and a female:male ratio of about 1.6–2:1.

Clinical and laboratory features at diagnosis

- Most patients with ET tend to be asymptomatic and the diagnosis is often suspected following a blood test for unrelated reasons.
- The existence of relatives with thrombocytosis, erythrocytosis, or with known MPN neoplasms should be elicited from the medical history; historical studies suggest about a 7-fold increased risk among

first-degree relatives. Likewise, symptoms of microvascular disturbances should also be interrogated.

- Palpable splenomegaly is present in 10% of patients and is usually of moderate size.
- The hallmark feature of ET is the presence of sustained thrombocytosis, with a platelet count > 450 × 10^9/L; leukocytosis >10 × 10^9/L, but <20 × 10^9/L, is present in about 25% of patients. Haemoglobin and haematocrit are within normal ranges; in those patients who present high values, PV must be excluded.
- Spurious hyperkalaemia is a common finding in patients with high platelet counts. Increased levels of uric acid, serum vitamin B_{12}, and lactate dehydrogenase can also be observed in a variable percentage of patients. Serum ferritin is normal except in patients with previous bleeding. Acute phase proteins are not increased unless the patient presents concomitant inflammation disorders.
- Other laboratory and test abnormalities include a low serum erythropoietin at diagnosis in 21–33% of patients. The *ex vivo* platelet function tests are usually abnormal due to qualitative platelet dysfunction, but they do not correlate with clinical bleeding or thrombotic tendency; *in vitro* endogenous growth of erythroid progenitors is seen at diagnosis in 70% of patients, particularly in those *JAK2*-mutated. Of note, about 15–20% of triple-negative patients (*JAK2*/*CALR*/*MPL* wild-type) may show *in vitro* growth of megakaryocytic and/or erythroid progenitors.

Thrombotic complications

- Overall, major thrombosis occurs in 7–29% of ET patients at diagnosis and in 5–30% of patients during follow-up; factors such as age, history of previous thrombosis, and cardiovascular risk may affect the incidence of thrombosis; thrombocytosis *per se* at diagnosis is not predictive, nor does it correlate with thrombosis.
- Arterial thrombotic events are more frequent than venous events (70–80% of total thrombosis) and include stroke, transient ischaemic attack, retinal artery occlusion, myocardial infarction, unstable angina, acute peripheral ischaemia, and digital ischaemia. The most frequently involved arterial site is the central nervous system.
- Venous thrombotic events encompass deep vein thrombosis, pulmonary embolism, and thrombosis at unusual sites: splanchnic veins (Budd–Chiari syndrome and portal vein thrombosis) and cerebral sinus veins; overall rate of fatal and non-fatal thrombotic events of 1.9% per patient-years (arterial 1.2% and venous 0.6%, respectively) have been reported in a large cohort of patients meeting the revised 2016 WHO diagnostic criteria for ET.
- The revised International Prognostic Score of Thrombosis for ET (IPSET-thrombosis) comprises three risk factors for thrombosis: age >60 years, thrombosis history, and the presence of *JAK2*V617F. It identifies four risk categories based on these adverse variables: very low (no adverse factors), low (presence of *JAK2*V617F), intermediate (age >60 years) and high (presence of thrombosis history or presence of both advanced age and *JAK2*V617F).

- *CALR*-mutated ET patients have a lower risk of thrombotic events compared with *JAK2*-mutated patients.
- The acquired thrombophilic state in ET includes, among other mechanisms, neutrophil activation with release of proteolytic enzymes, and increased expression of CD11b, platelet activation with expression of P-selectin and tissue factor, and release of microparticles after cellular interaction of neutrophils with platelets and endothelial cells. All these facts may play a role in thrombus formation.

Haemorrhagic complications

- Bleeding events occur in about 10% of ET patients, either at diagnosis or during the clinical course of their disease. The gastrointestinal site is often the most commonly affected, followed by the skin and mucous membranes, the urinary tract, and soft tissues.
- The risk of bleeding has been associated with the use of aspirin and with extreme thrombocytosis ($> 1000 \times 10^9$/L), and the emergence of the acquired von Willebrand disease, which is fully reversible once the platelet count is normalized.

Vasomotor symptoms

- About a third of ET patients show at diagnosis vasomotor symptoms, including headache, acral paraesthesias, and visual disturbances such as amaurosis fugax, scintillating scotomata, and blurred vision, which are often transient lasting for a few seconds or longer. Neurological symptoms of dizziness, vertigo, and transient unsteadiness are not uncommon and are due to platelet-induced arterial cerebral microcirculation ischaemia.
- Erythromelalgia, a painful burning, redness, and warm congestion of the extremities, may be the presenting symptom of ET. It is a platelet-mediated inflammatory condition of the end-arterial microvasculature that may progress to acrocyanosis or necrosis in toes or fingers if not treated. Aspirin achieves complete and immediate relief of symptoms and restoration of microvascular circulation.

Disease transformation

Myelofibrosis

- Transformation of ET to post-ET MF can often be heralded by progressive splenomegaly, anaemia, and leukoerythroblastic accompanied by bone marrow fibrosis. The median time to this transformation is about 10 years from first diagnosis of ET.
- In a series of 891 WHO-defined ET patients, that is, excluding early/prefibrotic PMF cases, the rates of progression to overt myelofibrosis (cumulative incidence) at 10 and 15 years were 0.8% and 9.3%, respectively.
- Currently the only post-ET MF prognostic models is the Myelofibrosis Secondary to PV and ET-Prognostic Model (MYSEC-PM); all others are extrapolated from PMF and might not have the same degree of accuracy.
- *CALR* type 1 mutated patients show a higher risk to evolve to MF than *JAK2*V617F and *CALR* type 2 mutated patients.

Acute leukaemia

- AML is an exceedingly rare event in the 2016 WHO-defined ET, with an estimated incidence of about 0.7% at 10 years. In retrospective clinical series, leukaemic transformation has been reported in 2–5% of patients at 10–15 years.
- A large Swedish population study comprising of 11 039 MPN patients, observed an increased risk of secondary AML/MDS in ET patients receiving ^{32}P or alkylating agents, but not hydroxyurea (hydroxycarbamide). The risk appears to be increased with the use of more than one cytoreductive drug. Of note, 25% of all classic MPN who evolved to AML/MDS had never been exposed to alkylating agents, ^{32}P, or hydroxyurea; anagrelide and interferon-alpha do not appear to be leukaemogenic.
- The survival of ET transforming to AML is poor with AML-type treatments in generally associated with a survival of <6 months (see Chapter 14).

Polycythaemia vera

- Some ET patients (2–5%) can evolve into a full clinical phenotype of PV during their clinical course. Acquisition of *JAK2*V617F homozygosity might play a role in those ET patients heterozygous for the mutation.

Diagnosis

Diagnostic criteria

- The diagnosis of ET is based on a composite assessment of clinical and laboratory characteristics (Box 10.1). The revised 2016 WHO major diagnostic criteria include mutations of *CALR* and *MPL* genes besides *JAK2*V617F mutation. It is important to exclude other classic MPN or myeloid malignancies with accompanying thrombocytosis, and no evidence of reactive thrombocytosis (Figure 10.1).

Differential diagnosis

- With other MPN.
- PV should be excluded in *JAK2*V617F patients presenting with thrombocytosis and high values of haemoglobin and/or haematocrit. According to some expert haematopathologists, this distinction can be established by bone marrow morphology, although there is no universal consensus about this issue. The confirmation of an increased red cell mass by isotopic methods may help to diagnose PV in this clinical setting. Current 2016 WHO diagnostic criteria for PV have lowered the former WHO 2008 Hb values for PV diagnosis and have also incorporated haematocrit values (see Chapter 8).
- Patients with prefibrotic PMF may present with isolated thrombocytosis as the only haematologic abnormality, without showing the characteristic features of PMF such as leukoerythroblastic syndrome, splenomegaly, and anaemia. Furthermore, bone marrow of prefibrotic patients may display minimal or even absence of reticulin fibrosis, which additionally makes this distinction difficult. According to an international

Box 10.1 2016 WHO diagnostic criteria for ET

Major criteria

- Platelet count ≥450 × 10^9/L
- Bone marrow biopsy showing proliferation mainly of the megakaryocytic lineage with increased numbers of enlarged, mature megakaryocytes with hyperlobulated nuclei. No significant increase or left shift in neutrophil granulopoiesis or erythropoiesis and very rarely minor (grade 1) increase in reticuline fibres
- Not meeting WHO criteria for *BCR-ABL1* + CML, PV, PMF, MDS, or other myeloid neoplasms
- Presence of *JAK2, CALR*, or *MPL* mutation

Minor criterion

- Presence of a clonal marker or absence of evidence for reactive thrombocytosis

Diagnosis requires meeting all four major criteria or, the first three major criteria and the minor criterion.

Adapted from Arber DA, et al. (2016). The 2016 revision to the World Health Organization classification of myeloid neoplasms and acute leukemia. *Blood*. 127(20):2391–405. https://doi.org/10.1182/blood-2016-03-643544. Reprinted with permission from the American Society of Hematology.

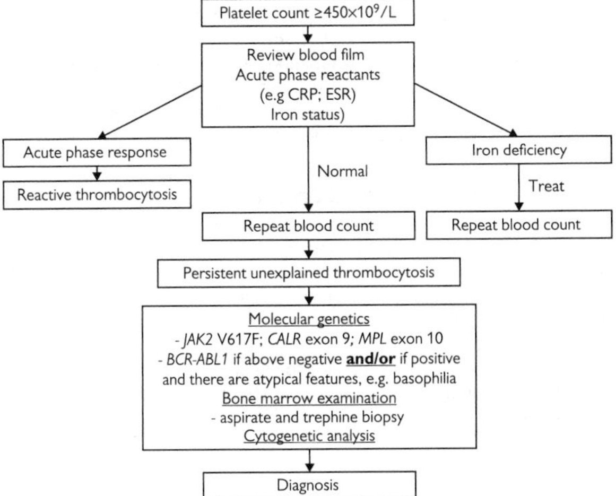

Figure 10.1 Diagnostic workflow for the investigation of thrombocytosis.

Reproduced with permission from Harrison CN, et al. (2014). Modification of British Committee for Standards in Haematology diagnostic criteria for essential thrombocythemia. *Br J Haematol*. 167(3):421–3. DOI: 10.1111/bjh.12986.

study of 891 ET and 180 prefibrotic PMF, the survival of the latter was considerably worse than that of ET patients, with higher rates of transformation to MF. However, the clinical significance of prefibrotic PMF diagnosis is still not conclusive because a large proportion of these patients do not develop myelofibrotic transformation and the impact on survival is small. Several bone marrow morphological features, including increased cellularity, granulocytic hyperplasia, and atypical megakaryocytes with hyperchromatic and irregularly folded nuclei forming dense clusters, among other characteristics, are postulated to be able for differentiating both entities. However, some investigators debate that the reproducibility of the distinct morphological features between prefibrotic PMF and ET is low due to interobserver variation and consequently, histology may not be a conclusive diagnostic criterion to distinguish them.

- Rarely ET should be excluded from the related MDS/MPN conditions, such as refractory anaemia with ring sideroblasts and marked thrombocytosis (RARS-T). The differentiation of ET from RARS-T is established by the presence in the latter of ring sideroblasts (≥15%) and presence of the *SF3B1* mutation (85% in RARS-T).
- The 5q-syndrome can often be associated with thrombocytosis and macrocytic anaemia. It can be distinguished by the presence of dysplasia and the specific chromosomal abnormality of 5q.
- Some patients with chronic myeloid leukaemia (CML) may present a thrombocythaemia onset with moderate leukocytosis, mimicking ET. The *BCR-ABL1* rearrangement (many cases with e14a2 transcript) allows establishing the proper diagnosis.
- In patients with reactive thrombocytosis, it is important to exclude iron deficiency, blood loss (acute or chronic), an absent spleen, surgery, bacterial infection, chronic inflammation, and several malignancies, represent the most frequent causes of secondary or reactive thrombocytosis. Generally, the clinical setting leads to the diagnosis, although in some cases the aetiology may remain unclear (Box 10.2).

Box 10.2 Practical tips on diagnosis

- Always check the existence of previous high platelet counts when assessing a patient with thrombocytosis.
- Discuss unexpected genetic results with the molecular biologist during the work-up of a patient with clinical suspicion of MPN.
- Do not overestimate nor underestimate the diagnostic value of bone marrow biopsy.
- Be sure of having performed a thorough differential diagnosis in patients with triple-negative molecular status (*JAK2*, *CALR*, and *MPL* wild-type).

Clinical management

Goals of therapy

- The principal goals of treatment in ET is the lowering of the risk of thrombosis and control of symptoms, and to reduce the risk of bleeding. It is important to avoid unnecessary treatment and treatment-related side effects, which might impact risk to transformation to MF or AML, and manage risk situations such as surgery and pregnancy.

Risk-adapted treatment approach

- The current risk stratification method is discussed earlier and depicted in Table 10.1. More recently a four categories risk stratification has been introduced into the clinics. It considers patients as very low risk if their age <60 years, with no thrombosis history with *JAK2*wild-type; low risk if age <60 years, no thrombosis history with *JAK2* mutation; intermediate risk if age >60 years, no thrombosis, *JAK2* wild-type; high-risk if *JAK2* mutation plus age >60 years or thrombosis history.
- Risk factors for ET to transform to AML include thrombosis and platelets >1000 × 10^9/L, and age and anaemia predict for transformation to MF; interestingly the presence of *JAK2*V617F is associated with a lower risk of transformation to MF.
- New prognostic systems, derived from retrospective data, such as the IPSET (International Prognostic Score in WHO-ET)-survival and the IPSET-thrombosis have been developed to refine the classical stratification system. They incorporate some clinical and biological variables such as the leucocyte count in the IPSET-survival model and cardiovascular risk factors and presence of *JAK2*V617F mutation in the IPSET-thrombosis system. *CALR* mutation status does not impact on the IPSET-thrombosis prognostic score.

High-risk patients

First-line cytoreduction options

- Hydroxyurea, an antimetabolite, has demonstrated to be effective in preventing thrombosis in a randomized prospective clinical trial which tested it against no cytoreductive therapy. Following a median follow-up of 27 months, the rate of thrombotic events was 3.6% *versus* 24% (p = 0.003). The cytoreductive options for patients with ET are depicted in Table 10.2.
- Another randomized prospective study (*UK-PT1*) tested low-dose aspirin (acetylsalicylic acid) in combination with either hydroxyurea or anagrelide, an imidazoquinazolin, in more than 800 high-risk patients diagnosed according to Polycythemia Vera Study Group (PVSG) criteria, and observed the combination of hydroxyurea and low-dose aspirin to be superior in terms of reducing the risk of arterial, but not venous thrombosis, major bleeding and fibrotic progression; anagrelide/low-dose aspirin combination was found to be superior in preventing venous thrombosis. Importantly there were no statistically significant differences in survival and death from thrombotic or bleeding, nor transformation to MF. The cohort with *JAK2*V617F-positive ET appeared to garner

Table 10.1 Risk stratification of ET. Classical thrombotic risk requires to fulfil at least one of the two variables: age >60 or history of thrombosis. History of haemorrhage and platelet count >1500 × 10^9/L are features of a high bleeding risk

	Classical		BCSH			IPSET-thrombosis	IPSET-survival
	HR	LR	HR	IR	LR		
Age >60 years[1]	+	–	+			1 point	2 points
Age 40–60 years				+			
Age <40 years					+		
History of thrombosis[1]	+	–	+	–	–	2 points	1 point
History of haemorrhage	+	–	+	–	–		
Cardiovascular risk factors[2]						1 point	
Diabetes or hypertension[3]			+	–	–		
Platelet count >1500 × 10^9/L[4]	+	–	+	–	–		
Leukocyte count >11 × 10^9/L							1 point
JAK2V617F mutation						2 points	
						Score (thrombosis risk, patients/year) LR: <2 (1.03%) IR: 2 (2.35%) HR: >2 (3.56%)	Score (median survival) LR: 0 (not reached) IR: 1–2 (24.5 years) HR: ≥3 (13.8 years)

BCSH, British Committee for Standards in Haematology; HR, high-risk; IR, intermediate-risk; LR, low-risk.

[1] high-risk of thrombosis; [2] smoking, hypertension, or diabetes; [3] requiring pharmacological therapy; [4] high-risk of bleeding.

Reproduced with permission from Besses C and Alvarez-Larrán A (2016). How to Treat Essential Thrombocythemia and Polycythemia Vera. *Clin Lymphoma Myeloma Leuk*. 16 Suppl: S114–23. DOI: 10.1016/j.clml.2016.02.029.

greater benefit and required lower hydroxyurea doses compared with those with *JAK2V617F*-negative patients; no such effect was noted in the anagrelide group. It was also of interest to observe higher rates of arterial events in the *JAK2V617F*-positive patients that received anagrelide showing higher rates of arterial thrombosis, compared with hydroxyurea. The rate of drug discontinuation was higher in the anagrelide arm.

- Anagrelide has also been tested as a monotherapy against hydroxyurea in 2008 WHO-defined high-risk ET patients (*ANAHYDRET* study), with

Table 10.2 Cytoreductive options in high-risk ET patients

	First line	Second line
<60 years	Hydroxycarbamide Interferon* Anagrelide*	Anagrelide Hydroxycarbamide Interferon*
≥60 years	Hydroxycarbamide	Anagrelide Interferon*
>75 years	Hydroxycarbamide Busulfan	Busulfan

* off-label indication.

no important differences in terms of incidences of major and minor arterial and venous thrombosis (3.3% *vs.* 3.4%), severe bleeding, nor rates of drug discontinuation. The study did observe a greater decrease in haemoglobin levels and cardiovascular side effects in the anagrelide cohort, whereas mucocutaneous abnormalities were higher in the patients receiving hydroxyurea.

- Hydroxyurea is administered orally at a dose of about 500 mg once or twice daily and titrated to achieve target platelet level (usually in 6–8 weeks) without reducing leukocyte values below 2.5×10^9/L. The drug is remarkably well tolerated with few side effects, which include mucocutaneous skin lesions, and rarely leg ulcers .

Second-line cytoreduction options

- Anagrelide reduces platelet production by inhibition of both megakaryocyte maturation and proplatelet formation. It inhibits AMP PDE-III causing positive inotropic and vasodilator effects, leading to common side effects such as headache, tachycardia, palpitations, diarrhoea, and fluid retention that are the cause of discontinuation in a significant proportion of patients. Congestive heart failure and arrhythmia are major contraindications to the use of anagrelide. A mild-to-moderate anaemia is observed in 24–35% of all treated patients. In contrast to chemotherapeutic drugs, anagrelide lacks leukaemogenic potential.

Interferon

- In patients with MPN interferon has been shown to suppress megakaryopoiesis, suppress bone marrow fibroblast progenitors, and reduce the *JAK2*V617F and the *CALR* allele burden. Three types of interferons have been tested in ET: interferon (IFN)-alpha-2b, pegylated IFN-alfa-2a, and pegylated IFN-alfa-2b. Overall, all types of IFN achieve about 60–80% of complete haematological responses (normalization of blood cell count), regression of splenomegaly, and in 5–15% of ET patients complete molecular response. In ET and PV patients resistant or intolerant to hydroxyurea, a phase 2 trial using pegylated interferon alfa-2a showed 69% overall response rates at 12 months in ET patients. CR rates were higher in *CALR*-mutated patients. Drug discontinuation due to chronic non-haematologic toxicity occurs in 20–50% of patients.

Busulfan

- In frail and elderly ET patients refractory or intolerant to hydroxycarbamide (HC), busulfan administered orally at 2 mg/d constitutes an adequate cytoreductive option, achieving complete haematologic response usually of long duration in 80% of patients. The risk of acute transformation may be increased in patients receiving busulfan after HC.

Antiplatelet therapy

- Low-dose aspirin is of benefit to prevent thrombotic events in most patients with ET. It suppresses thromboxane A2 biosynthesis as a consequence of the irreversible inactivation of platelet cyclo-oxygenase-1 and is remarkably effective in controlling microvascular symptoms. However, the effectiveness of low-dose aspirin in the primary prevention of thrombosis in ET has not been assessed in prospective randomized clinical trials (Figure 10.2).
- In high-risk patients, low-dose aspirin is offered as secondary prophylaxis to all patients who have had arterial thrombosis to prevent subsequent events. Oral anticoagulation is indicated in patients with venous thrombosis or embolic arterial thrombosis, and for those with unprovoked and/or recurrent venous thrombosis and those with history of two or more venous thrombotic events. When low-dose aspirin is combined with cytoreductive therapy, it is particularly beneficial for those aged over 60 years, those with cardiovascular risk factors, or those harbouring the *JAK2V617F* mutation. Despite aspirin being associated with bleeding, the risk:benefit ratio tends to support it reducing thrombotic events.

Treatment of ET

Secondary prophylaxis of thrombosis

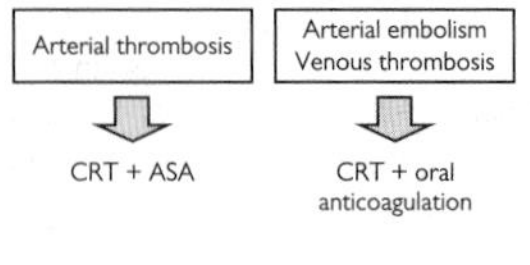

Primary prophylaxis of thrombosis

High-risk patients

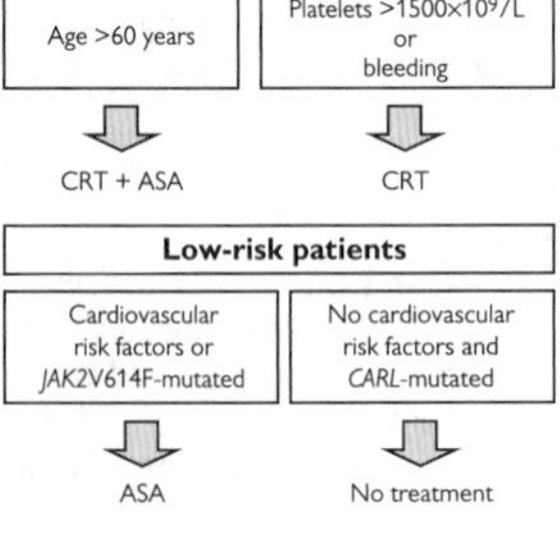

Contraindications to low-dose ASA

- Platelets >1500×10⁹/L
- History of bleeding
- Active bleeding
- Allergy to ASA
- Children <12 years (Reye syndrome)

HC: Hydroxycarbamide
ASA: Acetylsalicylic acid
CRT: cytoreductive therapy

Figure 10.2 Antiplatelet therapy in ET.

Low-risk patients

Watch and wait approach

- Most asymptomatic patients with ET do not require any specific therapy and the clinical management is largely based on risk stratification for vascular events, with prior vascular events and age >60 years, being the strongest indications for treatment; a small minority of patients might require reduction of platelet counts exceeding 1000–1500 × 10^9/L to reduce risk of bleeding.

Antiplatelet therapy

- In view of the excessive bleeding risk due to acquired von Willebrand's disease in low-risk patients, in particular those with extreme thrombocytosis (>1000 × 10^9/L), it is best to avoid aspirin. If possible, screening for ristocetin cofactor activity (which should be >20%) is desirable.
- Retrospective data, however, observes low-dose aspirin's usefulness in low-risk patients with cardiovascular risk factors and *JAK2*V617F-positive patients. Conversely, in patients with low-risk *CALR*-mutated ET, low-dose aspirin does not reduce the risk of thrombosis and may increase the risk of bleeding.
- Aspirin should always be used with caution in patients with history of bleeding and in those with prior history of peptic ulcer disease.

Intermediate-risk patients

- According to the British guidelines, an intermediate risk category is established for patients aged between 40 and 60 years lacking features of high-risk disease, as well as lacking diabetes and/or hypertension. Recent data suggest these patients should only be treated with aspirin alone until there is another clinical indication for cytoreduction.

Cardiovascular risk factors and symptom burden assessment

- In general, a healthy lifestyle, enabling suitable control of cardiovascular risk factors, such as hypertension, smoking, and diabetes should be encouraged. Recent studies have shown a significant symptom burden and diminished quality of life in MPN patients and impact on treatment decisions (see Chapter 18).

Evaluation of treatment efficacy and targets of treatment

- In contrast to most myeloid malignancies, ET appear to have a remarkable long natural history where many patients have an essentially normal survival. Such patients, when they require specific therapy, for example, to reduce thrombotic and/or bleeding events, it is important to use an algorithm that avoids unnecessary treatment, treatment-related side effects, and increase the risk of transformation to AML or MF. Currently there is no therapy which modifies the natural history of ET or reduce the transformation risk. Moreover, there is no firm evidence that reducing the platelet counts with cytoreductive therapy to a specific predetermined value, such as <600 × 10^9/L, or the reduction of leucocytosis to normal range, may be clinically useful. In this regard, the use of aspirin in particular with low-risk patients is often adequate.

- The ELN recently proposed standardized response criteria for the use of cytoreductive treatment in clinical trials for patients with ET. Complete remission is defined by achieving durable (≥12 weeks) normal platelet and leukocyte counts, symptom improvement according the MPN-SAF TSS (≥10 points decrease), impalpable spleen (if previously palpable), an absence of haemorrhagic or thrombotic events and signs of progressive disease, and bone marrow histological remission. Molecular response is not required in the definition of complete remission. This set of criteria is not usually employed in the routine assessment of response to cytoreductive therapy.

Resistance/intolerance to hydroxycarbamide

- At present there is a paucity of data to impact treatment decisions for patients with ET who are considered to be non-responsive or are intolerant to hydroxycarbamide. In this regard, the ELN has suggested definition of hydroxyurea resistance/intolerance, depicted in Box 10.3 and Box 10.4. Prospective trials addressing this clinically unmet need require studies which assess ET-specific endpoints, including thrombosis, bleeding, survival, and risk of transformation to AML and MF. Of note, the recent randomized phase 3 study which led to the licensing of ruxolitinib for hydroxyurea resistance/intolerance in PV patients failed to assess such important study endpoints; instead, the study focused on the control of haematocrit, splenomegaly, and symptom control as the principal study endpoints.
- The MAJIC-ET trial comparing ruxolitinib versus best available therapy in ET patients intolerant or resistant to hydroxyurea has shown no superiority of ruxolitinib over second-line treatments for ET.

Box 10.3 Criteria for resistance/intolerance to hydroxycarbamide (HC) in ET

1. Platelet count >600 × 10^9/L after 3 months of at least 2 g/day of HC (2.5 g/d in patients with a body weight >80 kg), **OR**
2. Platelet count >400 × 10^9/L and white blood cell (WBC) count <2.5 × 10^9/L at any dose of HC, **OR**
3. Platelet count >400 × 10^9/L and haemoglobin <100 g/L at any dose of HC, **OR**
4. Presence of leg ulcers or other unacceptable muccotaneous manifestations at any dose of HC, **OR**
5. HC-related fever

The definition of resistance/intolerance requires the fulfilment of at least one criterion.

Adapted with permission from Barosi G, et al. (2007). A unified definition of clinical resistance/intolerance to hydroxyurea in essential thrombocythemia: results of a consensus process by an international working group. *Leukemia.* 21(2):277–80. https://doi.org/10.1038/sj.leu.2404473.

Box 10.4 Practical tips on treatment

- Spend time to describe and discuss the pros and cons of all therapeutic options to all ET patients who need cytoreduction.
- My personal approach is to recommend a consultation with the dermatologist at the start of hydroxycarbamide and then every 6–12 months especially in patients with pre-existent skin lesions.
- In patients without history of cardiac disease who must start anagrelide, a normal electrocardiogram (ECG) is enough, and no extensive cardiac assessment is needed.
- Make slow and progressive dose escalation in patients who are going to be treated with any type of interferon.

Management of unusual and risk situations

Surgery

- About 7% of ET patients show haemorrhagic or thrombotic complications related to surgery. It is therefore important to discontinue antiplatelet therapy for about 1 week prior to elective surgery, and recommenced carefully postoperatively.
- For those ET patients who are on cytoreductive therapies, it is useful to aim for a platelet count of <600 × 109/L, and therefore monitor patients until they have recovered sufficiently from the surgery, when standardized thrombo-prophylaxis can be offered until full recovery and reassessment of ET risks in the clinics.
- Clearly all patients should be assessed carefully with regards to specific bleeding risks associated with any planned surgery, including assessment of acquired von Willebrand's disease and other coagulopathies.

Pregnancy

- Aspirin therapy is useful in preventing complications in pregnancy, in particular in *JAK2*V617F mutant ET. Several reports highlight the increased risk of about 30% or more in first trimester miscarriage, though these do not appear to be causally related to ET therapies.
- Thromboprophylaxis using low molecular weight heparin (LMWH) is useful if administered for at least 6 weeks post-partum, irrespective of the pregnancy risk group.
- In women with a previous history of thrombosis, LMWH is initiated in the first trimester at individual adjusted doses and is increased to twice daily from 16 weeks, besides ASA (aspirin). If cytoreduction is needed, recombinant interferon-alpha is the best option. Recent data show PEG-IFN as an effective and safe alternative to IFN for pregnant women requiring cytoreduction.
- Cytoreductive treatments, but not interferon or aspirin, are potentially teratogenic in the first trimester and must be avoided. Indeed, several reports have confirmed the efficacy and safety of the interferons, in particular the pegylated formulation, in pregnant women with MPN, including ET, who require MPN-directed therapies.
- Strict control of platelet count is mandatory in the post-partum period. Lactation is contraindicated with cytoreductive agents, but safe with LMWH.

Children

- The classical MPN, appear to be extremely rare in children, with ET and PV estimated to occur in 1–2 cases per 10 000 000 children annually. Recent efforts, however, suggest that with increasing awareness, the precise incidence is higher.
- There is considerable ambiguity with regards to the primary drivers of childhood MPN, including ET. Some studies suggest higher rates of triple-negative disease, which in turn impacts on the 2016 WHO diagnostic criteria for ET.
- In general, the risk of vascular events is very low. Therefore, a cautious approach should be the general rule when considering treating the patient. Extreme thrombocytosis is not a criterion to start treatment. There is no firm consensus on the optimal clinical management of children with ET. Hydroxyurea is used frequently, but its precise role, efficacy, and safety, remains unclear in children; and there is limited data on use of interferon in children.

Summary

- Patients diagnosed with the revised 2016 WHO diagnostic criteria for ET have a remarkably long natural history where many, if not most, patients, have a survival that is not dissimilar from that of the general population.
- Much has been learned about the genomic landscape of ET and its impact on the clinical characteristics, and how it informs on classification and personalized treatment.
- Most asymptomatic patients with ET do not require any specific therapy and in those that do, it is based on risk stratification, with prior vascular events and age of more than 60 years being the strongest indications for cytoreductive treatment.
- Since no current therapy for ET impacts on survival or transformation, the treatment emphasis remains on reducing the risk of thrombotic and bleeding events, or control of symptoms. It is also important to ensure the safety and efficacy of treatment, but safeguard against potential risk to transformation to AML or MF.

Further reading

Alvarez-Larrán A, Cervantes F, Pereira A, et al. Observation versus antiplatelet therapy as primary prophylaxis for thrombosis in low-risk essential thrombocythemia. *Blood*. 2010;116(8):1205–10.

Arber DA, Orazi A, Hasserjian R, et al. The 2016 revision to the World Health Organization classification of myeloid neoplasms and acute leukemia. *Blood*. 2016;127(20):2391–405.

Barbui T, Finazzi G, Falanga A. Myeloproliferative neoplasms and thrombosis. *Blood*. 2013;122(13):2176–84.

Barbui T, Tefferi A, Vannucchi AM, et al. Philadelphia chromosome-negative classical myeloproliferative neoplasms: revised management recommendations from European Leukemia Net. *Leukemia*. 2018;32(5):1057–69.

Barbui T, Thiele J, Gisslinger H, et al. The 2016 WHO classification and diagnostic criteria for myeloproliferative neoplasms: document summary and in-depth discussion. *Blood Cancer J*. 2018;8(2):15.

Barbui T, Thiele J, Passamonti F, et al. Survival and disease progression in essential thrombocythemia are significantly influenced by accurate morphologic diagnosis: an international study. *J Clin Oncol*. 2011;29(23):3179–84.

Beer PA, Erber WN, Campbell PJ, Green AR. How I treat essential thrombocythemia. *Blood*. 2011;117(5):1472–82.

Besses C, Alvarez-Larrán A. How to treat essential thrombocythemia and polycythemia vera. *Clin Lymphoma Myeloma Leuk*. 2016;16 Suppl:S114–23.

Cazzola M, Kralovics R. From Janus kinase 2 to calreticulin: the clinically relevant genomic landscape of myeloproliferative neoplasms. *Blood*. 2014;123(24):3714–19.

Harrison CN, Butt N, Campbell P, et al. Modification of British Committee for Standards in Haematology diagnostic criteria for essential thrombocythemia. *Br J Haematol*. 2014;167(3):412–13.

Hultcrantz M, Kristinsson SY, Andersson TM, et al. Patterns of survival among patients with myeloproliferative neoplasms diagnosed in Sweden from 1973 to 2008: a population-based study. *J Clin Oncol*. 2012;30(24):2995–3001.

Spivak JL. Myeloproliferative neoplasms. *N Engl J Med*. 2017;376:2168–81.

Tefferi A, Barbui T. Polycythemia vera and essential thrombocythemia: 2019 update on diagnosis, risk-stratification and management. *Am J Hematol*. 2019;94:133–43.

Tefferi A, Guglielmelli P, Larson DR, et al. Long-term survival and blast transformation in molecularly annotated essential thrombocythemia, polycythemia vera, and myelofibrosis. *Blood*. 2014;124(16):2507–13.

Chapter 11

Systemic mastocytosis

Jason Gotlib

Introduction *169*
Classification of systemic mastocytosis *169*
Diagnostic evaluation of mastocytosis *174*
Diagnostic decision-making *178*
Survival and prognostic factors *179*
Treatment *179*
Future directions *187*

Introduction

While normal mast cells (MCs) play important roles in allergy, infection, and inflammation, perturbation of their normal growth and function is reflected in the clinical sequelae of mastocytosis. The pathologic accumulation of MC in the skin only (cutaneous mastocytosis [CM]) and/or extracutaneous organs such as the bone marrow, lymph nodes, liver, spleen, and gastrointestinal tract (systemic mastocytosis [SM]), together with mast cell mediator release, can impose significant burdens on affected patients. Recent therapeutic developments have focused on small molecule inhibitors of KIT that demonstrate activity against the D816V oncogenic variant present in approximately 90% of patients. This chapter will highlight recent changes in the classification of SM, review the current landscape of conventional and novel therapies, and summarize future directions in the field.

Classification of systemic mastocytosis

In the 2017 World Health Organization (WHO) classification of haematolymphoid neoplasms, mastocytosis was removed as a disease subtype from the major category of 'myeloproliferative neoplasms (MPN)'. Instead, it now serves as its own major category with three broad subtypes: CM, SM, and the rare entity, mast cell sarcoma.

CM, which includes the variants maculopapular CM, diffuse CM, and more rarely, solitary mastocytoma, is more commonly encountered in children and is rarely accompanied by systemic involvement. Skin lesions typically regress by the time of puberty, but the reasons for this are not well understood. In adults, by contrast, skin lesions are almost always associated with systemic disease; in such cases, the nomenclature changes from CM to mastocytosis in the skin, or 'MIS' since a diagnosis of CM indicates a workup for SM has been undertaken and is negative.

The current WHO criteria for diagnosis of SM require one major plus one minor criterion or at least three minor criteria. The major criterion is the presence of multifocal dense aggregates of MCs (>15 MC in aggregates) in the bone marrow or other extracutaneous organ(s); minor criteria include: (1) >25% of the MCs in the infiltrate are of spindled or atypical morphology; (2) presence of an activating mutation at codon 816 in the *KIT* gene; (3) expression of CD25 with or without CD2 in addition to normal MC markers (e.g. CD117); and (4) serum tryptase level more than 20 ng/mL (unless there is an associated myeloid disorder which makes this parameter not valid) (Table 11.1).

SM is divided several subtypes that reflect the presence or absence of certain clinical or laboratory findings referred to as 'B-findings', indicating a higher burden of disease, and 'C-findings' indicating SM-related organ damage (Box 11.1), a feature of advanced SM which often mandates consideration of cytoreduction.

Indolent systemic mastocytosis (ISM)

The most common form of SM in adults is indolent SM (ISM), characterized by the presence of neoplastic MCs in the bone marrow and/or another

Table 11.1 World Health Organization diagnostic criteria for systemic mastocytosis*

Major criterion	Multifocal dense infiltrates of mast cells (>15 mast cells in aggregates) detected in sections extracutaneous organ(s)
Minor criteria	In biopsy sections of bone marrow or other extracutaneous organs, >25% of the mast cells in the infiltrate are spindle-shaped or have atypical morphology or, of all mast cells in bone marrow aspirate smears, >25% are immature or atypical
	Detection of an activating point mutation at codon 816 in *KIT* in bone marrow, blood, or another extracutaneous organ
	Mast cells in bone marrow, blood, or other extracutaneous organs express CD25 with or without CD2 in addition to normal mast cell markers
	Serum total tryptase persistently exceeds 20 ng/mL (unless there is an associated clonal myeloid disorder, in which case this parameter is not valid)

*Requires 1 major + 1 minor criteria or ≥3 minor criteria.

Reproduced from Arber DA, et al. (2016). The 2016 revision to the World Health Organization classification of myeloid neoplasms and acute leukemia. *Blood*. 127(20):2391–405. https://doi.org/10.1182/blood-2016-03-643544. Reprinted with permission from the American Society of Hematology.

Box 11.1 Major variants of systemic mastocytosis and 'B' and 'C' findings

Indolent systemic mastocytosis (ISM)

- Meets criteria for SM. No 'C' findings and no evidence of an AHN. The mast cell burden is low and skin lesions are frequently present.
- Bone marrow mastocytosis: ISM with bone marrow involvement, but no skin lesions.

Smouldering systemic mastocytosis (SSM)

- Two or more 'B' findings, but no 'C' findings. Usually with skin lesions.

*Systemic mastocytosis with associated haematologic neoplasm (SM-AHN)**, §

- Meets criteria for SM and criteria for an AHN (MDS, MPN, MDS/MPN, AML) or other WHO-defined myeloid haematologic neoplasm, with or without skin lesions.

Aggressive systemic mastocytosis (ASM)

- Meets criteria for SM. One or more 'C' findings. No evidence of mast cell leukaemia. Variable involvement by skin lesions.

*Mast cell leukaemia (MCL)*MAST CELL LEUKAEMIA (MCL)

- Meets criteria for SM. Bone marrow biopsy shows a diffuse infiltration, usually compact, by atypical, immature mast cells. Bone marrow aspirate smears show 20% or more mast cells. MCL: mast

Box 11.1 *Contd.*

cells comprise 10% or more of peripheral blood white cells.
Aleukemic MCL: <10% of peripheral blood white cells are mast cells. Usually without skin lesions.

B-findings

1. Bone marrow biopsy showing >30% infiltration by mast cells (focal, dense aggregates) AND serum total tryptase level >200 ng/mL.
2. Signs of dysplasia or myeloproliferation, in non-mast cell lineage(s), but insufficient criteria for definitive diagnosis of a haematopoietic neoplasm (AHN), with normal or only slightly abnormal blood counts.
3. Hepatomegaly without impairment of liver function, and/or palpable splenomegaly without hypersplenism, and/or lymphadenopathy on palpation or imaging (>2 cm).

*C-findings***

1. Bone marrow dysfunction manifested by one or more cytopenia (ANC< 1×10^9/L, or Hb <10 g/dL, or platelets <100×10^9/L).
2. Palpable hepatomegaly with impairment of liver function, ascites, and/or portal hypertension.
3. Skeletal involvement with large osteolytic lesions and/or pathological fractures.
4. Palpable splenomegaly with hypersplenism.
5. Malabsorption with weight loss due to gastrointestinal (GI) mast cell infiltrates.

* A lymphoproliferative disorder or plasma cell dyscrasia may rarely be diagnosed with SM.

§ The term SM with an associated haematologic neoplasm (SM-AHN) may be used in place of, or interchangeably with SM-AHNMD (SM with an associated haematologic non-mast cell lineage disease).

**Must be attributable to the MC infiltrate.

Reproduced from Gotlib J, et al. (2013). International Working Group-Myeloproliferative Neoplasms Research and Treatment (IWG-MRT) and European Competence Network on Mastocytosis (ECNM) consensus response criteria in advanced systemic mastocytosis. *Blood*. 121(13):2393–401. Reprinted with permission from the American Society of Hematology.

extracutaneous organ and less than two B-findings. ISM patients lack MC-related organ damage or an associated haematologic neoplasm, and the life expectancy of these patients is similar to an age-matched population. Bone marrow mastocytosis is a subtype of ISM with only bone marrow (BM) involvement without any skin lesions or other evidence of extracutaneous organ involvement. MIS is frequently present in patients with ISM.

Smouldering systemic mastocytosis (SSM)

SSM is defined by two or more 'B' findings, including higher mast cell disease burden compared to ISM, and no presence of an associated haematologic neoplasm (AHN). SSM patients often exhibit clonal multilineage involvement of the *KIT* D816V mutation. In the 2017 WHO classification, SSM was removed as a subtype of ISM and designated as its own variant, owing to the higher risk of progression to more advanced disease compared to ISM patients.

SM with an associated haematologic neoplasm (SM-AHN)

The 2017 WHO classification permits use of the new diagnosis label 'SM with associated haematologic neoplasm (SM-AHN)' to be used interchangeably with the term 'SM with an associated haematologic non-mast cell lineage disease (SM-AHNMD)'; however, the new term 'SM-AHN' is expected to supplant SM-AHNMD' given its relative simplicity. The overwhelming majority of AHNs are of myeloid origin and include myelodysplastic syndromes (MDS), myeloproliferative neoplasms (MPN), chronic eosinophilia leukaemia (CEL), acute myeloid leukaemia (AML), and most commonly, MDS/MPN overlap disorders such as chronic myelomonocytic leukaemia (CMML), or MDS/MPN-unclassifiable (MDS/MPN-U). Most studies indicate that the prognosis of SM-AHN usually relates to the AHN component; while often the case, the prognosis of the various AHNs can vary widely. For example, SM-MPN is associated with a significantly longer median survival (31 months) compared to SM-CMML (15 months), SM-MDS (13 months), and SM-AML (11 months). The rate of leukaemic transformation is more frequent in SM-MDS (29%) than in SM-MPN (11%) or SM-CMML (6%). In cases with a high burden SM and lower burden/stage AHN, prognosis may be driven by the mast cell component. Lymphoid neoplasms such as chronic lymphocytic leukaemia, lymphomas, or multiple myeloma are rarely diagnosed as the concomitant AHN. It can be challenging to ascertain whether organ damage (C-findings) are due to the SM or AHN component; in addition to a BM biopsy, directed biopsy of other organs may be required to ascertain the aetiology of non-haematologic organ damage (e.g. liver biopsy to clarify the basis for liver function abnormalities, portal hypertension, and/or ascites). A commonly used treatment approach has been to treat the SM component as if the myeloid neoplasm were not present, and to treat the myeloid neoplasm as if SM were not present. Because the KIT D816V mutation may be present in the cells of the SM and AHN, KIT inhibitors may provide clinical benefit for both diseases.

Aggressive systemic mastocytosis (ASM)

ASM is characterized by one or more C-findings as noted in Box 11.1. The term ASM-t (ASM in transformation) has been used for patients with an increased percentage of neoplastic MCs on a BM aspirate (e.g. 5–19%), and reflects a potential for higher risk of transformation to mast cell leukaemia (MCL) compared to ASM patients with <5% mast cells on a BM aspirate.

Mast cell leukaemia (MCL)

MCL is very rare form of SM and is defined histopathologically by ≥20% neoplastic MC on BM aspirate smears. On the core biopsy, MC typically form a diffuse, compact infiltrate with low levels of fibrosis. In MCL, the aleukemic variant (< 10% MC in the peripheral blood [usually no visible circulating MC] is more common than MCL with ≥10% mast cells in the peripheral blood. MCL can arise *de novo* or as a secondary MCL from less advanced forms of disease and may also coexist with an AHN. MCL has a poor prognosis that is often cited as 6 months or less; however, as in other SM subtypes, clinical and biologic heterogeneity contribute to variable outcomes with some patients exhibiting a survival in the range of 1–2 years. Although less common, 'chronic MCL' is a term used to describe MCL patients without C-findings and a more favourable prognosis compared to patients with C-findings, referred to as 'acute MCL'. Still, patients with chronic MCL are expected

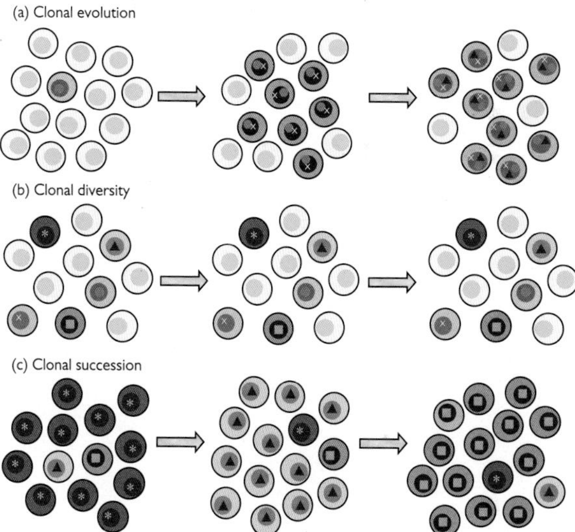

Figure 2.1 Concepts of clonality. (a) Clonal evolution. A single cell acquires a somatic mutation (mutation 1) and subsequently develops additional mutations during clonal expansion (mutations 2 and 3) resulting in a single clone with all three mutations. (b) Clonal diversity. Multiple diverse clones, each with a unique mutation (mutations 1, 2, 3, 4, or 5) coexist without significant change over time. (c) Clonal succession. Multiple diverse clones exist together with dominance of a single clone at different time points (mutation 3 or 4), e.g. related to selection on therapy.

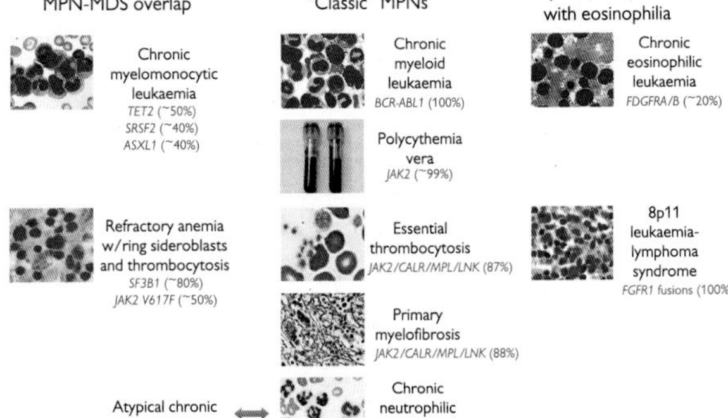

Figure 3.1 Molecular pathogenesis of MPN. The 'classic' MPN together with the MPN-MDS overlap syndromes and myeloid neoplasms with eosinophilia are depicted, with representative histopathology of blood, marrow, or lymph node. Specific mutations and their approximate frequencies in each disease are given in red. Note that atypical chronic myeloid leukaemia and chronic neutrophilic leukaemia are similar and overlapping diseases.

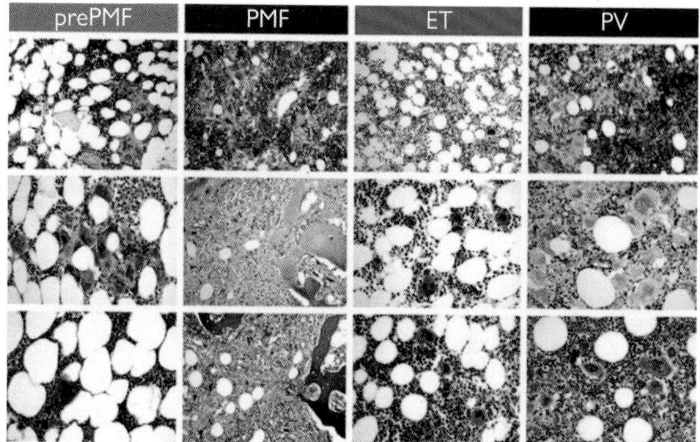

Figure 4.1 Bone marrow morphology in WHO-defined prefibrotic/early primary myelofibrosis (prePMF), advanced primary myelofibrosis (PMF), essential thrombocythaemia (ET), and polycythaemia vera (PV). **Prefibrotic/early primary myelofibrosis (prePMF):** remarkable hypercellularity for advanced age revealing large clusters of megakaryocytes abnormally dislocated towards the trabecular bone. In addition to megakaryocyte proliferation, there is a conspicuous increase in neutrophil granulopoiesis accompanied by reduction of nucleated erythroid precursors. Clustered small to giant megakaryocytes show a prevalence of striking maturation defects including cloud-like, hypolobulated, and hyperchromatic nuclei with only some irregular foldings. No significant increase in reticulin fibres. **Advanced primary myelofibrosis (PMF):** streaming-like pattern of haematopoiesis including atypical megakaryocytes in addition to initial osteosclerosis. Densely clustered megakaryocytes surrounded by neutrophil granulopoiesis but only a very few erythrocyte precursors. Clustered megakaryocytes are lying along a dilated sinus and reveal severe aberrations of maturation including cloud-like, dense, or abnormally lobulated nuclei. Overt myelofibrosis showing bundles of collagen between a dense network of reticulin and osteosclerosis. **Essential thrombocythaemia (ET):** age-matched cellularity, except for a prominent increase in large to giant megakaryocytes loosely clustered or dispersed throughout the bone marrow space. No proliferation or significant left shift of neutrophil granulopoiesis or erythropoiesis surrounding giant mature megakaryocytes. Conspicuous increase in large megakaryocytes without maturation defects showing hyperlobulated, occasionally staghorn-like nuclei. No increase in reticulin fibres, but giant megakaryocytes with deep foldings of their nuclei. **Polycythaemia vera (PV):** conspicuous hypercellularity for age with increase of all three cell lineages (panmyelosis) including extended islets of nucleated erythroid precursors and dispersed mature megakaryocytes. Prominent enlargement of erythropoiesis surrounded by left-shifted neutrophil granulopoiesis. Megakaryocytes of different size ranging from small to giant ones are increased and may be clustered, but fail to show maturation defects. No increase in reticulin fibres.

Reproduced courtesy of Prof. Dr. Hans Michael Kvasnicka, University Cancer Centre, Frankfurt, Germany.

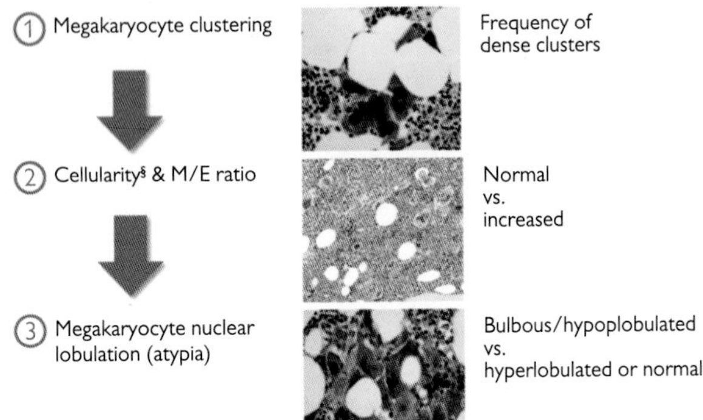

Figure 4.2 Relative importance of distinctive morphological features for the diagnosis of prefibrotic/early primary myelofibrosis (pre-MF).

Reproduced courtesy of Prof. Hans Michael Kvasnicka, University Cancer Centre, Frankfurt, Germany.

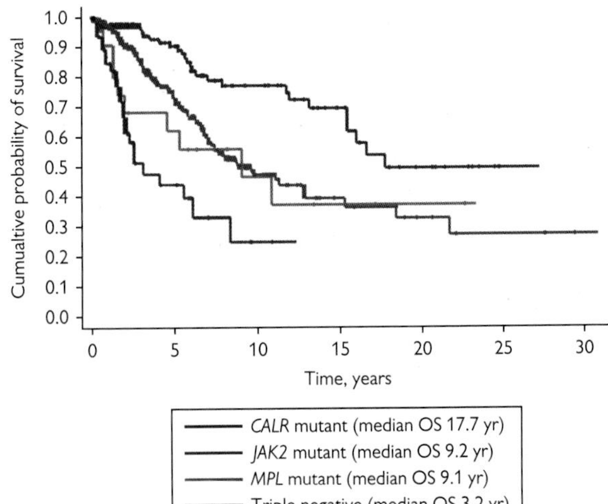

Figure 6.2 Kaplan–Meier analysis of the impact of phenotypic driver mutations (*JAK2*V617F, *MPL*W5151, and *CALR* mutations), and the condition of 'triple negativity', on overall survival in patients with PMF.

Adapted from Rumi E, et al. Clinical effect of driver mutations of JAK2, CALR or MPL in primary myelofibrosis. *Blood*. 124(7):1062–9. DOI: 10.1182/blood-2014-05-578435. Reprinted with permission from the American Society of Hematology.

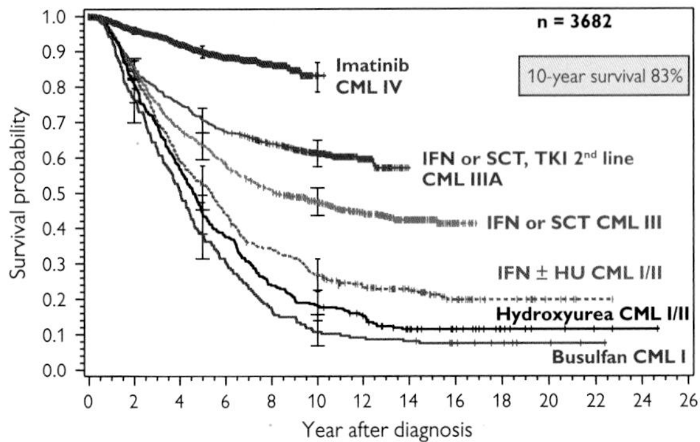

Figure 7.1 Survival with CML over time (1993–2013): the German CML-Study Group experience.

Reproduced with courtesy of Rüdiger Hehlmann, German CML Study Group, Germany.

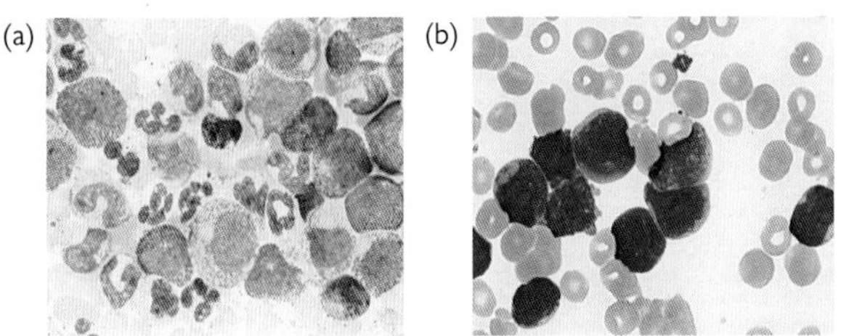

Figure 7.2 Peripheral blood appearances of a patient with CML at diagnosis. Note the increased number of leucocytes including immature granulocytes and occasional blast cells.

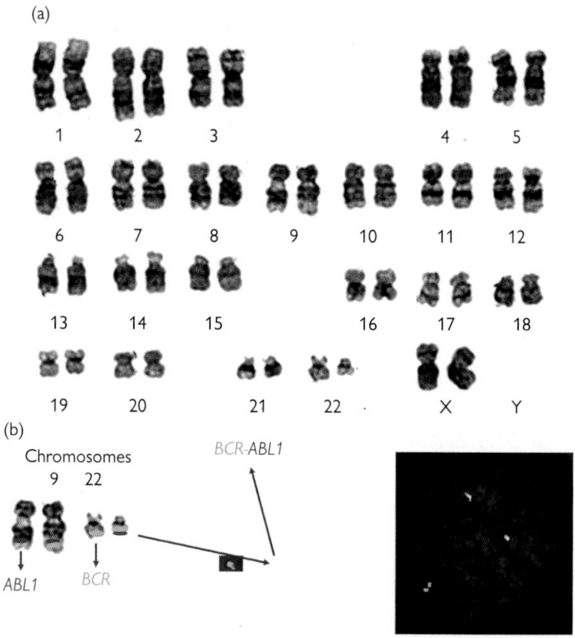

Figure 7.3 (a) Ph chromosome by conventional cytogenetics; (b) BCR-ABL1 by fluorescence in situ hybridization (FISH).

Reproduced with permission from Mughal TI, et al. (2016) Chronic Myeloid Leukemia: Reminiscences and Dreams. *Haematologica*. 101(5):541–58. DOI:10.3324/haematol.2015.139337.

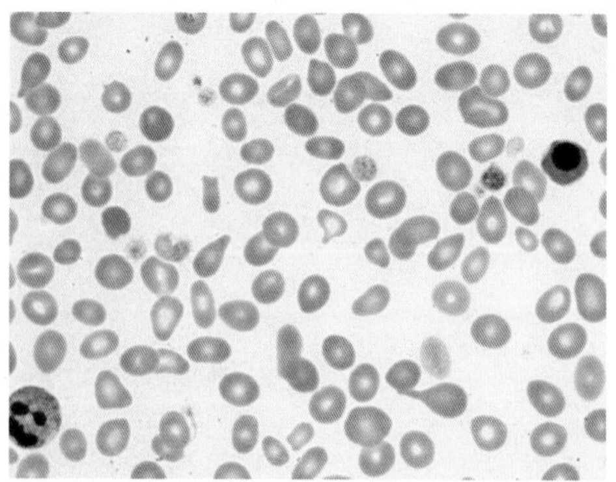

Figure 9.2 Blood film with typical teardrop cell and nucleated red cell.

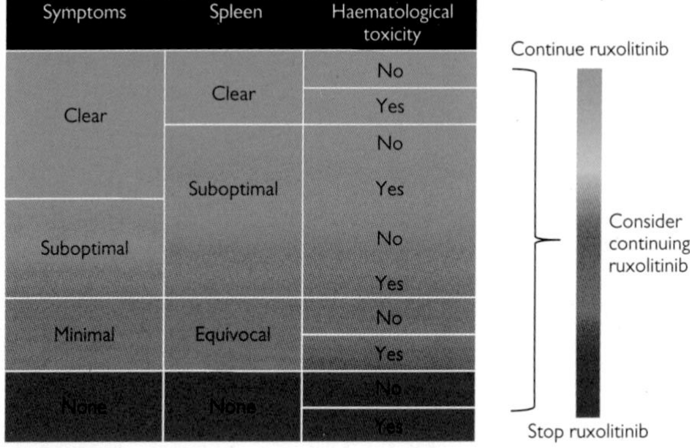

Figure 9.6 Considerations in the decision to continue or discontinue ruxolitinib therapy.

Reproduced with permission from Reilly JT, et al. (2014). Use of JAK inhibitors in the management of myelofibrosis: a revision of the British Committee for Standards in Haematology Guidelines for Investigation and Management of Myelofibrosis 2012. *Br J Haematol.* 167(3):418–20. DOI: 10.1111/bjh.12985.

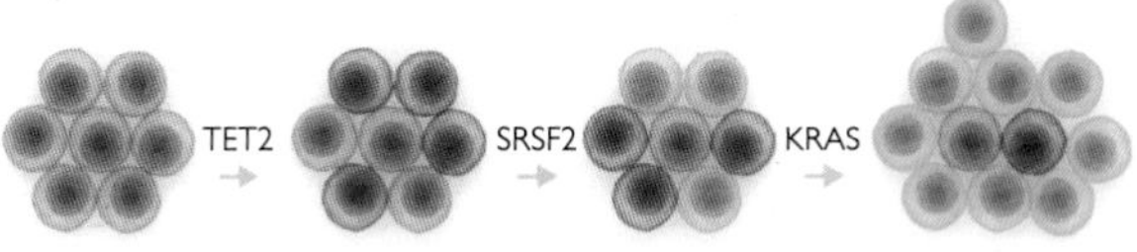

- Early clonal dominance in HSC compartment
- Linear acquisition of mutations, starting with epigenetic and splicing genes
- Growth advantage to the more mutated cells with differetiation

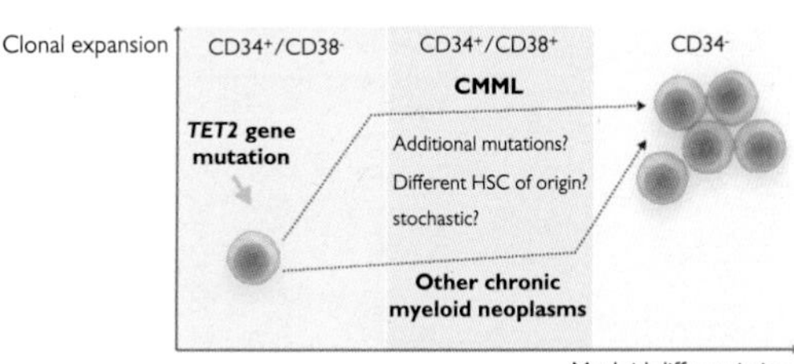

Figure 12.4 Early clonal dominance (CD34+/CD38−cells) in chronic myelomonocytic leukaemia (CMML) compared to myeloproliferative neoplasms (MPN).

Reproduced with permission from Mughal TI, et al. (2015). An International MDS/MPN Working Group's perspective and recommendations on molecular pathogenesis, diagnosis, and clinical characterisation of myelodysplastic/myeloproliferative neoplasms. *Haematologica.* 100(9):1117–1130. DOI: 10.3324/haematol.2014.114660. Copyright © 2015 Ferrata Storti Foundation. Source: data from Itzykson R, et al. (2013). Clonal architecture of chronic myelomonocytic leukemias. *Blood.* 121(12):2186-98. DOI: 10.1182/blood-2012-06-440347.

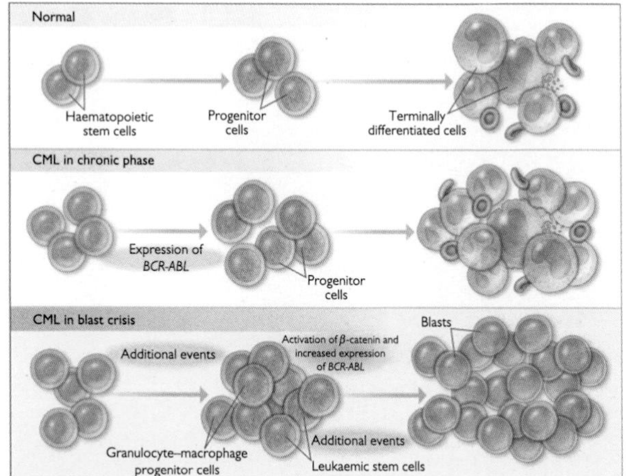

Figure 14.1 Schematic representation of the role of activated β-Catenin in the progression of CML.

Reproduced from Jamieson CH, et al. (2004). Granulocyte-macrophage progenitors as candidate leukemic stem cells in blast-crisis CML. *N Engl J Med.* 351(7):657–67. DOI: 10.1056/NEJMoa040258. Copyright © Massachusetts Medical Society. All rights reserved. Reprinted with permission from Massachusetts Medical Society.

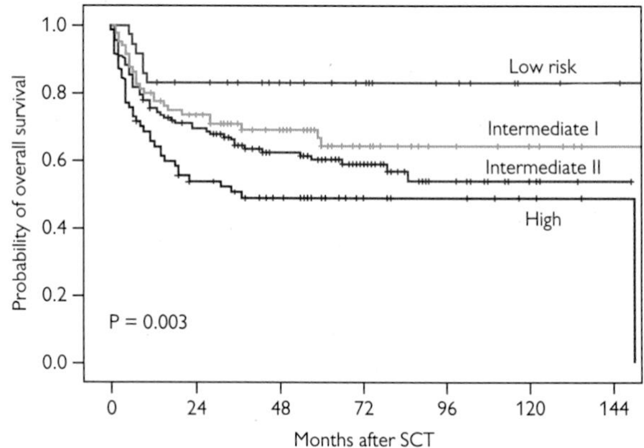

Figure 16.4 Outcome after allogeneic stem cell transplantation according to DIPSS.

Adapted with permission from Kröger N, et al. (2014). Dynamic of bone marrow fibrosis regression predicts survival after allogeneic stem cell transplantation for myelofibrosis. *Biol Blood Marrow Transplant.* 20(6):812–15. DOI: 10.1016/j.bbmt.2014.02.019.

to show progression within a short period of time. More data are needed to confirm whether the absence of presence of organ damage is an independent discriminator of prognosis between these two subtypes of MCL.

MC sarcoma is a rare MC tumour that can invade local tissues and has a high potential to develop advanced systemic disease with a fulminant course. Owing to its rarity, extracutaneous mastocytoma, which follows a benign course, was removed as a subtype of mastocytosis in the 2017 WHO classification.

Well-differentiated SM (WDSM)

WDSM is morphologic variant of SM characterized by round rather than atypical or spindle-shaped MC. MCs express either low or absent CD25. Cases usually demonstrate wild-type KIT, or exhibit mutations in the juxtamembrane or transmembrane region of KIT (e.g. KIT F522C mutation), which typically exhibit responsiveness to imatinib. WDSM is not a WHO subtype of SM, but instead can be found across a spectrum of WHO-defined SM subtypes, including ISM, SSM, and more advanced SM subtypes such as ASM or MCL.

Mast cell activation syndrome (MCAS)

MCAS refers to a group of disorders associated with mast cell mediator release. Defining MCAS criteria include: 1) episodic symptoms consistent with mast cell mediator release affecting ≥2 organ systems; 2) a decrease in the frequency or severity, or resolution of symptoms with antimediator therapy; and 3) elevation of a validated urinary or serum marker of mast cell activation, with the serum tryptase level being the marker of choice. MCAS is not considered a subtype of SM, nor is MCAS considered an entity with a well-defined rate of progression to frank SM.

MCAS can be divided into primary, secondary, and idiopathic. In patients without cutaneous involvement and diagnostic criteria for SM are not fulfilled (e.g. serum tryptase level less than 20 ng/mL and low mast cell burden) but clonality of mast cells is demonstrated by finding the KIT D816V mutation and/or mast cell expression of CD25, then patients are diagnosed with primary MCAS, also referred to as monoclonal mast cell activation syndrome (MMAS). In patients with mast cell activation symptoms, but with normal mast cell morphology/immunophenotype and no KIT D816V mutation, other causes of mast cell activation should be considered (e.g. secondary causes such as allergies, urticarias, and chronic inflammatory or neoplastic disorders). In patients with mast cell activation symptoms for whom no cause is identified, a provisional diagnosis of idiopathic MCAS is rendered until a specific cause of mast cell activation is identified.

Some patients with MCAS and/or other systemic symptoms have been diagnosed with hereditary alpha-tryptasemia, a recently characterized multisystem disorder associated with duplications and triplications in the *TPSAB1* gene encoding alpha-tryptase. This condition is associated with elevation of the basal serum tryptase level (which is found in 4–6% of the general population) as well as symptoms including cutaneous flushing and pruritus, dysautonomia, functional gastrointestinal symptoms, chronic pain, and connective tissue abnormalities, including joint hypermobility.

Diagnostic evaluation of mastocytosis

Close collaboration between the clinician and pathologist who have familiarity with mastocytosis, and referral to centres of expertise are critical for making the diagnosis of SM. In addition to obtain a complete blood count with differential, as well as chemistries and liver function tests, tests should be undertaken with the purpose of trying to establish WHO diagnostic criteria for SM. This testing includes a BM biopsy with special mast cell stains, serum tryptase level, and *KIT* D816V mutation analysis by a high sensitivity assay. In addition to the normal immunohistochemical (IHC) mast cell markers such as tryptase and CD117, CD25 is used to identify neoplastic MC as this surface marker is not expressed on normal MC. Multiparameter flow cytometry of the BM aspirate using CD117 and CD25, and CD2 may be useful in selected cases. Morphologic evaluation of the blood and BM aspirate are essential for assessing the presence of an AHN (e.g. dysplasia, monocytosis, eosinophilia, and/or increased blasts). CD34 quantification by IHC or flow cytometry may also be helpful in cases wherein myeloblasts express this marker. CD30 (Ki-1) is a cytoplasmic and membrane-bound antigen expressed on MCs in a proportion of SM cases. Although it was originally reported as an IHC marker specific to more advanced forms of SM, several studies indicate CD30 is expressed in both indolent and advanced forms of SM and may be sent as a complementary IHC and flow cytometric marker in the diagnostic workup of SM.

Serum tryptase level

†Tryptase is a serine protease primarily produced by MC, and to a lesser extent by mature basophils and myeloid progenitors. Commercially available ELISA-based assays measure total serum tryptase which consists of both mature tryptase (β-tryptase) and pro-tryptases (e.g. α-tryptase). The total serum tryptase level reflects MC burden and activation. Depending on the assay, the upper limit of the normal reference range for the serum tryptase level is <10 or <11.4 ng/mL. However, healthy individuals can rarely exhibit levels in the range of 15 ng/mL or higher, which may be confounded by the association between advancing age and increasing serum tryptase levels. Although a serum tryptase level > 20 ng/mL serves as a minor diagnostic criterion for SM, a minority of patients with biopsy-proven SM exhibit values lower than this threshold. In adult patients with MIS or *Hymenoptera* allergy, a serum tryptase level greater than 20 ng/mL suggests a diagnosis of SM. Conversely, patients with CM usually exhibit a serum tryptase level less than 20 ng/ml, or it may be within normal range. Besides SM and anaphylaxis, elevated tryptase levels may be observed with renal disease and myeloid neoplasms, including MDS, MPN, AML, and eosinophilia-associated myeloid neoplasms driven by the *FIP1L1-PDGFRA* fusion tyrosine kinase. Such cases may demonstrate an increase in loosely scattered, CD25$^+$ BM MC.

Serum tryptase levels generally reflect the subtype of SM. Although ISM patients typically exhibit only mild elevation of the serum tryptase level,

† Section 'Serum tryptase level' adapted with permission from Gotlib J, et al. (2018). 'Mast Cells and Mastocytosis' in Hoffman R, et al. (Eds.), *Hematology: Basic Principles and Practice, Seventh Edition*. Philadelphia, USA: Elsevier, Inc. https://doi.org/10.1016/C2013-0-23355-9.

they can vary widely. One of the B-findings that defines SSM is a BM MC burden more than 30% and serum tryptase level more than 200 ng/mL. Patients with ASM and MCL often exhibit serum tryptase levels in the several-hundred range to over 1000 ng/mL. In addition to serving as minor diagnostic criterion and general marker of MC burden, it has become a standard marker to measure response to cytoreductive therapy, including novel agents such as KIT inhibitors being evaluated in clinical trials.

KIT mutation analysis

The somatic mutation D816V is located in exon 17 of the *KIT* gene, and is a pathogenic drive of mastocytosis identified in approximately 90–95% of patients. D816F/H/I/Y are rare codon 816 *KIT* variants with functional similarity to *KIT* D816V; D820G and N822K are examples of additional exon 17 variants that have been identified in advanced forms of SM including ASM and mast cell sarcoma. Transmembrane *KIT* mutations in exons 8 to 9 of the extracellular region (del419, S451C, ITD 502–503), transmembrane region (exon 10; e.g. F522C), and juxtamembrane domain (exon 11; e.g. V560G/I) are rare *KIT* mutations that have been isolated in a few patients (Figure 11.1). These exon 8–11 mutations are more likely to exhibit sensitivity to imatinib, whereas exon 17 variants, including KIT D816V, are imatinib-resistant. The frequency of *KIT* D816V is less in MCL compared to other subtypes (range 40–80%) and reflects an increased frequency of wild-type *KIT* or other rare variants in the *KIT* gene.

The assay sensitivity of *KIT* mutation detection is critical and can lead to false negative results if a lower sensitivity method is used. Myeloid mutation panels are not recommended for screening of *KIT* D816V because of their relatively low sensitivity (~5%). Instead, allele-specific oligonucleotide quantitative reverse transcriptase polymerase chain reaction (AS-PCR), which has a high sensitivity in the range of 0.1% to 0.01%, should be used for screening of *KIT* D816V from the BM or peripheral blood. However, in patients with a very low MC burden, AS-PCR on the peripheral blood may lead to a negative result, warranting mutation analysis from the BM. Since AS-PCR is specific the D816V mutation, detection of alternative *KIT* D816 mutations, or variants in other domains of the *KIT* gene would necessitate alternative techniques such as peptide nucleic acid (PNA)-mediated PCR and sequencing of the whole *KIT* gene.

Whereas ISM tends to be driven by *KIT* D816V alone, advanced forms of SM, particularly SM-AHN, often harbour additional mutations that reflect the associated myeloid neoplasm. These mutated genes include *SRSF2, ASXL1, RUNX1, JAK2, DNMT3A, CBL, K/NRAS, UA2F1, ZRSF2 EZH2, ETV6,* and *SETBP1*. *JAK2* V617F has been found in SM with primary myelofibrosis, *BCR-ABL1* has been identified in rare cases of SM-CML, and the t(8;21)(q22;q22) *RUNX1/RUNX1T* rearrangement is a well-known association in SM-AML. Mutations in the ethanolamine kinase gene *ETNK1* are enriched in SM patients with eosinophilia, but are also found in patients with CMML or atypical chronic myeloid leukaemia at a frequency of 5–10%.

Biologic studies incorporating sequencing of granulocyte-macrophage colony-forming progenitor cells (CFU-GM) indicate that mutations in *TET2* often precede the acquisition of *KIT* D816V. Special research techniques have been used to interrogate the cell-specific distribution of mutations. For

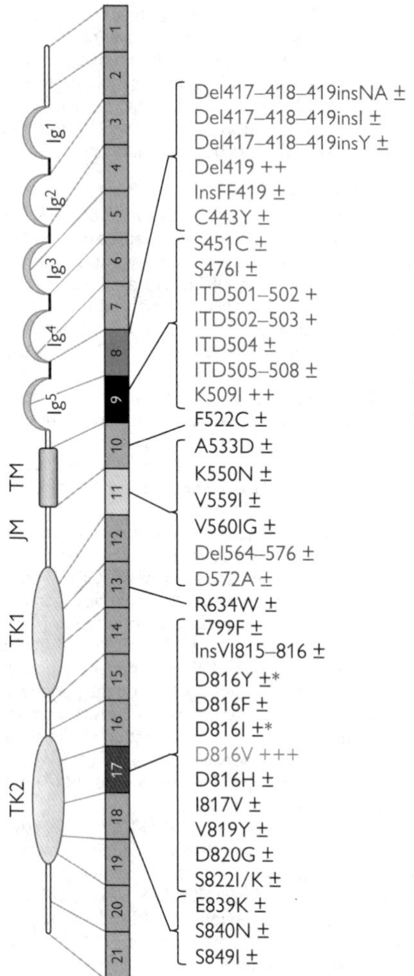

Figure 11.1 Structure of the *KIT* gene and mutations in mastocytosis. Representation of the structure of *KIT*, illustrating the localization of the more frequently observed mutations in the *KIT* sequence in paediatric and adult patients with mastocytosis. The receptor is presented under its monomeric form, whereas its WT counterpart dimerizes upon ligation with stem cell factor (SCF) before being activated in normal cells. In children, the *KIT* D816V PTD mutant (in red) is found in nearly 30% of the patients, whereas the ECD mutants (in blue) are found in nearly 40% of the affected children, the most frequent being the deletion 419. In adults,

example, *KIT* D816V and the *SRSF2* P95 mutation have been demonstrated in cell lineages of the MC and AHN component (e.g. MCs and monocytes in cases of associated CMML) by cell laser-microdissection or other techniques. Chromosome abnormalities may also be shared by cells derived from the SM and AHN; for example, t(8;21) has been identified by fluorescence in situ hybridization (FISH) in BM MCs and the leukaemic clone of a patient with SM-AML.

Additional diagnostic studies

Imaging studies are a key component of the diagnostic workup of SM, particularly in smouldering SM and advanced variants. Ultrasound, MRI, and/or computed tomography (CT) of the abdomen and pelvis can help establish the presence of B-findings such as hepatomegaly, splenomegaly, lymphadenopathy, as well as C-findings such as ascites and/or portal hypertension. Volumetric assessment of spleen and liver volumes by CT or MRI is now commonly incorporated into clinical trial assessment of novel agents. Upper and lower endoscopy with random biopsies can be useful to establish mast cell involvement of the gastrointestinal tract in patients with diarrhoea and/or malabsorption resulting in hypoalbuminemia and weight loss. Biopsy specimens should under immunohistochemistical staining to quantitate the number of lesional MCs and to determine whether they express neoplastic markers (e.g. CD25 in addition to the normal mast cell markers CD117 and tryptase). In patients with indolent and advanced disease, dual-energy X-ray absorptiometry density (DEXA) scanning should be undertaken to assess bone mineral density in light of the increased risk for osteoporosis in SM patients. The frequency of DEXA scans will be guided by the presence and severity of osteopenia or osteoporosis and the use of intercurrent therapy, but serial evaluation every 1 to 3 years may be considered. Metastatic skeletal survey may also be undertaken in individuals with severe focal bone pain who may be at risk for osteolysis and/or pathologic fractures. For patients with symptoms and signs of mast cell degranulation, 24-hour urine studies for biochemical evidence of mast cell activation, may also be considered in selected circumstances, including N-methylhistamine, prostaglandin D2, and 2,3-Dinor-11beta-prostaglandin F2 alpha. Release of heparin from activated MCs may account for the bleeding diathesis in some

---

depending of the category of mastocytosis, the *KIT* D816V mutant (in red) is found in at least 80% of all patients. The complete list of *KIT* mutants retrieved in the literature for mastocytosis is depicted here. In children, the structure of *KIT* is found WT in ~25% of the patients analysed, whereas in adults, *KIT* is found WT in <20% of all patients analysed so far. Some of the mutations are found only in a very few patients. Del, deletion; ECD, extracellular domain; Ins, insertion; ITD, internal tandem duplication; JMD, juxtamembrane domain; KI, kinase insert; PTD, phosphotransferase domain; TMD, transmembrane domain. The symbols indicate the following: ±, mutation found in <10% of the paediatric or adult patients; +, mutations found in 1 to 5% of paediatric patients; ++, mutation found in 5 to 20% of paediatric patients; +++, mutation found in ~30% of paediatric patients and in >80% of all adult patients. *Mutation also found in children at low frequency.

Adapted with permission from Arock M, et al. (2015). KIT mutation analysis in mast cell neoplasms: recommendations of the European Competence Network on Mastocytosis. *Leukemia*. 29(6):1223–32. DOI: 10.1038/leu.2015.24.

patients with SM; therefore, assessment of a heparin activity level may be considered in selected cases. Human leukocyte antigen (HLA) testing should be undertaken in patients with advanced disease who are candidates for, and are being considered for haematopoietic stem cell transplantation.

Symptom and quality-of-life assessments are increasingly being incorporated as secondary endpoints in clinical trials of novel therapies for patients with indolent and advanced SM. The Mastocytosis Symptom Assessment form (MSAF) and the Mastocytosis Quality of Life Questionnaire (MQLQ) have recently been validated in patients with ISM and SSM; their use of these patient-reported outcome (PRO) instruments is encouraged to enhance the understanding of the impact of both disease and treatments on the individual suffering from SM.

Diagnostic decision-making

For the patient suspected of having a mast cell disorder such as SM, the diagnostic workflow begins with evaluation of suspected signs or symptoms of mast cell activation (e.g. anaphylaxis, diarrhoea, flushing), and the presence of an increased serum tryptase level. The finding of MIS, B- or C-findings, or abnormal blood counts, are also part of the initial evaluation of mastocytosis. BM biopsy (or biopsy of another extracutaneous organ), molecular testing for *KIT* D816V by allele-specific PCR, and mast cell immunophenotyping by immunohistochemistry and/or by flow cytometry comprise the panel of tests needed to establish a WHO diagnosis of SM. If one major plus one minor criterion or at least three minor criteria are present, a diagnosis of SM can be made. In patients wherein WHO criteria for SM are not fulfilled but MIS is present, a diagnosis of CM is rendered. Individuals without the major criterion and less than three minor criteria (e.g. *KIT* D816V^{+} and/or CD25^{+} MC), a diagnosis of primary MCAS (monoclonal mast cell activation syndrome [MMAS]) should be considered. Secondary MCAS (e.g. due to allergies, urticarias, medications, infection) or idiopathic MCAS are considerations in patients presenting with the aforementioned signs and symptoms of mastocytosis but whose mutation analysis demonstrates wild-type *KIT* and normal mast cell morphology/immunophenotype. In this latter group, the presence of an elevated serum tryptase level should also merit consideration of a hereditary alpha-tryptasemia, a recently described multisystem disorder characterized by duplications and triplications in the *TPSAB1* gene encoding a-tryptase associated with elevation of the basal serum tryptase level and symptoms including cutaneous flushing and pruritus, dysautonomia, functional gastrointestinal symptoms, chronic pain, and connective tissue abnormalities, including joint hypermobility.

The large majority of adults with MIS will also be found to have SM when further testing is undertaken to assess for WHO criteria for systemic disease. However, in adult patients with MIS and mild elevation of the serum tryptase level, lack of blood count abnormalities, and absence of B- or C-findings, the utility of a BM should be discussed with the patient. While a BM may confirm a diagnosis of SM, a low mast cell burden will not typically trigger a change in treatment. Since children with CM rarely exhibit systemic disease, BM biopsies are typically only indicated in patients with abnormal blood counts, unusually high or progressively rising tryptase levels, and/or evidence of organ dysfunction.

Survival and prognostic factors

The WHO subtype of SM generally correlates with prognosis. In a Mayo series of 342 SM patients, those with ISM exhibited similar survival to age- and sex-matched populations controls. However, patients with more advanced SM exhibited markedly inferior median overall and leukaemia-free survivals: 41 months for ASM (n = 41), 24 months for SM-AHN (n = 138), and 2 months for MCL (n = 4). In their multivariable analysis, adverse prognostic factors included advanced age, anaemia, thrombocytopenia, hypoalbuminemia, weight loss, and excess BM blasts. A Spanish group found that multilineage involvement of the *KIT* D816V mutation (e.g. in additional myeloid lineages besides MCs) was associated with an increased risk of progression to advanced SM. The presence of eosinophilia in SM patients has been associated with variable outcomes, with one study demonstrating worse survival, and another study showing prognostically neutral outcomes.

A German group has identified an increased serum alkaline phosphatase and splenomegaly as adverse clinical variables. Cytogenetic/molecular variables contributing to worse outcomes include poor-risk karyotype (monosomy 7 or complex cytogenetics) as well as the number of mutations beyond *KIT* D816V. In particular, mutation of *SRSF2, ASXL1*, and/or *RUNX1* (so-called S/A/R panel) is associated with an inferior prognosis. A mutation-augmented prognostic scoring system (MAPSS) incorporating clinical and laboratory variables, as well as the *ASXL1* mutation has been developed to stratify patients with advanced SM into low, intermediate, and high risk with significantly different median survival (86 months, 21 months, and 5 months, respectively). More refined prognostic scoring systems that include the results of S/A/R profiling are currently being developed. Myeloid mutation panel testing should generally be performed on the BM, but may also be performed on the peripheral blood, especially in the presence of an AHN and/or circulating MCs.

Treatment

Therapy of mastocytosis often requires that patients be referred to specialized centres with expertise in SM given the rarity of the diagnosis and the challenges of managing symptoms of mast cell activation, and organ damage caused by neoplastic MCs in advanced disease. All patients should be counselled regarding signs and symptoms of disease and to avoid known triggers of mast cell activation/anaphylaxis. Examples of mediator symptoms related to degranulation of MC include pruritis, flushing, diarrhoea, abdominal cramping, and neuropsychiatric complaints. The triggers of these mediator symptoms are not always identified. Potential non-immunoglobulin E (IgE) and IgE-mediated causes of mast cell activation and/or anaphylaxis include emotional or physical stress; exercise; hot or cold stimuli; medications including aspirin, non-steroidal anti-inflammatory agents (NSAIDs), opioid analgesics, or antibiotics such as penicillins or cephalosporins;, alcohol; radiocontrast dye, and IgE-mediated *Hymenoptera* venom allergy. Notably, the presence of skin disease appears to portend a reduced risk of anaphylaxis, especially due to *Hymenoptera* envenomation.

All patients are advised to carry injectable epinephrine (2 auto injectors) to manage potential episodes of anaphylaxis. Emergency use of diphenhydramine and oral corticosteroids is less well established in mitigating symptoms of acute anaphylaxis. Management of MC activation follows a stepwise treatment algorithm that is first anchored to use of H1-antihistamines for flushing and pruritis, and H_2-antihistamines for gastrointestinal symptoms such as diarrhoea, abdominal discomfort/cramping, nausea, vomiting, and peptic ulcer disease. Standard doses need to be titrated to symptomology, and higher doses may be necessary for symptoms refractory to standard treatment. For breakthrough symptoms, addition of leukotriene receptor antagonists such as montelukast may help further alleviate flushing and pruritis. Although aspirin can be help mitigate refractory flushing, it should be used with caution because of its potential to precipitate MC activation. Cromolyn sodium (Gastrocrom) is used for refractoriness of the aforementioned gastrointestinal symptoms (and may also be used for persistent neurologic and naso-ocular mast cell activation symptoms), and proton pump inhibitors may be useful for patients with refractory GERD/peptic ulcer disease. Ketotifen (compounded for oral use) has purported antihistamine and mast cell stabilizing effects that may benefit mast cell activation symptoms affecting the skin, gastrointestinal, and neurologic systems. The anti-IgE antibody omalizumab has been used off-label for prophylactic management of cardiovascular (presyncope, tachycardia) and pulmonary symptoms (wheezing, throat swelling), and for: (1) prevention of unprovoked anaphylaxis; (2) anaphylaxis which is *Hymenoptera* or food-induced with negative specific IgE or negative skin testing; and (3) improving tolerance while on immunotherapy. While corticosteroids can mitigate symptoms of mast cell activation, longer-term use is limited by toxicities.

Bone disease (osteopenia, osteoporosis, osteolysis with or without pathologic fractures) is observed at an increased frequency across the spectrum of SM subtypes and also requires medical surveillance to determine the need for intervention. Supplemental calcium and vitamin D are recommended for osteopenia/osteoporosis. Bisphosphonates (e.g. alendronate, risedronate, pamidronic acid, and zoledronic acid) with continued use of antihistamines may improve bone pain and improve bone mineral density, particularly in the vertebral bones. Interferon-alpha (IFN-α) has been employed with bisphosphonates, and/or as single agent therapy, especially for patients with refractory bony pain, and/or MC-related osteoporosis and pathologic fractures. The published experience with interferons for bone disease is primarily limited to case reports and series. The anti-RANKL monoclonal antibody denosumab may also be considered for patients with bone pain not responding to bisphosphonates or who are not candidates for these agents because of renal insufficiency. In selected cases, vertebroplasty or kyphoplasty is employed for pain related to vertebral compression fractures that is refractory to other therapies.

For cutaneous lesions, or skin-related mediator symptoms unresponsive to the antimediator therapies described earlier, phototherapy (UVA_1, narrow-band UVB, and UVA plus psoralen) may be considered. In addition, occlusion dressings embedded with topical steroids with or without phototherapy, and both topical and oral forms of cromolyn sodium may provide benefit.

Because SM patients carry a risk of anaphylaxis in the perioperative period that is higher than the general population, multidisciplinary collaboration with allergy/immunology and/or anaesthesia subspecialty services is encouraged in anticipation of procedures/surgery. Management plans should be devised that minimize exposure to certain medications that carry an increased potential for provoking mast cell degranulation (e.g. certain anaesthetic or analgesic agents). Similarly, pregnant women, or women of childbearing age who are interested in becoming pregnant should seek consultation with a high-risk obstetrician, as well as anaesthesia and/or allergy specialists. Such consultation should span the preconception, pregnancy, and the peripartum period in order to minimize exposure to medications which may carry potential harm to the patient and fetus. Currently, insufficient evidence exists regarding whether SM results in increased rates of adverse maternal or fetal outcomes (e.g. spontaneous miscarriage, preterm infants, complications of labour and delivery) compared to the general population. A diagnosis of SM does not appear to affect fertility.

Figure 11.2 shows a treatment algorithm for indolent versus advanced stages of SM and the broad therapeutic strategies that are available based on the presence of mediator symptoms, organ damage, and a concomitant AHN.

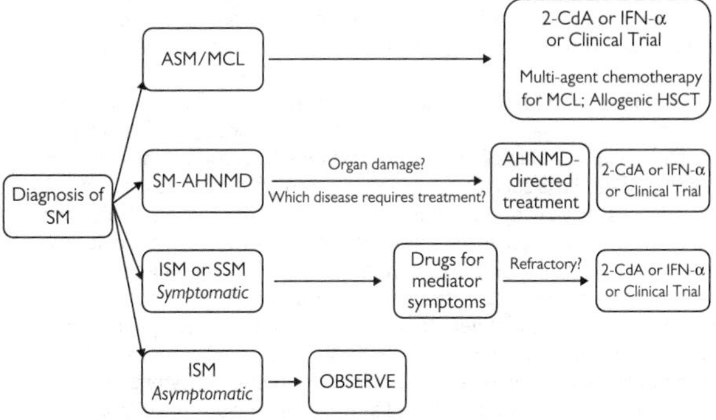

ISM: indolent systemic mastocytosis; SSM: smoldering systemic mastocytosis; ASM: aggressive systemic mastocytosis; MCL: mast cell leukemia; AHNMD: associated hematologic non-mast cell lineage disease; 2CdA: 2-chlorodeoxyadenosine; IFN-α; interferon-α, HSCT; hematopoietic stem cell transplantation

Figure 11.2 Treatment options based on subtype of systemic mastocytosis.

Reproduced with permission from Gotlib J, et al. (2018). 'Mast Cells and Mastocytosis' in Hoffman R, et al. (Eds.), *Hematology: Basic Principles and Practice, Seventh Edition*. Philadelphia, USA: Elsevier, Inc. DOI: https://doi.org/10.1016/C2013-0-23355-9.

Cytoreductive agents

Interferon-α

‡Different formulations of interferon-α (interferon-α-2b, PEG-interferon-α-2a, PEG-interferon-α-2a) with or without corticosteroids (prednisone or prednisolone 0.5–1 mg/kg) have been used as a cytoreductive strategy in ISM patients with refractory mediator symptoms, but primarily in individuals with advanced SM and organ damage. Severe and/or persistent mediator symptoms or organ damage may require a longer-term maintenance strategy and slower taper of corticosteroids.

Dosing of IFN-α has varied between studies and no optimal dose has been identified. Initial doses have ranged from 1 million units (MU)/day to 3 MU three times weekly (TIW) with median total weekly maintenance doses in the range of 15–30 MU. In the Mayo experience with IFN-α (with or without prednisone), 21 of 40 evaluable patients exhibited response (53%) which consisted of 6/10 ISM, 6/10 ASM, and 9/20 SM-AHN patients. The 21 responses consisted of 1 complete remission (CR), 6 major responses (MR), and 14 partial responses (PR). The median duration of response was 12 months (range 1–67 months) with no difference between responders and non-responders regarding prednisone use or the median weekly interferon-α dose. Lack of mediator symptoms was associated with a lower response rate. In the French experience with 20 SM patients (4 ISM and 16 ASM), IFN-α-2b was started at 1 MU daily and increased to 5 MU/m^2 daily as tolerated. Among 13 patients treated for 6 or more months, all had partial or complete resolution of systemic or cutaneous disease manifestations, but no significant reduction in BM MC burden. The lack of a substantive effect on tumour burden, and observation of rapid relapse in some responding patients after drug withdrawal indicates that interferon-α exerts a cytostatic effect on MC, and therefore may be more appropriate in patients with slowly progressive disease who are not in need of rapid debulking.

Responses to IFN-α have included reduction of MC mediator symptoms and laboratory markers of MC activation (e.g. levels of histamine or its metabolites), clearing of MIS, amelioration of osteoporosis, and improvement of C-findings such as cytopenias, liver dysfunction and/or ascites, and weight loss. However, tolerability to interferon-α can be challenging and may often require dose reduction and/or discontinuation. Toxicities such as such as flu-like symptoms, myelosuppression, liver function abnormalities, hypothyroidism, and depression, require close monitoring. For these reasons, interferon-α is generally only recommended for patients with advanced SM. However, it may also be useful in selected patients with indolent or smouldering SM with severe, refractory mediator symptoms, or bone disease not responsive to antimediator therapy or bisphosphonates.

‡ Section 'Cytoreductive agents' adapted with permission from Gotlib J, et al. (2018). 'Mast Cells and Mastocytosis' in Hoffman R, et al. (Eds.), *Hematology: Basic Principles and Practice, Seventh Edition*. Philadelphia, USA: Elsevier, Inc. https://doi.org/10.1016/C2013-0-23355-9.

Cladribine

§Cladribine (2-chlorodeoxyadenosine; 2-CdA) has been used off-label across a spectrum of SM subtypes. Following an initial report indicating that cladribine could elicit improvement of mediator symptoms, cutaneous lesions, and reduction of measures of mast cell burden), Kluin-Nelemans and colleagues published a series of ten patients (ISM, n = 3; SSM, n = 1; SM-AHN, n = 3; ASM, n = 3). Cladribine was given at a dose of 0.10–0.13 mg/kg over 2 hours IV for 5 days every 8 weeks. Among 9 evaluable patients, the drug improved mediator symptoms, decreased skin lesions, MC burden and serum tryptase levels, and reduced urine metabolites of MC activation.

In the Mayo Clinic experience, cladribine was dosed at 5 mg/m^2 (or 0.13–0.17 mg/kg) daily for 5 days intravenously. A median of three cycles (range 1–9) was administered. The overall response rate was 12/22 (55%), consisting of 1 CR, 7 MR, and 4 PR. Responses were observed in 5/9 ISM, 1/2 ASM, and 6/11 SM-AHN patients. Patients experienced improvement in mediator symptoms, organomegaly, C-findings such as ascites and anaemia, and markers of MC burden and/or activation. The median response duration was 11 months, and inferior outcomes were associated with leukocytosis, monocytosis, and circulating immature myeloid cells, the latter remaining statistically significant in a multivariable analysis.

The long-term French experience with cladribine has been reported in both indolent (n = 36) and advanced (n = 32) SM patients. Cladribine was administered subcutaneously at a dose of 0.14 mg/kg, for 1 to 5 days, every 4–12 weeks. A median of 3.7 courses was administered (range 1–9). The overall response rate was 72% (92% for indolent disease and 50% for advanced subtypes). Among patients with advanced SM, the respective CR, MR, and PR rates were 0%, 37.5%, and 12.5%. Significant decreases in serum tryptase levels were only observed among indolent SM patients. BM MC burden was evaluated in just nine patients, prohibiting interpretation of this endpoint. The median duration of response was 2.47 (0.5–8.6) years in advanced SM patients. Lymphopenia (82%), neutropenia (47%), and opportunistic infections (13%) were the most common grade 3/4 adverse events. Similar to interferon-α, cladribine's use in indolent disease (even those with refractory mediator symptoms) needs to be approached very cautiously because of the potential for high-grade toxicities. Cladribine is usually favoured over IFN-α in patients who require rapid cytoreduction.

Tyrosine kinase inhibitors

Dasatinib and nilotinib

Dasatinib and nilotinib are multikinase inhibitors with activity against KIT D816V *in vitro*. In a phase II trial of 33 patients (ISM, n = 18; ASM, n = 9; SM-AHN), dasatinib (140 mg daily) exhibited limited activity in SM with 11 (33%) of patients responding. Two complete responses occurred in patients with negative KIT D816V mutation status, including one patient with JAK2 V617F-positive SM with primary myelofibrosis (SM-PMF) and another

§ Section 'Cladribine' with permission from Gotlib J, et al. (2018). 'Mast Cells and Mastocytosis' in Hoffman R, et al. (Eds.), *Hematology: Basic Principles and Practice, Seventh Edition*. Philadelphia, USA: Elsevier, Inc. https://doi.org/10.1016/C2013-0-23355-9.

with SM with associated chronic eosinophilic leukaemia (SM-CEL). The other nine responses were of symptomatic benefit only. A phase II, open-label trial of nilotinib enrolled 61 patients; among the 37 patients with ASM, the overall response rate was 22% and there were no complete responses.

Imatinib

Imatinib is currently approved for adult patients with ASM without the *KIT* D816V mutation or with unknown *KIT* mutational status. Therefore, imatinib's therapeutic role is limited to 5–10% of SM patients without this canonical mutation and reinforces the need to use a highly sensitive assay to detect *KIT* D816V in order to avoid false negative results and inappropriate use of imatinib. However, imatinib does exert activity against mutated KIT with variants in the transmembrane and juxtamembrane domains (e.g. exons 8–10). For example, imatinib has generated high quality responses in cases well-differentiated SM variant with either the F522C transmembrane *KIT* mutation or wild-type *KIT*; in a patient with familial SM carrying the germline *KIT* K509I mutation; with deletion of codon 419 in exon 8 of *KIT* in paediatric CM; and in a case of MCL with mutation in exon 9 (p.A502_Y503dup).

Masitinib

Masitinib is an inhibitor of several kinases including Lyn, PDGFR-α/β, Lyn, and *wild-type* KIT; notably, however, it lacks activity against the D816V variant. Masitinib was evaluated in a phase II trial of patients with ISM or CM with symptoms unresponsive to prior therapy. Patients were randomized to receive 3 or 6 mg/kg/day for 12 weeks with the primary endpoint evaluating change in symptoms at week 12 compared to baseline. The overall clinical response rate was 56%, consisting of significant improvement in the frequency of flushing, pruritus, and Hamilton rating for depression by 64, 36, and 43%, respectively. During the 12-week period, 21 patients (84%) experienced at least one masitinib-related adverse events (AEs) which were graded as mild [n = 11], moderate [n = 19], and severe [n = 9]). The most common AE were nausea/vomiting (52%), oedema (44%), muscle spasms (28%), and rash (28%). The QLQ-C30 symptom score showed no significant improvement versus baseline, which may reflect drug-related AEs. In a multicentre randomized trial of 135 severely symptomatic patients with indolent SM or smouldering SM, masitinib reduced symptoms, tryptase levels, and skin lesions compared with placebo. Twenty-four percent of patients experienced side effects (e.g. diarrhoea, rash, and asthenia) that required drug discontinuation. The drug Committee for Medicinal Products for Human Use (CHMP) of the European Medicines Agency (EMA) adopted a negative opinion of the study results, ultimately denying marketing authorization of masitinib.

Midostaurin

Midostaurin (N-benzoylstaurosporine; PKC412) is an oral multikinase inhibitor that inhibits both wild-type and D816V-mutated KIT, as well as FLT3, PDGFR-α/β, and VEGFR2. In Ba/F3 cells transformed by *KIT* D816V, the IC_{50} of midostaurin was 30–40 nM, compared to > 1uM with imatinib. In a phase 2 investigator-initiated trial of 26 patients with advanced SM with one or more C-findings, treatment with midostaurin 100 mg twice daily on continuous cycles produced a response rate of 69% according to modified Valent and Cheson criteria. A MR; resolution of one or more C-findings) was observed in 50% of patients.

These encouraging data led to a global, multicentre, open-label trial of midostaurin, dosed in a similar fashion in a similar population of advanced SM patients with one or more signs of SM-related organ damage. The trial employed a study steering committee and central pathology review to adjudicate eligibility, response, and histopathology. An overall response rate of 60% was observed among 89 evaluable patients, including an overall MR rate of 45%. Responses were observed regardless of *KIT* mutation status, prior therapy, or the presence of an AHN. The median best reduction in serum tryptase level was –58%. In addition, the median change in BM MC burden was –59%, and 57% of patients had a ≥50% reduction in BM MCs. After a median follow-up of 26 months, the median duration of response (DOR), median overall survival (OS), and progression-free survival were respectively 24.1, 28.7, and 14.1 months. Median OS in responders was 44.4 months. Of the 16 patients with MCL, 8 responded, including 7 MR (44%). The median OS was 9.4 months among all patients with MCL, and was not reached among responding MCL patients. Symptoms and quality of life, measured by the Memorial Symptom Assessment Scale (MSAS) and Short-Form 12 (SF-12) survey, respectively, were significantly improved with midostaurin treatment. The drug was generally well tolerated with a manageable toxicity profile consisting mostly of grade 1–2 gastrointestinal side effects and myelosuppression, especially in patients with pre-existing cytopenias. The Food and Drug Administration (FDA) and EMA approved midostaurin in 2017 for the treatment of patients with advanced SM (e.g. ASM, SM-AHN, and MCL).

In a separate analysis of 38 advanced SM patients treated with midostaurin on the global trial or on a compassionate use basis, worse outcomes (e.g. response rate, DOR, and survival) were observed in patients with the S/A/R mutation profile, and in patients with a less than 25% reduction in *KIT* D816V mutant allele burden. Progression was observed in patients with the appearance of new mutations or increase in the allele frequency of non-*KIT* D816V mutations such as *K/N-RAS*, *RUNX1*, *IDH2*, and *NPM1*. In progressors, no acquired resistance mutations in *KIT* were identified on midostaurin therapy.

More recently, phase II trial data were published regarding the safety and efficacy of midostaurin in 20 patients with ISM. Midostaurin produced significant reductions in severity of symptoms measured by the MSAF. The greatest improvements were noted in fatigue and musculoskeletal pain. Skin lesions improved in 12 (80%) of the 15 patients with skin symptoms, resulting in a 40% reduction in median Scoring Mastocytosis Index score. In addition, 19 patients showed a reduction in serum tryptase level and the BM mast cell burden decreased in 8/16 patients (50%). Grade 1–2 nausea (80%), headache (50%), and diarrhoea (35%) were the most common AEs, consistent with the tolerability profile of the drug. After protocol-specified treatment period of 24 weeks, most patients experienced return of symptoms and an increase of tryptase levels off midostaurin. Ten patients were retreated; 8 individuals again experienced improvement of symptoms and reduction in serum tryptase levels.

Selective KIT D816 inhibitors in clinical trials

Avapritinib (BLU-285; Blueprint Medicines) is a potent and selective oral type I multikinase inhibitor with activity against KIT D816V (IC50 0.27 nM). Based on its activity in preclinical models such as HMC1.2 cell lines (V560G- and D816V-mutated) and mice xenografted with P815 mastocytoma cells, a multicentre phase 1 trial was initiated in advanced SM patients (ClinicalTrials.gov identifier NCT02561988).

Results of the phase I dose escalation and expansion phases have been reported, with the expansion component still enrolling patients. Responses in organ damage, MC burden, and spleen volume were observed regardless of advanced SM subvariant, prior therapy, or mutational profile (e.g. S/A/R status). Among 36 patients with bone marrow MCs ≥ 5% and availability of on-treatment BM and serum tryptase assessments, 29 (81%) experienced ≥ 50% reduction in both measures. In addition, 88% of patients exhibited ≥ 50% reduction of KIT D816V mutant allele burden early in the course of therapy. Among the 52 enrolled patients in the dose escalation and expansion cohorts, 23 patients were evaluable for response by IWG-MRT-ECNM criteria. The overall response rate was 83%, consisting of 17% CR + CRh (CR with partial recovery of peripheral blood counts), 53% PRs, and 13% with clinical improvement. Responses were also observed in patients who had experienced progression or intolerance on prior midostaurin therapy. The most commonly reported toxicities included periorbital oedema, fatigue, nausea, diarrhoea, peripheral oedema, and cognitive effects, primarily grade 1–2 in nature. Myelosuppression including thrombocytopenia and anaemia as well as some cases of nausea, vomiting, fatigue, ascites, and periorbital oedema were the most common grade 3–4 AEs. Dose reductions and interruptions due to AEs were reported in 56% of patients each, mostly occurring at doses greater than 200 mg daily. After a median follow-up of 14 and 5 months in the dose escalation and expansion groups, respectively, 42/52 (80%) enrolled patients remained on treatment. The phase II study in advanced SM has recently initiated accrual and a phase III randomized study of avapritinib vs. placebo in patients with indolent SM will also be undertaken.

DCC-2618 (Deciphera Pharmaceuticals) is a type II switch control kinase inhibitor with activity against multiple KIT and PDGFR-α mutants, with activity in preclinical models using KIT WT (IC50 11–61 nM) and D816V-transfected MC lines (IC50 133–256 nM). Enrolment of patients with advanced SM as part of an expanded phase 2 trial is currently ongoing with a recommended phase 2 dose of 150 mg daily (ClinicalTrials.gov identifier NCT02571036).

Haematopoietic stem cell transplantation (HSCT)

**The role of HSCT in advanced SM has not been well studied. However, in 2014, Ustun and colleagues published a large, multicentre retrospective

** Section 'Hematopoietic Stem Cell Transplantation (HSCT)' adapted with permission from Gotlib J, et al. (2018). 'Mast Cells and Mastocytosis' in Hoffman R, et al. (Eds.), *Hematology: Basic Principles and Practice, Seventh Edition*. Philadelphia, USA: Elsevier, Inc. https://doi.org/10.1016/C2013-0-23355-9.

analysis evaluating the outcomes of 57 SM patients (SM-AHN, n = 38 [AML = 20]; ASM, n = 7; and MCL, n = 12) who underwent allogeneic HSCT. Donor types included HLA-matched identical (n = 34), unrelated (n = 17), umbilical cord blood (n = 2), haploidentical (n = 1), and 3 unknown. Responses were observed in 70% of patients, including a 16% CR rate. The remaining 30% of responses were split between stable disease (21%) and primary refractory disease (9%). All 38 patients with SM-AHN achieved CR regarding the AHN component, but 10 subsequently relapsed with AHN, and half of these patients died.

The median 3-year OS for all patients was 57%, consisting of 74% for patients with SM-AHN, 43% for ASM, and 17% for MCL patients. The strongest risk factor for worse OS was a diagnosis of MCL; use of reduced intensity (versus myeloablative) conditioning was also associated with inferior outcomes. Patient age, donor age, donor type (sibling or unrelated donor), graft source (BM or peripheral HSCT), *KIT* mutation status, karyotype, and total body irradiation used in myeloablative conditioning had no impact on overall or progression-free survival. Treatment-related mortality at 6 months and 1 year was 11% and 20%, respectively, and was highest in MCL patients. Although a prospective trial is needed to better define the role of HSCT in advanced SM, these data suggest that transplantation may provide extended survival in selected patients, particularly those with SM-AHN.

Future directions

Recent next-generation sequencing (NGS) studies have lent substantial insight into the molecular pathogenesis of SM beyond *KIT* D816V. The co-occurrence of high-risk myeloid mutations such as *SRSF2, ASXL1*, and *RUNX1* in patients with advanced SM is providing an opportunity to generate clinical-molecular prognostic models that augment risk stratification of patients. Baseline and serial NGS monitoring of clonal dynamics during trial evaluation of novel agents such as KIT inhibitors will foster a better understanding of how to circumvent resistance with alternative therapies. Use of single cell genomic approaches and transcriptome and proteomic profiling of purified MC and AHN cell populations are future initiatives that should help further clarify the complicated biology of mast cell disease. It is already become standard approach to incorporate *KIT* mutant allele burden testing in clinical protocols as a biomarker of response.

Among the community of mast cell investigators, several ongoing collaborative initiatives are expected to generate further clarity regarding the various rare subtypes of SM. For example, the European Competency Network on Mastocytosis [ECNM]) has generated a multicentre registry containing over 3000 SM patients. These data should further buttress attempts to generate a prognostic scoring system that stratifies outcomes of different SM subtypes with larger numbers of patients in each disease variant. Efforts are also underway to validate advanced SM PRO instruments in addition to those currently available in indolent SM. Regulatory health agencies are increasingly focused on these patient measures for drug approval, and validated PROs are critical for stringent adjudication of treatment-related changes in the context of placebo-controlled, double blind study designs.

Encouraging data from the midostaurin studies and emerging data from trials of selective KIT D816 inhibitors such as BLU-285 have validated the paradigm of KIT inhibition in SM. However, numerous unmet clinical needs exist, and this is no more apparent than in patients with SM-AHN where KIT inhibition alone is unlikely to be an adequate strategy to address both disease components. In this regard, future clinical strategies will evaluate the value of combining KIT inhibitors with AHN-directed agents, such as the use of hypomethylating agents in patients with SM-MDS or SM-MDS/MPN. Clinical trials are under development to investigate targets and pathways relevant to SM. While a recent investigator-initiated trial of the anti-CD30 antibody drug immunoconjugate brentuximab vedotin failed to show clinical benefit in patients with CD30$^+$ advanced SM, other antibody drug immunoconjugates should be studied. For example, gemtuzumab ozogamicin, an anti-CD33 antibody immunoconjugate linked to calicheamicin, elicited a CR in a patient with multiply refractory/relapsed MCL. Inhibitors of JAK2, PI3 kinase, and BCL-2 warrant further investigation based on their involvement in mast cell differentiation and survival signalling pathways. The IWG-MRT-ECNM consensus response criteria are now being used by the FDA and EMA to harmonize adjudication of responses across trials of patients with advanced SM. Finally, newly released National Comprehensive Cancer Network (NCCN) treatment guidelines for systemic mastocytosis will encourage more standardized treatment approaches for these rare neoplasms.

Further reading

Alvarez-Twose I, Martinez-Barranco P, Gotlib J, et al. Complete response to gemtuzumab ozogamicin in a patient with refractory mast cell leukemia. *Leukemia*. 2016;*30*(8):1753–6.

Alvarez-Twose I, Zanotti R, González-de-Olano D, et al., on behalf of the Spanish Network on Mastocytosis (REMA) and the Italian Network on Mastocytosis (RIMA). Nonaggressive systemic mastocytosis (SM) without skin lesions associated with insect-induced anaphylaxis shows unique features versus other indolent SM. *J Allergy Clin Immunol*. 2014;133(2):520–8.

Anderson DM, Lyman SD, Baird A, et al. Molecular cloning of mast cell growth factor, a hematopoietin that is active in both membrane bound and soluble forms. *Cell*. 1990;63(1):235–43.

Arber D, Orazi A, Hasserjian R, et al. The 2016 revision to the World Health Organization (WHO) classification of myeloid neoplasms and acute leukemia. *Blood*. 2016;*127*(20):2391–405.

Arock M, Sotlar K, Akin C, et al. KIT mutation analysis in mast cell neoplasms: recommendations of the European Competence Network on Mastocytosis. *Leukemia*. 2015;29(6):1223–32.

Barete S, Lortholary O, Damaj G, et al. Long-term efficacy and safety of cladribine (2-CdA) in adult patients with mastocytosis. *Blood*. 2015;126(8):1009–16.

Bonadonna P, Perbellini O, Passalacqua G, et al. Clonal mast cell disorders in patients with systemic reactions to Hymenoptera stings and increased serum tryptase levels. *J Allergy Clin Immunol*. 2009;123(3):680–6.

Erben P, Schwaab J, Metzgeroth G, et al. The KIT D816V expressed allele burden for diagnosis and disease monitoring of systemic mastocytosis. *Ann Hematol*. 2014;93(1):81–8.

Escribano L, Alvarez-Twose I, Sánchez-Muñoz L, et al. Prognosis in adult indolent systemic mastocytosis: a long-term study of the Spanish Network on Mastocytosis in a series of 145 patients. *J Allergy Clin Immunol*. 2009;124(3):514–21.

Garcia-Montero AC, Jara-Acevedo M, Teodosio C, et al. KIT mutation in mast cells and other bone marrow haematopoietic cell lineages in systemic mast cell disorders: a prospective study of the Spanish Network on Mastocytosis (REMA) in a series of 113 patients. *Blood*. 2006;108(7):2366–72.

Georgin-Lavialle S, Lhermitte L, Dubreuil P, et al. Mast cell leukemia. *Blood*. 2013;121(8):1285–95.

Gotlib J, Akin C. Mast cells and eosinophils in mastocytosis, chronic eosinophilic leukemia, and non-clonal disorders. *Semin Hematol*. 2012;49(2):128–37.

Gotlib J, Berubé C, Growney JD, et al. Activity of the tyrosine kinase inhibitor PKC412 in a patient with mast cell leukemia with the D816V KIT mutation. *Blood*. 2005;106(8):2865–70.

Gotlib J, Kluin-Nelemans HC, George TI, et al. Midostaurin (PKC412) demonstrates a high rate of durable responses in patients with advanced systemic mastocytosis: results from the fully accrued global phase 2 CPKC412D2201 trial. *Blood*. 2014;124:636.

Horny HP, Akin C, Metcalfe DD, et al. Mastocytosis. In: Swerdlow SH, Campo E, Harris NL, et al. (eds.) WHO Classification of Tumors of Hematopoietic and Lymphoid Tissues. Lyon, France: International Agency for Research and Cancer (IARC), 2008, pp. 54–63.

Huang E, Nocka K, Beier DR, et al. The hematopoietic growth factor KL is encoded by the Sl locus and is the ligand of the c-kit receptor, the gene product of the W locus. *Cell*. 1990;63(1):225–33.

Jawhar M, Schwaab J, Schnittger S, et al. Molecular profiling of myeloid progenitor cells in multi-mutated advanced systemic mastocytosis identified KIT D816V as a distinct and late event. *Leukemia*. 2015. 29:1115–22.

Kirshenbaum AS, Kessler SW, Goff JP, et al. Demonstration of the origin of human mast cells from CD34+ bone marrow progenitor cells. *J Immunol*. 1991;146(5):1410–15.

Kristensen T, Vestergaard H, Bindslev-Jensen C, et al. Sensitive KIT D816V mutation analysis of blood as a diagnostic test in mastocytosis. *Am J Hematol*. 2014;89(5):493–8.

Lim KH, Pardanani A, Butterfield JH, et al. Cytoreductive therapy in 108 adults with systemic mastocytosis: outcome analysis and response prediction during treatment with interferon-alpha, hydroxyurea, imatinib mesylate or 2-chlorodeoxyadenosine. *Am J Hematol*. 2009;84(12):790–4.

Lim KH, Tefferi A, Lasho TL, et al. Systemic mastocytosis in 342 consecutive adults: survival studies and prognostic factors. *Blood*. 2009;113(23):5727–36.

Metcalfe DD. Mast cells and mastocytosis. *Blood*. 2008;112(4):946–56.

Nagata H, Worobec AS, Oh CK, et al. Identification of a point mutation in the catalytic domain of the protooncogene c-kit in the peripheral blood mononuclear cells of patients who have mastocytosis with an associated hematologic disorder. *Proc Natl Acad Sci U S A*. 1995;92(23):10560–4.

Pardanani A, Lim KH, Lasho TL, et al. Prognostically relevant breakdown of 123 patients with systemic mastocytosis associated with other myeloid malignancies. *Blood*. 2009;114(18):3769–72.

Pardanani A. How I treat patients with indolent and smoldering mastocytosis (rare conditions but difficult to manage). *Blood*. 2013;121(16):3085–94.

Pardanani A. Systemic mastocytosis in adults: 2015 update on diagnosis, risk stratification, and management. *Am J Hematol*. 2015;90(3):250–62.

Schwaab J, Schnittger S, Sotlar K, et al. Comprehensive mutational profiling in advanced systemic mastocytosis. *Blood*. 2013;122(14):2460–6.

Schwartz LB, Metcalfe DD, Miller JS, et al. Tryptase levels as an indicator of mast-cell activation in systemic anaphylaxis and mastocytosis. *N Engl J Med*. 1987;316(26):1622–6.

Sotlar K, Cerny-Reiterer S, Petat-Dutter K, et al. Aberrant expression of CD30 in neoplastic mast cells in high-grade mastocytosis. *Mod Pathol*. 2011;24(4):585–95.

Sotlar K, Fridrich C, Mall A, et al. Detection of c-kit point mutation Asp-816 → Val in microdissected pooled single mast cells and leukemic cells in a patient with systemic mastocytosis and concomitant chronic myelomonocytic leukemia. *Leuk Res*. 2002;26(11):979–84.

Sperr WR, Horny HP, Valent P. Spectrum of associated clonal hematologic non-mast cell lineage disorders occurring in patients with systemic mastocytosis. *Int Arch Allergy Immunol*. 2002;127(2):140–2.

Sperr WR, Jordan JH, Fiegl M, et al. Serum tryptase levels in patients with mastocytosis: correlation with mast cell burden and implication for defining the category of disease. *Int Arch Allergy Immunol*. 2002;128(2):136–41.

Ustun C, Reiter A, Scott BL, et al. Hematopoietic stem-cell transplantation for advanced systemic mastocytosis. *J Clin Oncol*. 2014;32(29):3264–74.

Valent P, Akin C, Arock M, et al. Definitions, criteria and global classification of mast cell disorders with special reference to mast cell activation syndromes: a consensus protocol. *Int Arch Allergy Immunol*. 2012;157(3):215–25.

Valent P, Akin C, Escribano L, et al. Standards and standardization in mastocytosis: consensus statements on diagnostics, treatment recommendations and response criteria. *Eur J Clin Invest*. 2007;37(6):435–53.

Valent P, Escribano L, Broesby-Olsen S, et al. Proposed diagnostic algorithm for patients with suspected mastocytosis: a proposal of the European Competence Network on Mastocytosis. *Allergy*. 2014;69(10):1267–74.

Valent P, Horny HP, Escribano L, et al. Diagnostic criteria and classification of mastocytosis: a consensus proposal. *Leuk Res*. 2001;25(7):603–25.

Valent P, Sotlar K, Sperr WR, et al. Refined diagnostic criteria and classification of mast cell leukemia (MCL) and myelomastocytic leukemia (MML): a consensus proposal. *Ann Oncol*. 2014;25(9):1691–700.

Valent P, Sperr WR, Akin C. How I treat patients with advanced systemic mastocytosis. *Blood*. 2010;116(26):5812–17.

Valent P, Sperr WR, Sotlar K, et al. The serum tryptase test: an emerging robust biomarker in clinical hematology. *Expert Rev Hematol*. 2014;7(5):683–90.

Verstovsek S, Tefferi A, Cortes J, et al. Phase II study of dasatinib in Philadelphia chromosome-negative acute and chronic myeloid diseases, including systemic mastocytosis. *Clin Cancer Res*. 2008;14(12):3906–15.

Zsebo KM, Wypych J, McNiece IK, et al. Identification, purification, and biological characterization of hematopoietic stem cell factor from buffalo rat liver-conditioned medium. *Cell*. 1990;63(1):195–201.

Chapter 12

Myelodysplastic syndromes/ myeloproliferative overlap neoplasms

Eric Padron, Tariq I. Mughal, David Sallman, and Alan F. List

Introduction and classification *192*
Chronic myelomonocytic leukaemia *195*
Juvenile myelomonocytic leukaemia *199*
Atypical chronic myeloid leukaemia *200*
MDS/MPN-RS-T *201*
MDS/MPN-U *202*
Concluding thoughts *202*
Key learning points *202*

Introduction and classification

The myelodysplastic/myeloproliferative (MDS/MPN) overlap neoplasms are a collection of haematologic malignancies characterized by myeloid proliferation, bone marrow dysplasia, and ineffective haematopoiesis (Figure 12.1). The 2016 World Health Organization (WHO) classification of the MDS/MPN group comprises chronic myelomonocytic leukaemia (CMML), juvenile myelomonocytic leukaemia (JMML), atypical chronic myeloid leukaemia, *BCR-ABL1*-negative (aCML), MDS/MPN with ring sideroblasts and thrombocytosis (MDS/MPN-RS-T) and MDS/MPN, unclassifiable (MDS/MPN-U) (Table 12.1). The current classification defines distinct biological entities with myelodysplastic and myeloproliferative features, considerable molecular heterogeneity, and the lack of specific genotypic markers. While monocytosis or eosinophilia foster recognition of CMML/JMML or chronic eosinophilic leukaemia, (CEL) respectively, the differentiation between aCML, MDS/MPN-U, and MPN-U is often difficult.

Incidence and aetiology

Currently there is a paucity of published registry data on the precise incidence of the various subtypes of MDS/MPN, with the notable exception of CMML. Estimates from the US Surveillance, Epidemiology, and End Results (SEER) Program that relies solely upon hospital registry data, indicate the relative incidence of MDS/MPN is low and significantly underestimated, the annual incidence of CMML is estimated at 1/100 000 adults, with a median age of 70 years and a male predominance. Like many haematological

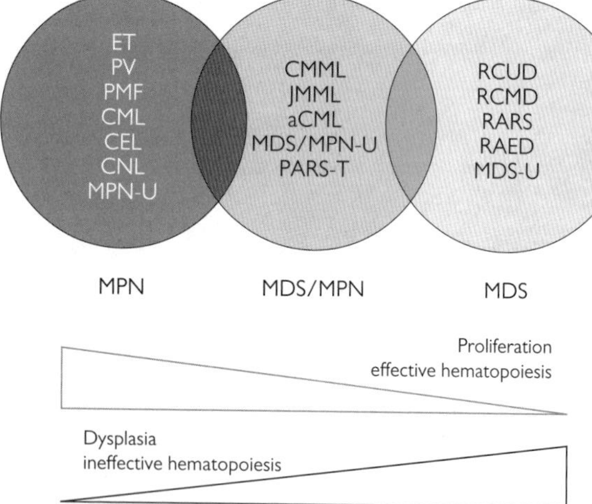

Figure 12.1 Myeloproliferative neoplasms and myelodysplastic syndromes.

Reproduced with permission from Mughal TI, et al. (2015). An International MDS/MPN Working Group's perspective and recommendations on molecular pathogenesis, diagnosis, and clinical characterisation of myelodysplastic/myeloproliferative neoplasms. *Haematologica*. 100(9):1117–30. DOI: 10.3324/haematol.2014.114660. Copyright © 2015 Ferrata Storti Foundation.

Table 12.1 WHO-defined diagnostic criteria for MDS/MPN classification

CMML	aCML	JMML	MDS/MPN-U
Persistent peripheral blood monocytosis $>1 \times 10^9$	WBC $\geq 13 \times 10^9$ with increased and dysplastic neutrophils	Peripheral blood monocytosis $>1 \times 10^9$	Features of one MDS category *and*
No *BCR-ABL1* or *PDGFR* fusion gene	No *BCR-ABL1* or *PDGFR* fusion gene	No BCR-ABL1 or PDGFR fusion gene	Prominent myeloproliferative features *and*
Fewer than 20% blasts in the blood and bone marrow	Fewer than 20% blasts in the blood and bone marrow	Fewer than 20% blasts in the blood and bone marrow	No preceding history of MPN or MDS and no BCR-ABL1 or PDGFR fusion and no isolated del(5q), chr 3 inversion *or*
Dysplasia in one more lineages, if no dysplasia then:	Minimal absolute basophilia	Two of the following must be present:	features of mixed MDS and MPN and cannot be assigned MDS, MPN, or MDS/MPN category
> an acquired clonal cytogenetic or genetic abnormality	No or minimal monocytosis	> Haemoglobin F increase	
> the monocytosis is has persisted for >3 months *and*	Hypercellular BM with granulocyte dysplasia	> Immature granulocytes in peripheral blood	
> all causes of monocytosis have been excluded	Neutrophil precursors ≥10% of peripheral blood WBC	> WBC greater than 10×10^9/L	
		> Clonal chromosome abnormality	
		> GM-CSF hypersensitivity of myeloid progenitors *in vitro*	

Adapted from Arber DA, et al. (2016). The 2016 revision to the World Health Organization classification of myeloid neoplasms and acute leukemia. *Blood*. 127(20):2391–405. https://doi.org/10.1182/blood-2016-03-643544. Reprinted with permission from the American Society of Hematology.

malignancies, there is a trend towards older age for MDS/MPN, with the exception of JMML, which has a median age of occurrence of 2 years, and an incidence of 0.12 per 100 000 children with a disproportionate male preponderance. This bias, and the observations that in some subtypes, like CMML, there seems to be a relationship with clonal haematopoiesis of indeterminate potential (CHIP), suggesting that CMML might represent the leukaemic transformation of the myelomonocytic lineage-biased aged haemopoiesis.

Genetics

Chromosome abnormalities, in particular aneuploidies (trisomy 8, monosomy 7) or deletions [del(7q), del(13q), del(20q)], and translocations involving tyrosine kinase fusions leading to constitutive activation of the kinases predominate occur in approximately 30% of cases. As an illustration, *PDGFRA, PDGFRB, ABL1, JAK2* and *FGFR1* are found in >70% of the patients. In addition, somatic mutations may include growth factor receptors (*CSF3R*), downstream cytokine receptor signalling intermediates (*JAK2, NRAS, KRAS*) and negative regulators of signalling pathways (*PTPN11, CBL, NF1*) (Table 12.2). Mutations deregulating *RAS* are found in almost all patients with JMML. Signalling mutations occur in ~50% of CMML patients and correlate with a myeloproliferative phenotype and enhancement of *in vitro* sensitivity to GM-CSF. Up to 80% of patients with MDS/MPN-RS-T have activated JAK-STAT signalling as a consequence of the presence of *JAK2*V617F, *CALR*, or *MPL* mutations, in addition to mutations in epigenetic genes such as *TET2* and *ASXL1, IDH1/2, EZH2, SUZ12, EED*, and *UTX* (Figure 12.2). Approximately 50% of CMML patients have mutations involving *SRSF2*, with 20% exhibiting mutations in other splicing complex genes (*SF3B1, U2AF35, U2AF65*, and *SF3A1*). Clonal architecture analysis in CMML has demonstrated linear acquisition of candidate mutations with limited branching through loss of heterozygosity. Additionally, *SF3B1* mutations are present in about 70% of patients with MDS/MPN-RS-T. These *SF3B1* mutations are not always mutually exclusive and may be accompanied by *DNMT3, JAK2, ASXL1*, and *TET2* mutations, but not other splicing complex genes. Functionally, disruption of *SF3B1* function leads to the formation of ring sideroblasts; however, its exact role in malignant transformation remains unclear. The *RUNX1* gene is mutated in 15–30% of CMML patients. SET binding protein 1 (*SETBP1*) was recently identified as a novel oncogene mutated in 25% of aCML cases, and less frequently in other MDS/MPN. A small minority of MDS/MPN have calreticulin (*CALR*) mutations.

Clinical features

In general, most patients present with non-specific features, not distinguishable from MDS or MPN. The respective MDS/MPN subtypes are typically identified by the type of myeloid subset that predominates in the peripheral blood. For example, CMML and JMML are characterized by a unique expansion of peripheral blood monocytes, while aCML is associated with highly dysplastic granulocyte predominance. Multiparameter flow cytometry helps to characterize patients with CMML who have a specific expansion of 'classical' monocytes ($CD14^{hi}/CD16^{neg}$). As a general rule the clinical heterogeneity in MDS/MPN vastly exceeds the genetic heterogeneity. The constellation of features that can occur include symptoms of ineffective haemopoiesis (anaemia, infections, bleeding) or constitutional symptoms

Table 12.2 Frequencies of recurrent genetic mutations in WHO-defined MDS/MPN

(%)	CMML	JMML	aCML	MDS/MPN-U	RARS-T
ASXL1	40	0	69	?	15
CALR	0	0	0	0	<1
CBL	10	15	0	?	4
CSF3R	0	0	variable	0	0
DNMT3A	2	0	?	?	15
ETV6	<1	0	?	?	3
EZH2	5	0	?	10	?
IDH1/2	6	0	?	?	?
JAK2	8	0	7	19	57
JAK3	n/a	12	?	?	?
K/N RAS	19	39	35	14	?
NF1	<1	13	?	?	?
PTPN11	<1	44	?	?	?
RUNX1	15	0	?	14	?
SETBP1	9	8	48	10	1
SF3B1	6	0	?	?	93
SRSF2	46	0	?	?	7
TET2	58	0	?	?	25
TP53	<1	0	?	?	?
U2AF1	5	0	?	?	5
ZRSF2	8	0	?	?	3

Distinction between '0' and '?' is that data exists that mutation has been profiled or not, respectively.

Reproduced with permission from Padron E (2015). Surveying the landscape of MDS/MPN research: overlap among the overlap syndromes? *Hematology Am Soc Hematol Educ Program*. 2015(1):349–54. DOI: 10.1182/asheducation-2015.1.349.

and splenomegaly associated with myeloproliferation. MDS/MPN-RS-T is hallmarked by thrombocytosis and medullary ring sideroblasts while MDS/MPN-U has no clear association with a specific myeloid subset, but instead is identified by the presence of clinical and/or pathologic manifestations of myeloproliferation and bone marrow failure.

Chronic myelomonocytic leukaemia

Genetics

Cytogenetic abnormalities observed in patients with CMML include trisomy 8, monosomy 7, del(7q) and rearrangements with a 12p breakpoint; in contrast, del(5q) is almost never found. The unfolding genomic landscape includes mutations involving *TET2* (50–60%), *SRSF2* (40–50%), *ASXL1* (35–40%), and *RUNX1* (15%), as well as less frequently occurring mutations in

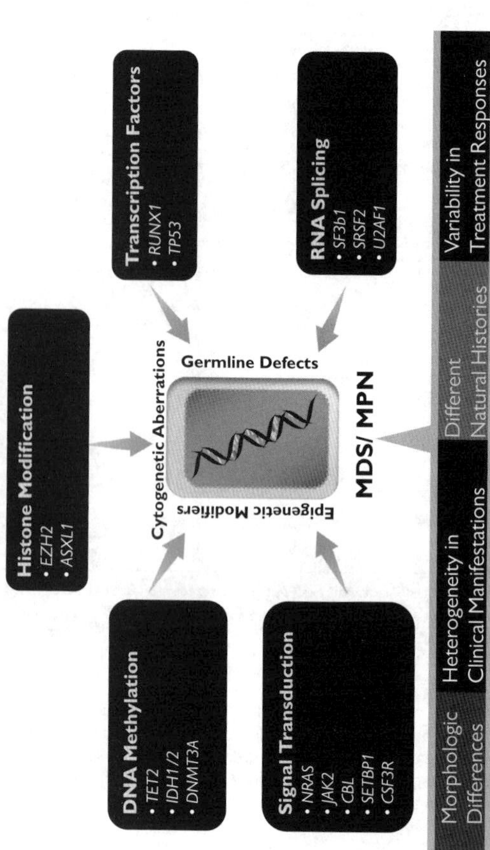

Figure 12.2 A schematic description of genotypic diversity in patients with myelodysplastic syndromes (MDS) and myeloproliferative neoplasms (MPN).

cytosine methylation genes (*DNMT3A and IDH2*), RNA splicing (*SF3B1, U2AF35, ZRSR2*), chromatin remodelling genes (*UTX, EZH2*) and signalling pathway genes (*NRAS, KRAS, CBL, JAK2, FLT3, CSF3R*). A *MAFB*-associated regulatory network has also been described in CML, which distinguishes it further from other MDS/MPN subtypes.

Diagnosis

The diagnosis of CMML is based upon haematologic and pathologic features, and complemented by cytogenetic and molecular abnormalities. The 2016 WHO classification defines CMML by the presence of monocytosis, that is relative (>10% of WBC) and absolute (> 1×10^9/L) and must persist for > 3 months, and marrow findings that typically meet MDS diagnostic criteria, hypercellularity with dysplasia in >1 cell lineage and <20% blasts. The classification divides CMML into a 'proliferative type' with a total WBC >13×10^9/L and a 'dysplastic type', with a WBC below this threshold, to reflect clinical and genetic distinctions.

Clinical features include splenomegaly, skin and lymph node infiltration, and serous membrane effusions. Cytological dysplasia is often subtle in the bone marrow, however, expansion of myeloid precursors, and myelocytes in particular is routine. Rarely, CMML can be therapy-related or a secondary neoplasm, arising from a background of MDS or as a progression of myelofibrosis, in particular in the presence of an *SRSF2* mutation. CMML is divided by the WHO into three groups based upon blast percentage: CMML-0 with 2% blasts in peripheral blood (PB) and 5% blasts in the bone marrow (BM); CMML-1 with 2–4% blasts in PB and/or 5–9% blasts in BM; and CMML-2 with 5–19% blasts in PB and 10–19% in BM, and/or presence of Auer rods (Figures 12.3 and 12.4). Clonal architecture analysis in CMML has demonstrated linear acquisition of candidate mutations with limited branching through loss of heterozygosity.

CMML is molecularly characterized by early clonal dominance arising within the CD34 positive/CD38 negative cells, and the subsequent granulomonocytic differentiation skewing of progenitors. Another important biological feature is the unique hypersensitivity to GM-CSF, as measured by haematopoietic colony formation and GM-CSF-dependent phosphorylation of STAT5. Mouse models recapitulating mutations in *TET2, JAK2, CBL*, and *NRAS* have also been reported to up regulate the STAT5 signalling pathway and/or enhance granulocyte/macrophage-colony formation in a cytokine-dependent fashion. These novel observations support the candidacy of JAK2 inhibitors for the treatment of CMML.

Risk stratification

Multiple prognostic scoring systems, based on monocyte counts, genetic lesions, clinical features, and risk to transform to acute myeloid leukaemia (AML) have been proposed and validated. As illustration, Solary (Paris) proposed a prognostic score based on *ASXL1* mutations, age, haemoglobin, WBC, and platelet counts defined three prognostic groups with varied overall survival.

Therapy

The management of patients with CMML is often a challenge with a small subset of patients having an indolent course with median survival in excess of 10 years, while others progress rapidly to AML. Allo-SCT remains the only treatment modality associated with long-term remissions and a long-term (10 year) overall survival of about 40%. Factors associated with favourable outcomes appear to be CMML risk group (CMML-0 vs. CMML-1 vs. CMML-2), pretransplant haematocrit, cytogenetic risk category, comorbidity index, presence of splenomegaly, and age. At present there are no satisfactory non-transplant options, and symptom-directed therapy with either cytoreductive therapy, such as hydroxyurea (hydroxycarbamide) or hypomethylating agents (HMAs), such as azacitidine or decitabine are useful to treat some patients, in particular those with significant proliferative and dysplastic components, respectively. However, these agents do not alter the natural history.

Investigational approaches include sapacitabine, JAK2, MEK, and BCL-2 inhibitors and other targeted agents, such as tagraxofusp, a CD123-targeted drug. Tagraxofusp is being tested as a monotherapy and in combination with HMAs or venetoclax.

There is additional interest in tagraxofusp in view of the finding of islands of CD123^{high} cells in the BM of patients with CMML. There is also emerging evidence of the heterogenous expression of cytokines, such as IL-10, which can be targeted.

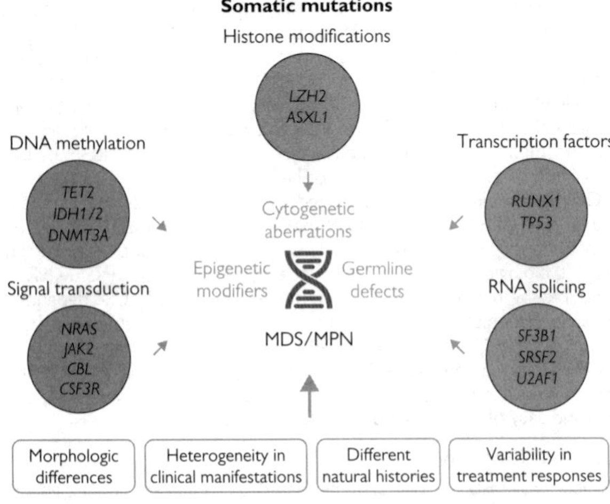

Figure 12.3 A photomicrograph from a patient with chronic myelomonocytic leukaemia (CMML)-1. (a) Peripheral blood smear showing three abnormal monocytes and one neutrophil. (b and c) Bone marrow aspirate and the corresponding naphthyl butyrate esterase image of the aspirate. (d) Bone marrow trephine biopsy.

Reproduced with permission from Mughal TI, et al. (2015). An International MDS/MPN Working Group's perspective and recommendations on molecular pathogenesis, diagnosis, and clinical characterisation of myelodysplastic/myeloproliferative neoplasms. *Haematologica*. 100(9):1117–1130. DOI: 10.3324/haematol.2014.114660. Copyright © 2015 Ferrata Storti Foundation.

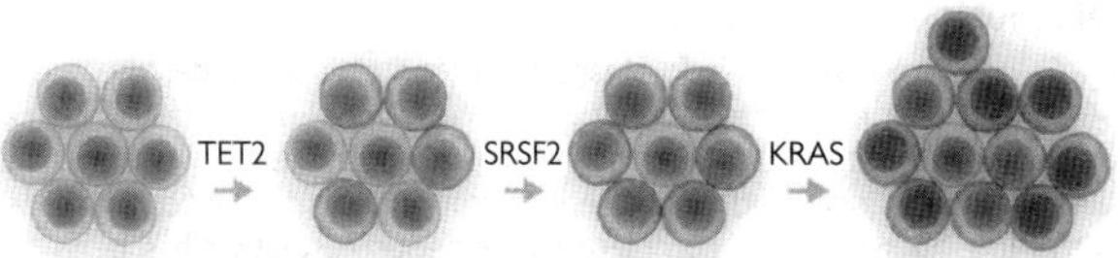

- Early clonal dominance in HSC compartment
- Linear acquisition of mutations, starting with epigenetic and splicing genes
- Growth advantage to the more mutated cells with differetiation

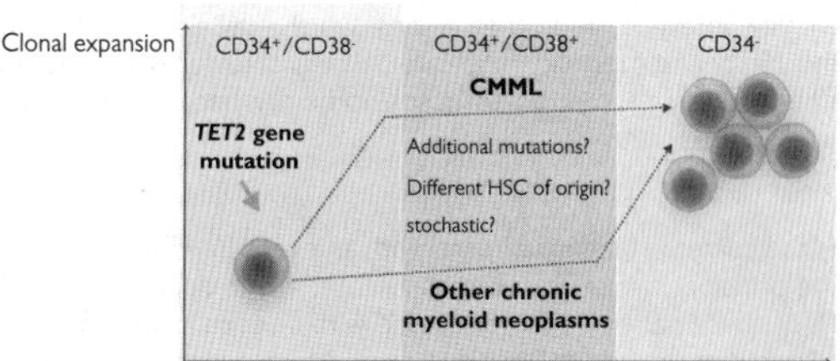

Figure 12.4 Early clonal dominance (CD34+/CD38−cells) in chronic myelomonocytic leukaemia (CMML) compared to myeloproliferative neoplasms (MPN) (also see plate section).

Reproduced with permission from Mughal TI, et al. (2015). An International MDS/MPN Working Group's perspective and recommendations on molecular pathogenesis, diagnosis, and clinical characterisation of myelodysplastic/myeloproliferative neoplasms. *Haematologica*. 100(9):1117–1130. DOI: 10.3324/haematol.2014.114660. Copyright © 2015 Ferrata Storti Foundation. Source: data from Itzykson R, et al. (2013). Clonal architecture of chronic myelomonocytic leukemias. *Blood*. 121(12):2186–98. DOI: 10.1182/blood-2012-06-440347.

Juvenile myelomonocytic leukaemia

Genetics

It is generally believed that juvenile myelomonocytic leukaemia (JMML) develops when a single pluripotent haematopoietic cell acquires somatic mutations in a *PTPN11, NF1, NRAS, KRAS*, or *CBL* gene resulting in hyperactivation of the RAS pathway. In some patients, the pathogenetic event can be monosomy 7 (-7), carrying a mutation in the *SETBP1* or *JAK3* gene. Rarely the disease may arise as a consequence of germline mutations in one or more of the aforementioned candidate genes. The notable absence of global mutations, in particular affecting epigenetic and splicing genes, often seen in myeloid malignancies, is noteworthy. Recently a novel fetal-like molecular subgroup with LIN28B overexpression with high age-adjusted fetal haemoglobin (HbF) levels was described. Uniquely, most patients with JMML exhibit an increased *in vitro* sensitivity to GM-CSF, which appears to augment signalling of other downstream effectors, in particular JAK/STAT5.

Diagnosis

JMML is a rare disease predominantly affecting children under the age of 3 years, with a male preponderance and accounting for about 1% of all childhood leukaemias. It shares some clinical and molecular features with CMML. Interestingly, and importantly, in some patients, particularly those with Noonan syndrome, complete spontaneous resolution has been observed, despite identification of clonal haematopoiesis, in contrast to other patients who have a poor prognosis characterized by a fulminant clinical course. The precise reason for this unique characteristic remains an enigma. Leukaemic transformation is relatively uncommon in JMML. Clinically JMML is characterized by an overproduction of monocytes that infiltrate liver, spleen lung, intestine, and other organs, which may also lead to considerable morbidity and mortality. The cardinal clinical features also include fever, thrombocytopaenia, monocytosis, splenomegaly, hepatomegaly, HbF elevation, and failure to thrive.

Therapy

Allo-SCT is the current standard of care, with an event-free 5-year survival of 52%. The principal cause for failure is relapse, which approaches 50%, though 50% of these patients can be rescued with a second allograft. It has been speculated that the high relapse rate might be related to an underlying fundamental immune defect or incomplete eradication of resistant disease prior to myeloablation. Strategies to rescue children post-relapse remain suboptimal, with limited success of donor lymphocyte infusions. Current non-transplant alternatives are limited, and many efforts to develop molecularly targeted treatments are urgently required.

Atypical chronic myeloid leukaemia

Genetics

Although no one specific molecular abnormality occurs in atypical chronic myeloid leukaemia (aCML), it is associated with *CSF3R* mutations in 10% of cases, whereas *SETBP1* and/or *ETNK1* gene mutations are demonstrable in nearly a third of cases. MPN-associated driver mutations such as *JAK2*, *CALR*, and *MPL* are typically absent in aCML. There are some clinical and morphological similarities between aCML and CNL, which is typically associated with a mutated *CSF3R* gene, occasionally found in aCML.

Diagnosis

The diagnosis of aCML requires the exclusion of not only *BCR-ABL1*, but also rearrangement of *PDGFRA*, *PDGFRB*, or *FGFR1*. The differential diagnosis includes CNL, CMML, and MDS/MPN-U. Patients tend to have severe anaemia, thrombocytopaenia, neutrophilia with prominent granulocytic dysplasia (uncommon in CNL), and splenomegaly; monocytosis and basophilia are usually absent or minimally present in the PB. The hallmark features include a hypercellular BM with marked granulocytic dysplasia accompanied by leukocytosis composed predominantly of neutrophilic precursors.

Therapy

There are no current aCML-specific treatment guidelines and at present allo-SCT is the only therapy that can afford patients the potential to achieve long-term remission, and possible cure. Many efforts are assessing the potential benefit of targeted therapies, such as dasatinib and ruxolitinib. The CSF3R truncating mutations result in constitutive activation of SRC kinases, which can be targeted by drugs such as dasatinib, and the membrane proximal mutations activate JAK/STAT signalling that are reported to be highly responsive to the JAK2 inhibitors, such as ruxolitinib. Interferon alpha has been tested in a small series of aCML with modest activity.

MDS/MPN-RS-T

Genetics

Somatic mutations in *SF3B1* have been described in about 90% of patients with myelodysplastic syndrome/myeloproliferative neoplasm with ringed sideroblasts and thrombocytosis (MDS/MPN-RS-T) and have generally been considered to be responsible for mitochondrial iron overload in sideroblasts, ineffective erythropoiesis, and anaemia (myelodysplastic features). In contrast, somatic mutations in *JAK2* or *MPL* are thought to drive thrombocytosis (myeloproliferative features). *JAK2* ^{V617F} mutation occurs in approximately 50% of cases with mutated patients having significantly higher platelet counts. Mutation of *JAK2* ^{V617F} is important as it typically does not occur in patients with refractory anaemia with ringed sideroblasts (RARS). Patients with wildtype *SF3B1* often harbour comutation of *JAK2* ^{V617F} and *ASXL1* or other spliceosome mutations, such as *U2AF1* or *SRSF2*, often with *ASXL1*. Together, mutations of one of these five mutations will be seen in almost all cases of MDS/MPN-RS-T. In very rare cases, *CALR* mutations have also been observed.

Diagnosis

MDS/MPN-RS-T, previously known as refractory anaemia with ring sideroblasts and thrombocytosis (RARS-T), is a new entity recognized in the 2016 revised WHO classification, with a median age of diagnosis of 73 years. The disease has MDS features with ring sideroblasts (≥15% of erythroid precursors) in addition to sustained thrombocytosis (>450 000/μL) and megakaryocyte cytological features resembling essential thrombocythaemia. There is some interesting clinical evidence suggesting that patients with SF3B1 and/or JAK2 V617 may have a better prognosis compared to wildtype patients, with overall survival of 6.9 versus 3.3 years, respectively, in untreated patients.

Therapy

There is no firm consensus regarding optimal clinical management and supportive care remains the cornerstone. Since the thrombotic risk appears low, platelet-suppressive therapy or aspirin prophylaxis is not indicated, and patients are managed primarily for symptomatic anaemia as per standard approaches for lower risk MDS. Anecdotal reports have described small numbers of cases with robust responses to imatinib or lenalidomide. Investigational therapies include JAK2 inhibitors and spliceosome inhibitors which can potentially exploit the haplodeficient state with the prospect of selective synthetic lethality.

MDS/MPN-U

MDS/MPN-Unclassifiable (MDS/MPN-U) is the most heterogeneous subgroup of MDS/MPN and includes patients who lack defining characteristics of the other MDS/MPN subtypes. It probably accounts for less than 5% of MDS/MPN patients. There is genetic, such as *SETBP1*, and clinical overlap with some patients with aCML as a distinct subgroup with unique clinical features and inferior survival. Clinically, patients often present with constitutional symptoms and splenomegaly. About 20% of patients demonstrate the presence of trisomy 8 and/or a *JAK2*V617F mutation. Treatment is often empiric, but occasionally can be guided by molecular features such as the presence of a *CSF3R* mutation. Suitable clinical trials should be pursued whenever possible.

Concluding thoughts

Remarkable progress over the past decade in discerning the cellular and molecular genetic mechanisms involved in MDS/MPN overlap neoplasms have provided significant insights into the genomic complexity and clonal evolution, including transformation to AML. Some of these findings are now being integrated into treatment algorithms to guide diagnosis, prognosis, and treatment decisions. Several novel targeted agents are currently being tested. For patients with no specific mutations that stringently define particular subtypes, clear associations have emerged, including *SF3B1* and *JAK2* mutations in MDS/MPN-RS-T and *SETBP1* in aCML. Understanding clonal hierarchies should serve as a cornerstone for development of a more robust molecular classification of these neoplasms in the future, as well as molecular predictors of prognosis and therapeutic response. An immediate initiative is the generation of large registries for many of these rare disorders, where the lack of clinical trials, small numbers reported, and clinical heterogeneity make it impossible to offer definitive recommendations. Efforts are also required to boost collaborative efforts to define risk models and suitable endpoints for clinical trials. Outside of clinical trials, at present, allo-SCT remains the most viable treatment options for the eligible patients with many of these myeloid malignancies, particularly where an effective targeted approach is currently not available.

Key learning points

- MDS-MPN represent a heterogeneous group of disorders.
- A key feature of MDS-MPN are the paradoxical presentation of myeloid proliferation in the context of ineffective haematopoiesis.

- Molecular profiling may assist in the clinical management of specific MDS-MPN.
- CMML is defined by monocytosis and next generation sequencing of nine genes identifies clonality in greater than 90% of cases.
- In CMML, allo-HCT is the only curative option with hydroxyurea and hypomethylating agents used for proliferative symptoms and cytopenias, respectively.
- JMML presents in early childhood with a molecular hallmark of increased *in vitro* sensitivity to GM-CSF.
- Allo-HCT is standard of care for JMML patients although relapse occurs in 50% of patients.
- Leukocytosis and granulocytic dysplasia define aCML.
- SETBP1 mutations occur in 24% of aCML patients and are associated with inferior survival.
- Specific CSF3R mutations in aCML support clinical investigation of SRC/JAK inhibition.
- Diagnosis of RARS-T requires ring sideroblasts (≥15% of erythroid precursors) and thrombocytosis ($\geq 450 \times 10^9/L$).
- RARS-T is defined by spliceosome mutations, particularly SF3B1 occurring in up to 90% of patients.
- JAK2 V617F mutation occurs in 50% of RARS-T cases.
- Lenalidomide, JAK inhibitors, and spliceosome inhibitors represent potential therapeutic strategies in RARS-T.
- MDS-MPN-U have myeloproliferation and dysplasia without meeting specific WHO-defined MDS/MPN.
- Further genetic characterization will allow for re-classification of many MDS-MPN-U cases.

Further reading

Arber DA, Orazi A, Hasserjian R, et al. The 2016 revision to WHO classification of myeloid neoplasms and acute leukemias. *Blood*. 2016;127(20):2391–405.

Gotlib J, Maxson JE, George TI, Tyner JW. The new genetics of chronic neutrophilic leukemia and atypical CML: implications for diagnosis and treatment. *Blood*. 2013;122:1707–11.

Locatelli F, Niemeyer CM. How I treat juvenile myelomonocytic leukemia (JMML). *Blood*. 2015;25:1083–90.

Malcovati L, Papaemmanuil E, Ambaglio I, et al. Driver somatic mutations identify distinct disease entities within myeloid neoplasms with myelodysplasia. *Blood*. 2014;124:1513–21.

Maxson JE, Gotlib J, Pollyea DA, et al. Oncogenic CSF3R mutations in chronic neutrophilic leukemia and atypical CML. *N Engl J Med*. 2013;368:1781–90.

Mughal TI, Cross NCP, Padron E, et al. An International MDS/MPN Working Group's perspective and recommendations on molecular pathogenesis, diagnosis, and clinical characterisation of myelodysplastic/myeloproliferative neoplasms. *Haematologica*. 2015;100:1117–30.

Nicolosi M, Mudireddy M, Vallapureddy R, et al. Lenalidomide therapy in patients with myelodysplastic syndrome/myeloproliferative neoplasm with ring sideroblasts and thrombocytosis (MDS/MPN-RS-T). *Am J Hematol*. 2018;93(1):E27–E30.

Padron E, Komrokji R, List AF. The clinical management of chronic myelomonocytic leukemia. *Clin Adv Hematol Oncol*. 2014;12:172–8.

Savona M, Malcovati L, Komrokji R, et al. An international consortium of uniform response criteria for MDS/MPN in adults. *Blood*. 2015;125:1857–65.

Vardiman JW, Thiele J, Arber, et al. The 2008 revision of the World Health Organization (WHO) classification of myeloid neoplasms and acute leukemia: rationale and important changes. *Blood*. 2009;114:937–51.

Chapter 13

Eosinophilia-associated myeloproliferative neoplasms

Andreas Reiter and Nicholas C.P. Cross

Introduction *205*
Clonal eosinophilia in myeloid neoplasms *207*
Clinical features *210*
Cytogenetics and molecular analyses *212*
Treatment *214*

Introduction

- The cut-off level for the normal eosinophil count in peripheral blood ranges between 0.4 and 0.75 × 10^9/L.
- Significant and persisting hypereosinophilia, defined as a persistent eosinophil count of at least 1.5 × 10^9/L, is commonly observed in a wide range of disparate reactive/non-clonal and neoplastic/clonal disorders.
- In the absence of a final diagnosis, the term 'hypereosinophilia of unknown significance (HE_{US})' was recently suggested by an expert panel at a Working Conference in Vienna.
- There are no robust immunological markers for the delineation of mature and immature eosinophils or for the differentiation between normal, reactive/non-clonal and neoplastic/clonal eosinophils.
- Reactive/non-clonal eosinophilia is usually a response to overproduction of eosinophilopoietic cytokines such as IL-3, IL-5, or GM-CSF[3] and is most frequently observed in association with atopic conditions, allergies, or autoimmune disorders, rarely in other haematological malignancies (e.g. T-cell lymphomas, or solid tumours).
- Neoplastic/clonal eosinophilia is a rare but recurrent morphologic feature of various myeloid neoplasms, e.g. myeloproliferative neoplasms (MPN-eo) or myelodysplastic/myeloproliferative neoplasms (MDS/MPN-eo), in many cases in strong association with distinct tyrosine kinase (TK) fusion genes or less frequently point mutations.
- Clinically most relevant is potentially life-threatening and irreversible organ damage due to tissue infiltration and consequent displacement of original tissue and/or the effects of eosinophil-derived mediators through release of granular contents. Organ damage may involve the heart, lungs, gastrointestinal tract, nervous system, or skin and is independent of the clonal status of eosinophils.
- The term 'hypereosinophilic syndrome (HES)' is used after exclusion of clear reactive and neoplastic conditions and in presence of organ infiltration and consequent dysfunction by non-clonal eosinophils (e.g. 'lymphocytic variant of HES').
- The proposed term 'myeloproliferative variant of HES (M-HES)' is generally not used by haematologists because the World Health Organization (WHO) classification provides a different and rather distinct categorization of various entities (Table 13.1). In the absence of a final diagnosis, the term 'hypereosinophilia of unknown significance (HE_{US})' was recently suggested by an expert panel at a Working Conference in Vienna.

Table 13.1 WHO 2016 classification of myeloproliferative neoplasms with eosinophilia (MPN-eo). MLN-eo (myeloid and lymphoid neoplasms with eosinophilia and abnormalities of *PDGFRA, PDGFRB*, or *FGFR1*), CEL-NOS (chronic eosinophilic leukaemia, not otherwise specified)

MLN-eo (WHO)	MPN with prominent eosinophilia and *FIP1L1-PDGFRA* fusion gene
	Acute myeloid leukaemia, lymphoblastic leukaemia/lymphoma with eosinophilia and *FIP1L1-PDGFRA* fusion gene
	MPN often with prominent eosinophilia and sometimes with neutrophilia or monocytosis and presence of t(5;12)(q31-q33;p12) or a variant translocation or demonstration of an *ETV6-PDGFRB* fusion gene or of rearrangements of *PDGFRB*
	MPN often with prominent eosinophilia and sometimes with neutrophilia or monocytosis or acute myeloid leukaemia or precursor T-cell or precursor B-cell lymphoblastic leukaemia/lymphoma (usually associated with peripheral blood or bone marrow eosinophilia) and presence of t(8;13)(p11;q12) or a variant translocation leading to *FGFR1* rearrangement demonstrated in myeloid cells, lymphoblasts, or both
CEL-NOS (WHO)	Eosinophil count $\geq 1.5 \times 10^9$/L
	No Ph chromosome or *BCR-ABL* or other MPN (PV, ET, PMF) or MDS/MPN (CMML or aCML)
	No t(5;12)(q31–35;p13) or other rearrangement of *PDGFRB*
	No *FIP1L1-PDGFRA* fusion gene or other rearrangements of *PDGFRA*
	No rearrangement of *FGFR1*
	The blast count in peripheral blood and bone marrow <20% and no inv(16)(p13q22) or t(16;16)(p13;q22) or other feature diagnostic for AML
	No clonal cytogenetic or molecular genetic abnormality, or blast cells are >2% in the peripheral blood or >5% in bone marrow
MPN-eo or MDS/MPN-eo	This term should also be used when cytogenetic or molecular data are not (yet) available
	Clear presence of myeloproliferative features, e.g. marked leukocytosis/eosinophilia with or without left shift, hypercellular marrow, and splenomegaly
	No cytogenetic or molecular marker (or not yet known)
	No increased blasts

Reproduced from Arber DA, et al. (2016). The 2016 revision to the World Health Organization classification of myeloid neoplasms and acute leukemia. *Blood*. 127(20):2391–2405. https://doi.org/10.1182/blood-2016-03-643544. Reprinted with permission from the American Society of Hematology.

Clonal eosinophilia in myeloid neoplasms

Tyrosine kinase fusion genes

- The WHO 2008 classification defines a rare subgroup characterized by selected TK fusion genes: '*myeloid and lymphoid neoplasms with eosinophilia (MLN-eo) and abnormalities of PDGFRA, PDGFRB, or FGFR1*'.[1]
- The abbreviation 'MLN-eo' was not formally introduced by the WHO but is used in this article.
- In daily clinical practice, the majority of physicians still uses the terms chronic eosinophilic leukaemia (CEL) or eosinophilia-associated myeloproliferative neoplasm (MPN-eo).
- By far the most common of these TK fusion genes is *FIP1L1-PDGFRA*, generated by a cytogenetically cryptic 800 kb interstitial deletion on chromosome 4q12.
- Retrospective series have suggested that *FIP1L1-PDGFRA* is identified in approximately 5–15% of patients with eosinophilia.
- In addition, cytogenetic analysis has identified four distinct recurrent breakpoint clusters that target *PDGFRA* at 4q12 and other TK such as *PDGFRB* at 5q31-33, *FGFR1* at 8p11-12, and *JAK2* at 9p24.
- As a consequence of balanced reciprocal translocations or rarely insertions or complex translocations, fusion genes similar to *FIP1L1-PDGFRA* are created, e.g. *ETV6-PDGFRB* in t(5;12)(p31-33;p12), *ZNF198-FGFR1* in t(8;13)(p11;q12), or *PCM1-JAK2* in t(8;9)(p11;p24).
- Alternative rare and structurally similar fusions involving other TK include *ETV6-ABL1* associated with a t(9;12)(q33;p12) or *ETV6-FLT3* associated with a t(12;13)(p11;q14).
- Overall, more than 50 different fusion genes (all indicated by cytogenetic analysis with the exception of *FIP1L1-PDGFRA*) encoding constitutively activated TK as the consequence of various chromosomal and molecular abnormalities TK have meanwhile been identified within the broad spectrum of MPN-eo or MDS/MPN-eo (Figure 13.1).
- In fusion proteins, the C-terminal part of a partner protein is fused to the N-terminal part of the TK, thus retaining the entire catalytic domain of the kinase.
- The vast majority of partner genes contain one or more dimerization domains that are required for the transforming activity of the fusion proteins.
- Homotypic interaction between specific domains of the partner protein leads to dimerization or oligomerization of the fusion protein mimicking the normal process of ligand-mediated dimerization and resulting in constitutive activation of the TK moiety.
- Of note, FIP1L1 does not contain any self-association motifs and it was shown that the FIP1L1 moiety is dispensable for the transforming activity of the truncated PDGFRα protein.
- With exception of *FIP1L1-PDGFRA*, TK fusion genes are present in less than 3% of patients with eosinophilia.

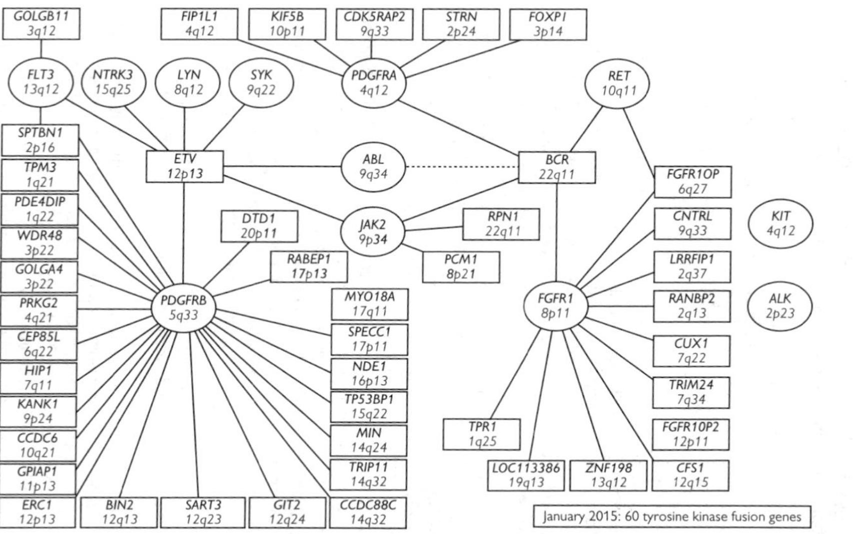

Figure 13.1 Tyrosine kinase fusion genes in MLN-eo and CEL-NOS (*PDGFRA*, n = 7; *PDGFRB*, n = 25; *FGFR1*, n = 13).

Reproduced with permission from Cross NCP, et al. (2016). 'Practical approaches to molecule testing and diagnosis of mastocytosis, hypereosinophilia, and MDS/MPN overlap syndromes', pp. 9–16, in Mesda R and Harrison C (Eds.). *Managing Myeloproliferative Neoplasms: A Case-Based Approach*. Cambridge, UK: Cambridge University Press.

Chronic eosinophilic leukaemia—not otherwise specified (CEL-NOS)

- For cases without TK fusion gene, proof of clonality by the finding of increased numbers of blasts >2% in peripheral blood (PB) and/or >5% in bone marrow (BM), and/or the presence of an alternative chromosomal aberration (e.g. a reciprocal translocation, monosomy, trisomy or deletion), leads to diagnosis of chronic eosinophilic leukaemia, not otherwise specified (CEL-NOS).
- Overall, both characteristics are only evident in a very small cohort of unselected patients with eosinophilia (T. Haferlach, Munich Leukemia Lab, personal communication).
- Formally, CEL-NOS would also be the adequate subcategory for patients with *JAK2*, *ABL1*, and *FLT3* fusion genes, although the morphologic phenotype and the disease-initiating pathogenetic mechanisms are similar to MLN-eo.
- Two recurrent chromosomal translocations are associated with non-clonal eosinophilia due to involvement and subsequent overexpression of the eosinophilopoietic cytokine IL-3.
- In MPN-eo or MDS/MPN-eo like disease, a t(5;12)(q32;p13) may result in an *ETV6-ACSL6* fusion gene in which eosinophils are non-clonal through overproduction of IL-3 via positional effects of ETV6 or other as yet unknown mechanisms. Because the karyotype of cases with *ETV6-PDGFRB* or *ETV6-ACSL6* fusion is indistinguishable, FISH analysis for identification of a rearrangement of *PDGFRB* or RT-PCR for identification of an *ETV6-PDGFRB* fusion gene should be performed in all patients with a t(5;12)(q31-33;p13).
- In acute lymphoblastic leukaemia, a t(5;14)(q31;q32) gives rise to overexpression of IL-3 by juxtaposition to the immunoglobin H (IgH) locus.
- Other cases, which do not (yet) fulfil the criteria for MLN-eo or CEL-NOS but have clear clinical and morphologic signs of a myeloid neoplasm, should be referred to MPN-eo or MDS/MPN-eo.

Clonal eosinophilia as consequence of point mutations

- Important to recognize are cases that do not fulfil the diagnostic criteria for MLN-eo or CEL-NOS but who may harbour TK point mutations (e.g. *KIT* D816V positive systemic mastocytosis), which would then be referred to as systemic mastocytosis with associated CEL (SM-CEL).
- Without representative BM histology/immunohistochemistry and molecular genetics, the clinical presentation may be indistinguishable between MLN-eo, CEL-NOS, and SM-CEL.
- Rarely, MPN- eo may test positive for *JAK2* V617F, JAK2 exon 13 indels or STAT5B N642H.
- Some cases test positive for myeloid-neoplasia associated mutations in genes such as *TET2, SRSF2, SETBP1, CSF3R, ASXL1, RUNX1, RAS, CBL, EZH2*, and others.

Clinical features

- The dominant clinical feature of cases with *PDGFRA*, *PDGFRB*, or *JAK2* fusion genes, but not *FGFR1*, is the male predominance, which exceeds a 9:1 male/female ratio in FIP1L1-PDGFRA positive patients.
- At diagnosis, pathogenetically relevant TK fusion genes are frequently missed or not considered in patients with eosinophilia and supposed AML and T-cell lymphoma. In such cases, either diagnosis would not be correct, as 'AML' is in fact 'myeloid blast phase', while 'T-cell lymphoma' reflects a stem cell disorder in which TK fusion gene positive T-lymphoblasts predominantly reside in the lymph node ('extramedullary lymphoid blast phase').
- 'Extramedullary lymphoid blast phase/lymphoma' is significantly more frequent in patients with *FGFR1* fusion genes, particularly *ZNF198-FGFR1* as consequence of a t(8;13)(p11;q13).
- Careful attention should therefore be paid to the potential presence of these TK fusion genes in myeloid and lymphoid malignancies of all subtypes which may be suggested by distinct additional clinical (e.g. splenomegaly), biochemical (e.g. elevated serum tryptase), morphological (e.g. fibrosis and increased numbers of loosely scattered mast cells) and molecular genetic features of MPN-eo.

Peripheral blood

- In addition to the qualitative (e.g. nuclear dyssegmentation, vacuoles, abnormal granulation) and quantitative evaluation of eosinophils, PB smears should also be screened for blasts, monocytes, basophils, dysplastic features, and leukoerythroblastosis which have repeatedly been reported in association with *PDGFRB*, *FGFR1*, and *JAK2* fusion genes.
- Patients can present with any level of haemoglobin or platelets from normal to significantly decreased values.
- The formal morphologic phenotype may resemble MDS/MPN-eo rather than MPN-eo in a substantial proportion of patients and eosinophils may be rather low if not absent in association with distinct fusion genes.
- Useful serum markers indicating an underlying TK fusion gene and particularly *FIP1L1-PDGFRA* are elevated levels of serum tryptase (normal value <11.4 ng/mL) and vitamin B12.
- A tryptase level of >100 ng/mL would generally be indicative of SM-CEL. In SM-CEL, significant monocytosis ($>1 \times 10^9$/L) is frequently also present.
- Elevated immunoglobin E (IgE) in the absence of allergies is suggestive for reactive/non-clonal eosinophilia.
- Cardiac enzymes (CK, TNI, pro-BNP) should be routinely monitored as indicators of, potentially clinically silent, cardiac involvement.

BM morphology

- Although there is a lack of validated primary morphologic features and antibodies for the differentiation between clonal and non-clonal eosinophilia, BM examinations should include cytomorphology and histology with reticulin staining and immunohistochemistry for mast cells and blasts.
- The term hypereosinophilia should be applied when more than 20% of all nucleated cells in the BM are eosinophils.
- Marrow fibrosis and loose aggregates of mast cells identified by immunostaining with tryptase and CD117 are important characteristics of *FIP1L1-PDGFRA* positive disease although similar features have also been seen in patients with rearrangements of *PDGFRB* and *JAK2*.
- In contrast to SM, the pronounced mast cells in *FIP1L1-PDGFRA* positive disease are loosely scattered but not found in dense infiltrates.

Organ involvement

- Clinical investigation, ultrasound, X-ray, echocardiography, CT/MRI, and endoscopies should be individually used for the identification of additional involvement of organs such as heart, lungs, gastrointestinal tract, lymph nodes, skin, central/peripheral nervous system, and others.
- There is no typical pattern of organ involvement that allows differentiation between non-clonal and clonal eosinophilia.
- Yet unpublished data of the 'German Registry of Disorders of Eosinophils and Mast Cells' have shown that the more organs are involved the less likely is a diagnosis of an MPN-eo in contrast to HES.
- Splenomegaly represents the most frequently and also solely observed organ involvement in MPN-eo.
- The prevalence of cardiac involvement in *FIP1L1-PDGFRA* positive disease is approximately between 5% and 20%. Typical cardiac findings and strong indicators for heart involvement include ventricular thrombus and endocardial thickening/fibrosis while the diagnostic value of valve abnormalities, ventricle dilatation and impaired ventricle function must be evaluated in consideration of other potentially underlying heart diseases (e.g. coronary heart disease, particularly in older patients with a respective cardiac disease history).
- Whenever possible, a biopsy and histologic evaluation of potentially involved organs (e.g. skin, lungs, hearts, etc.) should be undertaken. Biopsies of the heart are notorious to reveal negative results, in these cases the extracellular matrix should be carefully checked for deposits of eosinophil-derived by immunostaining.
- There is paucity of reports on sole eosinophilic gastrointestinal or pulmonary infiltration in MPN-eo.
- Skin involvement is more frequently observed in non-clonal eosinophilia but is also seen in MPN-eo.

- If present, a biopsy of enlarged lymph nodes should be performed for diagnosis of potentially underlying extramedullary lymphoid blast phase, which is frequently primarily diagnosed as T-cell lymphoma.
- In these cases, the molecular aberration can usually be identified contemporaneously in myeloid cells derived from BM and lymphoblasts in lymph node biopsies indicating a stem cell disorder with multilineage involvement and a disparate morphologic appearance in BM and lymph node.
- There is a strikingly high incidence of lymphoid blast phase/lymphoma that may be either of B or, more commonly, T-cell phenotype in patients with the t(8;13)(p11;q12) and a *ZNF198-FGFR1* fusion gene. There are also reports on individual patients and presence of *FIP1L1-PDGFRA* in cases initially diagnosed with myeloid sarcoma.

Cytogenetics and molecular analyses

- Screening for the cytogenetically invisible *FIP1L1-PDGFRA* fusion gene from mononuclear cells of PB (equal to BM) by nested RT-PCR, genomic DNA PCR or FISH (through deletion of *CHIC2*, a gene that lies between *FIP1L1* and *PDGFRA* on 4q12) should be performed at an early stage.
- If negative, cytogenetic analysis from a BM aspirate may indicate a rearrangement and the involved TK at hot spots such as 4q12 (*PDGFRA*), 5q31-33 (*PDGFRB*), 8p11 (*FGFR1*), and 9p24 (*JAK2*).
- If the fusion partner is unknown, techniques such as RACE-PCR, long-distance inverse PCR, or RNA-seq can be used to identify fusions formed by novel cytogenetic abnormalities.
- RT-PCR or FISH should be used to confirm the presence of a suspected fusion gene, not only for diagnosis but also for improved monitoring of residual disease at low levels by nested RT-PCR.
- If cytogenetic analysis has failed (e.g. because of dry tap and lack of progenitors in PB), quantitative RT-PCR for the expression of *PDGFRA* and *PDGFRB* because significantly may indicate elevated levels are associated with the presence of respective fusion genes.
- Other chromosomal aberrations (e.g. trisomies, monosomies or deletions) are rare and not useful as indicators for targeted treatment.
- *FIP1L1-PDGFRA* negative patients with normal karyotype should be screened for *KIT* D816V because eosinophilia is also a frequent feature in advanced *KIT* D816V positive SM.
- If positive, serum tryptase levels and the morphologic assessment of a BM biopsy with aggregates of spindle-shaped tryptase/CD117 positive mast cells with atypical expression of CD25 informs the correct diagnosis (e.g. SM-CEL).
- Patients who are negative for *FIP1L1-PDGFRA*, *KIT* D816V, and chromosomal aberrations should be screened for *JAK2* V617F.

- A key challenge remains the characterization of molecular aberrations underlying the majority of MPN-eo patients where the causative pathogenetic lesion is unknown.
- Because the clinical phenotype of TK fusion gene negative cases is frequently indistinguishable from those in whom a fusion gene is present, it is likely that as yet uncharacterized mutations or rearrangements that activate intracellular signalling pathways remain to be identified.
- The recent identification of genes involved in epigenetic regulators, the spliceosomal machinery, cohesins, calreticulin, etc. in myeloid neoplasms has highlighted the benefit of high-throughput screening for mutations by targeted or exome screens.
- This will, however, not identify cryptic rearrangements and other approaches such as RNA-seq or paired end whole genome sequencing will be required.
- Imatinib is active in only a small minority of these patients and usually haematologic responses are only transient; it thus appears that uncharacterized truly imatinib-responsive abnormalities are uncommon.
- Because the clone size may be relatively small, sequencing coverage needs to be high and/or the analysis may need to be performed on purified cell populations.

Analyses of T-cell clonality

- Clonal T-lymphocytes can induce non-clonal eosinophil proliferation through overproduction of eosinophilopoietic cytokines such as IL-3, IL-5, or GM-CSF.
- Flow cytometric analysis (through detection of T-cells with aberrant phenotype, e.g. CD3–/CD4+, CD3–CD8+ or CD3+/CD4–/CD8–) or PCR analysis (through detection of T-cell receptor gene rearrangement) has been recommended for proof of T-cell clonality as potentially underlying disease mechanism for non-clonal eosinophilia.
- Both methods and particularly PCR analysis have identified clonal T cells also in reactive conditions (e.g. infections or autoimmune disorders), and a substantial subset of patients with *FIP1L1-PDGFRA* positive disease.
- In addition to the proof of *FIP1L1-PDGFRA* positive CD3-positive lymphoblasts in lymph node biopsies, these results indicate that *FIP1L1-PDGFRA* may present as a stem cell disorder with multilineage involvement.
- A summary of the diagnostic procedures is provided in Table 13.2.

Table 13.2 Important diagnostic procedures in the diagnostic work-up of HE_{US}

	Feature	Indicative for
Peripheral blood	Elevated vitamin B12	MPN-eo
	Elevated immunoglobin E	Non-clonal/reactive eosinophilia
	Creatine kinase, troponin I	Heart involvement
Bone marrow	Increased numbers of blasts and mast cells, fibrosis	MPN-eo, MLN-eo, CEL-NOS
	T-cells	Lymphoma
Genetics	*FIP1L1-PDGFRA* (PB) by RT-PCR or FISH	MLN-eo
	Cytogenetic analysis (BM) with reciprocal translocations involving 4q12, 5q31-35, 8p11, or 9p24	MLN-eo, CEL
	Mutation analysis (*KIT* D816V, *JAK2* V617F)	SM-CEL, CEL
	T-cell clonality (FACS, PCR)	e.g. CD3-/CD4+, CD-/CD8+, CD3+/CD4-/CD8-(FACS) or T-cell clonality (PCR)
Organ involvement	Histology	Proof of organ infiltration and dysfunction
	MRI (e.g. heart)	Not indicative for the differentiation between clonal vs. non-clonal eosinophilia but important for treatment decisions and prognosis

Treatment

For treatment decisions, disease stage (chronic/blast phase), potential clinical course (indolent/aggressive), sensitivity to imatinib, or alternative TK inhibitors (*de novo*/resistant disease) and eligibility for allogeneic stem cell transplantation need to be taken into account on an individual basis (Table 13.3).

FIP1L1-PDGFRA positive MLN-eo in chronic phase

- Imatinib at a dose of 100 mg/day (PDGFRα and PDGFRβ are 100 times more sensitive to imatinib than to BCR-ABL) induces complete and durable clinical and haematological remissions (CHR) in more than 90–95% of *FIP1L1-PDGFRA* positive patients within the first 3 months.
- Complete molecular remissions (CMR), as determined by nested RT-PCR, are seen in more than 80–95% of patients within 12 months

Table 13.3 Treatment of MPN-eo

Molecular aberration	Phase	Treatment
FIP1L1-PDGFRA	Chronic phase	Imatinib 100 mg/d
	Blast phase	Imatinib 100–400 mg/d
	Maintenance	Imatinib 100 mg 1–3×/week
	Secondary resistance	Allogeneic SCT (possibly after initial trial with potentially only weakly effective second generation TKI)
Other *PDGFR* fusion genes	Chronic phase	Imatinib 100–400 mg/d
	Blast phase	Imatinib 100–400 mg/d
	Maintenance	Imatinib 100–400 mg/d
	Secondary resistance	Allogeneic SCT (possibly after initial trial with potentially only weakly effective second generation TKI)
FGFR1 fusion genes	Chronic phase	Allogeneic SCT (possibly after initial trial with potentially effective TKI, e.g. ponatinib*)
	Blast phase	Allogeneic SCT after ponatinib* with or without intensive chemotherapy
JAK2 fusion gene	Chronic phase	Allogeneic SCT (possibly after initial trial with potentially effective TKI, e.g. Janus kinase (JAK) inhibitor*)
	Blast phase	Allogeneic SCT after JAK inhibitor* with or without intensive chemotherapy
KIT D816V	Advanced SM [(A)SM/MCL-AHNMD]	Midostaurin (PKC412)
		Cladribine (4–6 cycles)
		IFN
		Allogeneic SCT
JAK2 V617F	Chronic/blast phase	JAK inhibitor (indication like for myelofibrosis)
		Allogeneic SCT (indication like for myelofibrosis)
No genetic aberration	Chronic/blast phase	Hydroxyurea
		Interferon-alpha
		Allogeneic SCT

*off-label use.

(frequently much earlier in individual patients), conferring high rates of progression-free and overall survival.

- No primary resistance was yet reported by the study groups.
- Secondary resistance has only been reported in a few cases, all of whom had the appearance of a T674I or a D842V point mutation in *PDGFRA* which was shown functionally to confer resistance to imatinib (Figure 13.2).
- These mutations are analogous to T315I in the ABL kinase in imatinib-resistant CML (T674I) and to the D816V in the KIT kinase in SM (D842V). The T674I mutant is *in vitro* effectively inhibited by PKC412, sorafenib, nilotinib, and ponatinib. However, clinical responses may only be partial or transient at best and the prognosis overall is dismal. Allogeneic stem cell transplantation (SCT) should therefore be considered early. To the best of our knowledge, there is only one long-term surviving patient who relapsed with resistant disease and underwent allogeneic SCT.
- The low frequency of clinical resistance might be related to the limited repertoire of possible PDGFRA kinase domain mutations *in vitro*.
- After achievement of CHR or CMR the dose is frequently reduced to (A) 100 mg three times per week or every other day, respectively, or (B) 100 mg to 200 mg once weekly. Both schedules seem to be sufficient to maintain durable CHR and CMR at low toxicity.

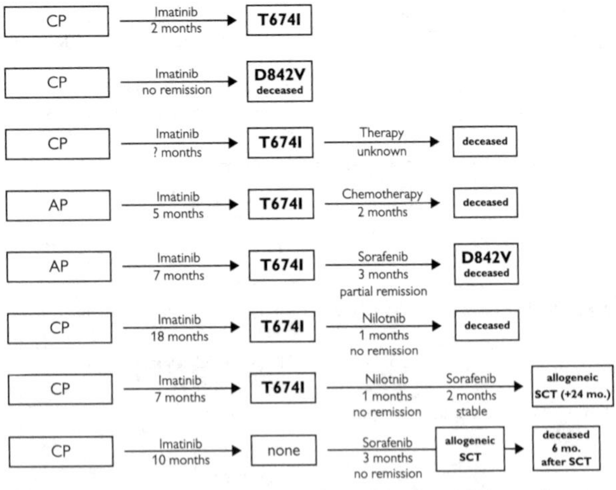

Figure 13.2 Secondary resistance in *FIP1L1-PDGFRA* positive MLN-eo in chronic (CP) and advanced phase (AP).

Source: data from Cools J, et al. 2003; Score J, et al. 2009; Metzgeroth G, et al. 2012; Griffin JH, et al. 2003; Gotlib J, et al. 2008; Lierman E, et al. 2009; Ohnishi H, et al. 2006; and von Bubnoff N, et al. 2005.

- Because the natural history of *FIP1L1-PDGFRA* positive MLN-eo is not well known, it remains challenging whether or not to treat an asymptomatic and young patient. Early initiation of therapy is reasonable because (i) development of transformation to blast phase seems inevitable, and (ii) targeted therapy results in complete remissions and can therefore prevent complications, including leukaemic transformation.
- Initial reports indicated that imatinib discontinuation or dose de-escalation leads to molecular relapse in all patients. Patients achieved a second CMR following reinstatement of imatinib, although an increased dose was needed in some patients to achieve and maintain remission.
- However, durability of CMR after cessation of imatinib has meanwhile been reported in several cases.
- Until there are data from more patients with adequate follow-up under controlled conditions, the cessation of imatinib cannot be generally recommended (also because the sensitivity with which *FIP1L1-PDGFRA* can be detected is relatively low and the PCR methodologies are not standardized).

Other *PDGFR* fusion genes in chronic phase

- Excellent clinical and haematological responses to imatinib have also been reported in cases with other *PDGFRA* and *PDGFRB* fusion genes.
- Patients with *PDGFRB* fusions are more often treated in the same way as patients with *BCR-ABL* positive CML (i.e. imatinib 400 mg/day). Meanwhile, we have however also observed rapid and durable responses using the same dosing schedules as for patients with *FIP1L1-PDGFRA* positive disease (unpublished).
- When investigated in due course, the majority of patients also achieved complete cytogenetic response or disappearance of fusion transcripts as measured by RT-PCR.

PDGFR fusion genes in blast phase

- Patients with various *PDGFR* fusion genes can also present with either i) myeloid blast phase (>20% blasts in PB and/or BM), ii) extramedullary lymphoid blast phase/lymphoma (lymph node infiltration by lymphoblasts of T-cell origin) or iii) chloroma (extramedullary tissue infiltration by myeloid blasts) (Figure 13.3).
- We have recently reported on 17 patients. Nine patients received primary chemotherapy or even subsequent allogeneic SCT (n = 2) but all patients were resistant or relapsed. Seven patients received imatinib as second-line treatment after the underlying fusion genes were identified as consequence of persisting eosinophilia while 8 patients were primarily treated with imatinib. Rapid CHR was achieved in all 15 patients and CMR was observed in all 12 *FIP1L1-PDGFRA* positive patients after a median of 5.4 months (2.9–32.0). One patient died of disease-independent causes. Eleven *FIP1L1-PDGFRA* positive patients are in sustained CMR for a median 65 months (7–103) and three patients with a *PDGFRB* fusion gene are in sustained CHR for median 56 months.

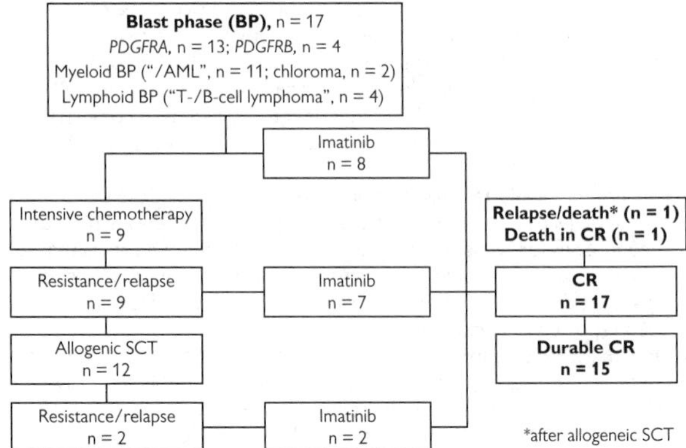

Figure 13.3 Imatinib in advanced MLN-eo as primary or secondary treatment after failure to intensive chemotherapy or allogeneic SCT.[31] CR (complete clinical and haematological remission, patients with *PDGFRB* fusion genes in complete cytogenetic remission, *FIP1L1-PDGFRA* positive patients in complete molecular remission).

Source: data from Metzgeroth G, et al. (2013). Long-term follow-up of treatment with imatinib in eosinophilia-associated myeloid/lymphoid neoplasms with PDGFR rearrangements in blast phase. *Leukemia*. 27(11):2254–6. DOI: 10.1038/leu.2013.129.

Other TK fusion genes

- MPN-eo with involvement of *FGFR1* and *JAK2* are frequently associated with an aggressive clinical course due to rapid transformation to blast phase, usually of myeloid phenotype.
- FGFR1 and JAK2 fusion proteins are unaffected by imatinib and due to the poor prognosis, early allogeneic SCT should be considered for eligible patients with a suitable donor.
- The JAK1/JAK2 inhibitor ruxolitinib has successfully been used in some *PCM1-JAK2* positive patients with achievement of CHR and complete cytogenetic responses (CCyR) but relapse may occur early.
- *In vitro* data suggest potential activity of ponatinib in *FGFR1* fusion genes and first results on the efficacy of ponatinib in patients with *FGFR1* fusion genes are awaited. Molecular confirmation of all candidate fusions should be obtained as cytogenetics alone may not be sufficient.
- Individual patients with *ETV6-ABL1* and *ETV6-FLT3* positive MPN-eo or MDS/MPN-eo achieved CHR and CCyR on imatinib and nilotinib or the FLT3 inhibitors sunitinib and/or sorafenib, respectively. Of note, one *ETV6-FLT3* positive patient developed secondary resistance due to a secondary N841K point mutation.

Reference

1. Vardiman JW, Thiele J, Arber DA, et al. The 2008 revision of the World Health Organization (WHO) classification of myeloid neoplasm and acute leukaemia: rational and important changes. *Blood*. 2009;114(5):937–51.

Further reading

Aguiar RC, Chase A, Coulthard S, et al. Abnormalities of chromosome band 8p11 in leukemia: two clinical syndromes can be distinguished on the basis of MOZ involvement. *Blood*. 1997;90:3130–5.

Apperley JF, Gardembas M, Melo JV, et al. Response to imatinib mesylate in patients with chronic myeloproliferative diseases with rearrangements of the platelet-derived growth factor receptor beta. *N Engl J Med*. 2002;347:481–7.

Arefi M, Garcia JL, Briz MM, et al. Response to imatinib mesylate in patients with hypereosinophilic syndrome. *Int J Hematol*. 2012;96:320–6.

Baccarani M, Cilloni D, Rondoni M, et al. The efficacy of imatinib mesylate in patients with FIP1L1-PDGFRalpha-positive hypereosinophilic syndrome. Results of a multicenter prospective study. *Haematologica*. 2007;92:1173–9.

Baxter EJ, Kulkarni S, Vizmanos JL, et al. Novel translocations that disrupt the platelet-derived growth factor receptor beta (PDGFRB) gene in BCR-ABL-negative chronic myeloproliferative disorders. *Br J Haematol*. 2003;120:251–6.

Capovilla M, Cayuela JM, Bilhou-Nabera C, et al. Synchronous FIP1L1-PDGFRA-positive chronic eosinophilic leukemia and T-cell lymphoblastic lymphoma: a bilineal clonal malignancy. *Eur J Haematol*. 2008;80:81–6.

Chen D, Bachanova V, Ketterling RP, Begna KH, Hanson CA, Viswanatha DS. A case of nonleukemic myeloid sarcoma with FIP1L1-PDGFRA rearrangement: an unusual presentation of a rare disease. *Am J Surg Pathol*. 2013;37:147–51.

Cools J, DeAngelo DJ, Gotlib J, et al. A tyrosine kinase created by fusion of the PDGFRA and FIP1L1 genes as a therapeutic target of imatinib in idiopathic hypereosinophilic syndrome. *N Engl J Med*. 2003;348:1201–14.

Cools J, Mentens N, Odero MD, et al. Evidence for position effects as a variant ETV6-mediated leukemogenic mechanism in myeloid leukemias with a t(4;12)(q11-q12;p13) or t(5;12)(q31;p13). *Blood*. 2002;99:1776–84.

Cross NCP, Hoade Y, Tapper WJ, et al. Recurrent activating STAT5B N642H mutation in myeloid neoplasms with eosinophilia. *Leukemia*. 2019 Feb;33(2):415–25. doi:10.1038/s41375-018-0342-3.

Dasari S, Naha K, Hande M, Vivek G. A novel subtype of myeloproliferative disorder? JAK2V617F-associated hypereosinophilia with hepatic venous thrombosis. *BMJ Case Rep*. 2013;2013:pii: bcr2013200087.

David M, Cross NC, Burgstaller S, et al. Durable responses to imatinib in patients with PDGFRB fusion gene-positive and BCR-ABL-negative chronic myeloproliferative disorders. *Blood*. 2007;109:61–4.

Elling C, Erben P, Walz C, et al. Novel imatinib-sensitive PDGFRA-activating point mutations in hypereosinophilic syndrome induce growth factor independence and leukemia-like disease. *Blood*. 2011;117:2935–43.

Erben P, Gosenca D, Muller MC, et al. Screening for diverse PDGFRA or PDGFRB fusion genes is facilitated by generic quantitative reverse transcriptase polymerase chain reaction analysis. *Haematologica*. 2010;95:738–44.

Galimberti S, Ciabatti E, Ottimo F, et al. Cell clonality in hypereosinophilic syndrome: what pathogenetic role? *Clin Exp Rheumatol*. 2007;25:17–22.

Gotlib J, Akin C. Mast cells and eosinophils in mastocytosis, chronic eosinophilic leukemia, and non-clonal disorders. *Semin Hematol*. 2012;49:128–37.

Gotlib J, Cools J. Five years since the discovery of FIP1L1-PDGFRA: what we have learned about the fusion and other molecularly defined eosinophilias. *Leukemia*. 2008;22:1999–2010.

Griffin JH, Leung J, Bruner RJ, Caligiuri MA, Briesewitz R. Discovery of a fusion kinase in EOL-1 cells and idiopathic hypereosinophilic syndrome. *Proc Natl Acad Sci U S A*. 2003;100:7830–5.

Helbig G, Kyrcz-Krzemien S. Cessation of imatinib mesylate may lead to sustained hematologic and molecular remission in FIP1L1-PDGFRA-mutated hypereosinophilic syndrome. *Am J Hematol*. 2013;89(1):115.

Helbig G, Moskwa A, Hus M, et al. Clinical characteristics of patients with chronic eosinophilic leukaemia (CEL) harbouring FIP1L1-PDGFRA fusion transcript--results of Polish multicentre study. *Hematol Oncol*. 2010;28:93–7.

Helbig G, Moskwa A, Hus M, et al. Heterogeneity among characteristics of hypereosinophilic syndromes. *J Allergy Clin Immunol*. 2010;125:1399–401.e2.

Jones AV, Kreil S, Zoi K, et al. Widespread occurrence of the JAK2 V617F mutation in chronic myeloproliferative disorders. *Blood*. 2005;106:2162–8.

Jovanovic JV, Score J, Waghorn K, et al. Low-dose imatinib mesylate leads to rapid induction of major molecular responses and achievement of complete molecular remission in FIP1L1-PDGFRA-positive chronic eosinophilic leukemia. *Blood*. 2007;109:4635–40.

Klion AD, Noel P, Akin C, et al. Elevated serum tryptase levels identify a subset of patients with a myeloproliferative variant of idiopathic hypereosinophilic syndrome associated with tissue fibrosis, poor prognosis, and imatinib responsiveness. *Blood*. 2003;101:4660–6.

Klion AD, Robyn J, Akin C, et al. Molecular remission and reversal of myelofibrosis in response to imatinib mesylate treatment in patients with the myeloproliferative variant of hypereosinophilic syndrome. *Blood*. 2004;103:473–8.

Klion AD, Robyn J, Maric I, et al. Relapse following discontinuation of imatinib mesylate therapy for FIP1L1/PDGFRA-positive chronic eosinophilic leukemia: implications for optimal dosing. *Blood*. 2007;110:3552–6.

Krause DS, Van Etten RA. Tyrosine kinases as targets for cancer therapy. *N Engl J Med*. 2005;353:172–87.

Legrand F, Renneville A, Macintyre E, et al. The Spectrum of FIP1L1-PDGFRA-associated chronic eosinophilic leukemia: new insights based on a survey of 44 cases. *Medicine (Baltimore)*. 2013;92(5):e1–9.

Lierman E, Folens C, Stover EH, et al. Sorafenib is a potent inhibitor of FIP1L1-PDGFRalpha and the imatinib-resistant FIP1L1-PDGFRalpha T674I mutant. *Blood*. 2006;108:1374–6.

Lierman E, Michaux L, Beullens E, et al. FIP1L1-PDGFRalpha D842V, a novel panresistant mutant, emerging after treatment of FIP1L1-PDGFRalpha T674I eosinophilic leukemia with single agent sorafenib. *Leukemia*. 2009;23:845–51.

Lierman E, Smits S, Cools J, Dewaele B, Debiec-Rychter M, Vandenberghe P. Ponatinib is active against imatinib-resistant mutants of FIP1L1-PDGFRA and KIT, and against FGFR1-derived fusion kinases. *Leukemia*. 2012;26:1693–5.

Macdonald D, Reiter A, Cross NC. The 8p11 myeloproliferative syndrome: a distinct clinical entity caused by constitutive activation of FGFR1. *Acta Haematol*. 2002;107:101–7.

Metzgeroth G, Erben P, Martin H, et al. Limited clinical activity of nilotinib and sorafenib in FIP1L1-PDGFRA positive chronic eosinophilic leukemia with imatinib-resistant T674I mutation. *Leukemia*. 2012;26:162–4.

Metzgeroth G, Schwaab J, Gosenca D, et al. Long-term follow-up of treatment with imatinib in eosinophilia-associated myeloid/lymphoid neoplasms with PDGFR rearrangements in blast phase. *Leukemia*. 2013;27:2254–6.

Metzgeroth G, Walz C, Erben P, et al. Safety and efficacy of imatinib in chronic eosinophilic leukaemia and hypereosinophilic syndrome: a phase-II study. *Br J Haematol*. 2008;143:707–15.

Metzgeroth G, Walz C, Score J, et al. Recurrent finding of the FIP1L1-PDGFRA fusion gene in eosinophilia-associated acute myeloid leukemia and lymphoblastic T-cell lymphoma. *Leukemia*. 2007;21:1183–8.

Ohnishi H, Kandabashi K, Maeda Y, Kawamura M, Watanabe T. Chronic eosinophilic leukaemia with FIP1L1-PDGFRA fusion and T6741 mutation that evolved from Langerhans cell histiocytosis with eosinophilia after chemotherapy. *Br J Haematol*. 2006;134:547–9.

Pardanani A, D'Souza A, Knudson RA, Hanson CA, Ketterling RP, Tefferi A. Long-term follow-up of FIP1L1-PDGFRA-mutated patients with eosinophilia: survival and clinical outcome. *Leukemia*. 2012;26:2439–41.

Pardanani A, Ketterling RP, Brockman SR, et al. CHIC2 deletion, a surrogate for FIP1L1-PDGFRA fusion, occurs in systemic mastocytosis associated with eosinophilia and predicts response to imatinib mesylate therapy. *Blood*. 2003;102:3093–6.

Patel AB, Franzini A, Leroy E, et al. JAK2 ex13InDel drives oncogenic transformation and is associated with chronic eosinophilic leukemia and polycythemia vera. *Blood*. 2019 Dec 26;134(26):2388–98.

Perna F, Abdel-Wahab O, Levine RL, Jhanwar SC, Imada K, Nimer SD. ETV6-ABL1-positive 'chronic myeloid leukemia': clinical and molecular response to tyrosine kinase inhibition. *Haematologica*. 2011;96:342–3.

Reiter A, Grimwade D, Cross NC. Diagnostic and therapeutic management of eosinophilia-associated chronic myeloproliferative disorders. *Haematologica*. 2007;92:1153–8.

Reiter A, Walz C, Cross NC. Tyrosine kinases as therapeutic targets in BCR-ABL negative chronic myeloproliferative disorders. *Curr Drug Targets*. 2007;8:205–16.

Reiter A, Walz C, Watmore A, et al. The t(8;9)(p22;p24) is a recurrent abnormality in chronic and acute leukemia that fuses PCM1 to JAK2. *Cancer Res*. 2005;65:2662–7.

Rumi E, Milosevic JD, Casetti I, et al. Efficacy of ruxolitinib in chronic eosinophilic leukemia associated with a PCM1-JAK2 fusion gene. *J Clin Oncol*. 2013;31:e269–71.

Sadovnik I, Lierman E, Peter B, et al. Identification of Ponatinib as a potent inhibitor of growth, migration and activation of neoplastic eosinophils carrying FIP1L1-PDGFRA. *Exp Hematol.* 2014;42(4):282–93.e4.

Schwaab J, Knut M, Haferlach C, et al. Limited duration of complete remission on ruxolitinib in myeloid neoplasms with PCM1-JAK2 and BCR-JAK2 fusion genes. *Ann Hematol.* 2015;94:233–8.

Score J, Curtis C, Waghorn K, et al. Identification of a novel imatinib responsive KIF5B-PDGFRA fusion gene following screening for PDGFRA overexpression in patients with hypereosinophilia. *Leukemia.* 2006;20:827–32.

Score J, Walz C, Jovanovic JV, et al. Detection and molecular monitoring of FIP1L1-PDGFRA-positive disease by analysis of patient-specific genomic DNA fusion junctions. *Leukemia.* 2009;23:332–9.

Steer EJ, Cross NC. Myeloproliferative disorders with translocations of chromosome 5q31-35: role of the platelet-derived growth factor receptor Beta. *Acta Haematol.* 2002;107:113–22.

Stover EH, Chen J, Folens C, et al. Activation of FIP1L1-PDGFRalpha requires disruption of the juxtamembrane domain of PDGFRalpha and is FIP1L1-independent. *Proc Natl Acad Sci U S A.* 2006;103:8078–83.

Tang TC, Chang H, Chuang WY. Complete response of myeloid sarcoma with FIP1L1-PDGFRA-associated myeloproliferative neoplasms to imatinib mesylate monotherapy. *Acta Haematol.* 2012;128:83–7.

Tefferi A, Gotlib J, Pardanani A. Hypereosinophilic syndrome and clonal eosinophilia: point-of-care diagnostic algorithm and treatment update. *Mayo Clin Proc.* 2010;85:158–64.

Tefferi A, Pardanani A, Li CY. Hypereosinophilic syndrome with elevated serum tryptase versus systemic mast cell disease associated with eosinophilia: 2 distinct entities? *Blood.* 2003;102:3073–4; author reply 4.

Valent P, Gleich GJ, Reiter A, et al. Pathogenesis and classification of eosinophil disorders: a review of recent developments in the field. *Exp Rev Hematol.* 2012;5:157–76.

Valent P, Horny HP, Bochner BS, Haferlach T, Reiter A. Controversies and open questions in the definitions and classification of the hypereosinophilic syndromes and eosinophilic leukemias. *Semin Hematol.* 2012;49:171–81.

Valent P, Klion AD, Horny HP, et al. Contemporary consensus proposal on criteria and classification of eosinophilic disorders and related syndromes. *J Allergy Clin Immunol.* 2012;130:607–12.e9.

Vardiman JW, Thiele J, Arber DA, et al. The 2008 revision of the World Health Organization (WHO) classification of myeloid neoplasm and acute leukaemia: rational and important changes. *Blood.* 2009;114(5):937–51.

von Bubnoff N, Gorantla SP, Engh RA, et al. The low frequency of clinical resistance to PDGFR inhibitors in myeloid neoplasms with abnormalities of PDGFRA might be related to the limited repertoire of possible PDGFRA kinase domain mutations *in vitro*. *Oncogene.* 2011;30:933–43.

von Bubnoff N, Gorantla SP, Thone S, Peschel C, Duyster J. The FIP1L1-PDGFRA T674I mutation can be inhibited by the tyrosine kinase inhibitor AMN107 (nilotinib). *Blood.* 2006;107:4970–1; author reply 2.

von Bubnoff N, Sandherr M, Schlimok G, Andreesen R, Peschel C, Duyster J. Myeloid blast crisis evolving during imatinib treatment of an FIP1L1-PDGFR alpha-positive chronic myeloproliferative disease with prominent eosinophilia. *Leukemia.* 2005;19:286–7.

Walz C, Chase A, Schoch C, et al. The t(8;17)(p11;q23) in the 8p11 myeloproliferative syndrome fuses MYO18A to FGFR1. *Leukemia.* 2005;19:1005–9.

Walz C, Cross NC, Van Etten RA, Reiter A. Comparison of mutated ABL1 and JAK2 as oncogenes and drug targets in myeloproliferative disorders. *Leukemia.* 2008;22:1320–34.

Walz C, Curtis C, Schnittger S, et al. Transient response to imatinib in a chronic eosinophilic leukemia associated with ins(9;4)(q33;q12q25) and a CDK5RAP2-PDGFRA fusion gene. *Genes Chromosomes Cancer.* 2006;45:950–6.

Walz C, Erben P, Ritter M, et al. Response of ETV6-FLT3-positive myeloid/lymphoid neoplasm with eosinophilia to inhibitors of FMS-like tyrosine kinase 3. *Blood.* 2011;118:2239–42.

Walz C, Haferlach C, Hanel A, et al. Identification of a MYO18A-PDGFRB fusion gene in an eosinophilia-associated atypical myeloproliferative neoplasm with a t(5;17)(q33-34;q11.2). *Genes Chromosomes Cancer.* 2009;48:179–83.

Walz C, Metzgeroth G, Haferlach C, et al. Characterization of three new imatinib-responsive fusion genes in chronic myeloproliferative disorders generated by disruption of the platelet-derived growth factor receptor beta gene. *Haematologica.* 2007;92:163–9.

Chapter 14

Transformation of myeloproliferative neoplasms to acute leukaemia

Omar Abdelwahab, Raajit Rampal, Catriona Jamieson, and Tariq I. Mughal

Introduction *223*
Incidence and risk factors *223*
Genetics and biology of transformation *225*
Clinical features *228*
Treatment *229*
Conclusion *231*

Introduction

The natural history of chronic myeloproliferative neoplasms (MPN), both Philadelphia-chromosome positive [chronic myeloid leukaemia (CML)] and negative [essential thrombocythaemia (ET), polycythaemia vera (PV), and primary myelofibrosis (PMF)] has been well documented but the mechanism underlying the apparently inexorable progression from an initial, rather indolent or chronic phase (CP) to advanced phase, a term including accelerated phase (AP) and blast crisis (BC), remains obscure. Most patients with MPN present in the indolent phase, during which myeloid progenitor numbers are greatly increased in the bone marrow and blood. This phase may continue for as little as 1 year or as long as 20 years or more, but eventually it transforms into acute leukaemia (BC), in which an increasing proportion of blast cells are found in the marrow and peripheral blood. The risk associated with the development of advanced-phase disease differs depending on the MPN subtype and is influenced by a number of factors such as duration of disease, clinical factors, the presence of certain mutations, and in some cases, the therapeutic interventions. ET probably carries the low rate of transformation to acute myeloid leukaemia (AML), whereas myelofibrosis (MF) may carry a relatively high risk; lymphoid transformation has been reported in rare cases. The risk of transformation in CML to BC in the protein tyrosine kinase inhibitors (TKI) era appears to be quite low at <2% per annum. Transformation to AML is a challenging complication in myelodysplastic syndrome (MDS) and myelodysplastic/myeloproliferative syndrome also. Transformed disease in general tends to be difficult to manage and is associated with a poor prognosis. This chapter will address recent translational research efforts which enhance our understanding of the underlying mechanisms for transformation, and also the emerging genetic landscape and investigational therapies.

Incidence and risk factors

For patients with CML, there are at least two definitions of BC, both of which rather arbitrary. The European LeukemiaNet (ELN) requires the presence of more than 30% blasts in the blood or marrow or the demonstration of extramedullary blastic infiltrates, while the World Health Organization (WHO) proposed a blast count of more than 20%, in keeping with the definition of AML. With this *caveat*, current estimates suggest about 10–15% of CML patients are diagnosed in advanced phase, and small numbers of CP cases, perhaps less than 2% per annum, experience disease progression each year during TKI treatment. A small minority of CML patients present in 'sudden' BC following having achieved an optimal response. In the interferon era, this was defined as onset of BC within 3 months of previously documented complete haematological response, while in the TKI era as BC arising after a documented complete cytogenetic response, and within 3 months of a documented complete haematological response. These patients present a rare but significant dilemma as the BC arises abruptly in the setting of optimal disease control. Currently no suitable biomarkers have been identified which might help identify these patients at diagnosis and potentially considered for more effective therapies, including an allogeneic stem cell transplantation.

In the *BCR-ABL1*-negative MPN, the risk of developing leukaemic transformation is in part dependent on the chronic-phase disease subtype, with MF carrying the highest risk of transformation. The estimated rate of leukaemic transformation from MF is approximately 20–30% during the first 10 years of diagnosis, with a median time to diagnosis of 2–4 years. ET and PV carry a lower risk of leukaemic transformation with a median time to diagnosis of acute leukaemia, respectively, of 15 and 14 years. Retrospective analyses have identified a number of risk factors associated with leukaemic transformation. Blood count parameters such as elevated white blood cell count, markedly elevated platelet count, anaemia, thrombocytopenia, and the presence of circulating blasts have all been linked to an elevated risk of leukaemic transformation in various retrospective series (Table 14.1). In addition, cytogenetic abnormalities such as monosomal karyotype and chromosome 17p deletions have been associated with increased risk of transformation. Some of the factors have been incorporated into prognostic scoring systems such as the Dynamic International Prognostic Scoring System (DIPSS and DIPSS-plus). Several treatment modalities for chronic-phase disease (some of which are more historic than utilized currently) have been associated with a risk of leukaemic progression. For example, the use of pipobroman, busulfan, radioactive phosphorus (P^{32}), danazol, and even erythropoiesis-stimulating agents have been demonstrated to increase risk of leukaemic transformation. Moreover, there has been considerable debate regarding the possible contribution of hydroxyurea (hydroxycarbamide) to leukemogenesis. Similarly, the impact of splenectomy on leukaemic transformation has been a subject of debate, with some studies demonstrating an increased risk of transformation and others not. Regardless of the risk factors, transformation to secondary AML carries a poor prognosis.

Table 14.1 Clinical risk factors for MPN to transform to acute leukaemia

MPN subtype	Risk factor
ET	Anaemia (<10 g/dL) or thrombocytosis (>1000 × 10^9/L)
PV	Age >70 years or prior exposure to P^{32}, busulfan, or pipobroman
MF	Leucocytosis >30 × 10^9/L, peripheral blood blasts >3% or platelets <100 × 10^9/L
	Abnormal cytogenetics, in particular monosomal or high-risk karyotype
	Bone marrow blasts >10%
	Previous splenectomy
	Time to development of anaemia (<10 g/dL), leucocytosis (>30 × 10^9/L), platelets <150 × 10^9/L

The rate and incidence of AML transformation in MDS/MPN is unknown, except for chronic myelomonocytic leukaemia (CMML) and MDS/MPN-RS-T. The incidence of CMML transforming to AML ranges between 15% and 52%, with ASXL1 or RUNX1, higher white blood counts, marrow cellularity, karyotype risk score, and revised International Prostate Symptom Score (IPSS) score increasing risk. The frequency of MDS/MPN-RS-T transforming to AML appears higher than that in ET. Collectively, MDS/MPN appears to have a higher risk of transformation compared to MPN, akin to that in MDS.

Genetics and biology of transformation

The observations of age-related clonal haematopoiesis of indeterminate potential, comprising of recurrent somatic mutations in several genes, such as *ASXL1*, *DNMT3A*, *JAK2*, and *TET2*, and an increased risk of myeloid malignancies, have led to the hypothesis that, in some cases, secondary AML might also arise because of sequential acquisition of mutations in chronic myeloid malignancies that are senescence-dependent.

In CML, despite the very substantial reduction of CML cells following treatment with *ABL1* TKI, genomic *BCR-ABL1* persists in the bone marrow of most, if not all, patients with CML, including those with sustained complete molecular responses. Progression to BC probably arises in the progenitor cells and involves additional mutations, involving genetic and epigenetic events, *BCR-ABL1* amplification, escape from adaptive and innate immune responses, and activation of additional molecular pathways, such as β-catenin pathway in granulocyte-macrophage progenitors (Figure 14.1). This enhances the self-renewal activity and leukaemic potential of these progenitors. Recent efforts have identified overexpression of *SETBP1*, *HOXA9*, or *HOXA10* and *MYB*, to play a pivotal role in the immortalization of the granulocyte-macrophage progenitors and progression of CML in CP to myeloid BC. Other candidate genes involved include *MYC*, *Cyclin D1*, *SRC*, *BMI-1*, *HOXB4*, *PRAME*, *ARG*, *ABL2*, *BCL2* family, and notch.

Work done by Skorski, Perrotti, and others suggests candidate trigger mechanisms for BC to include an overproduction of reactive oxygen species (ROS), corruption of the efficiency and/or fidelity of DNA repair, and continued *BCR-ABL*1 activity. More recently, Jamieson and her colleagues performed whole-transcriptome ribonucleic acid (RNA) sequencing of BC leukaemic stem cells (LSC) and confirmed the role of adenosine deaminase acting on double-stranded RNA (ADAR) family of editases in the survival and self-renewal of the LSC. This seminal observation may indeed serve as a tool to predict for transformation and therapy. CML cells also acquire additional cytogenetic abnormalities (ACA), which can worsen the genomic instability and trigger BC.

Cytogenetic analysis of a cohort of post-MPN AML patients has revealed recurrent deletions on chromosome 7p, with mapping of the deleted region to *IKZF1*. High-resolution single nucleotide polymorphism analysis has revealed that the number of genomic changes in patients with post-MPN AML is significantly greater than in chronic-phase patients (Figure 14.2).

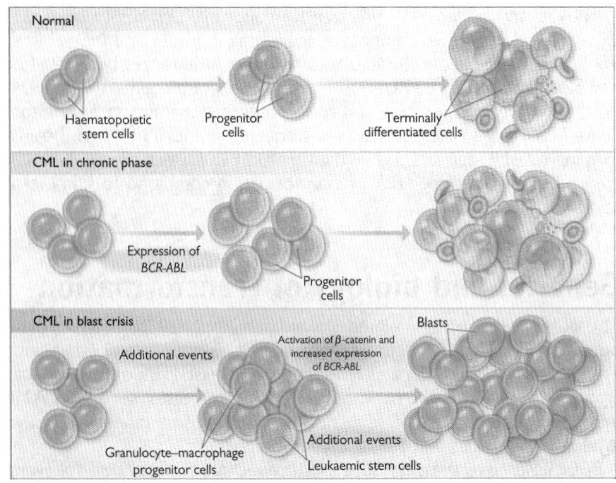

Figure 14.1 Schematic representation of the role of activated β-Catenin in the progression of CML (also see plate section).

Reproduced from Jamieson CH, et al. (2004). Granulocyte-macrophage progenitors as candidate leukemic stem cells in blast-crisis CML. *N Engl J Med.* 351(7):657–67. DOI: 10.1056/NEJMoa040258.

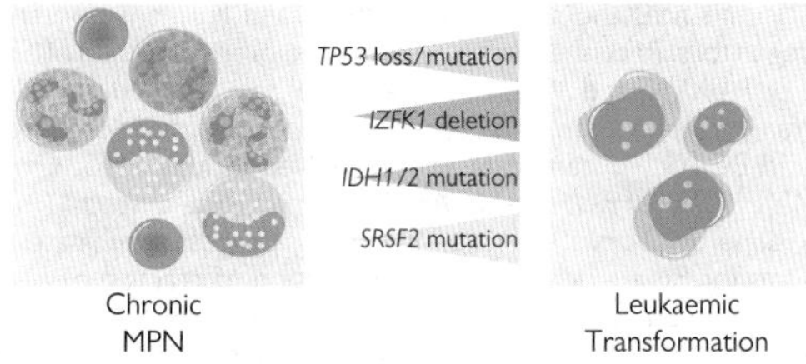

Figure 14.2 Genetic alterations associated with transformation of BCR/ABL-negative myeloproliferative neoplasms (MPN) to acute myeloid leukaemia (AML). Deletions of *IKZF1* and *TP53* have been reported to have high association with AML transformation as have mutations in *TP53, IDH1, IDH2*, or *SRSF2*.

This work also revealed alterations in regions containing known drivers of leukemogenesis, such as *MYC, ETV6*, p53, and *RUNX1*, as well as regions containing genes, such as *CUTL1, SH2B2, PIN1, ICAM1, CDC37*, and *ERG*. Numerous candidate gene sequencing studies have also been performed to identify possible mutational drivers of *BCR-ABL*1-negative MPN transformation to AML. These studies have revealed recurrent mutations in several pathways, including mutations in splicing factors, such as *SRSF2, ZRSR2, U2AF1*, and *SF3B1*. Importantly, *SRSF2* mutations are associated with a significantly impaired survival in this population, and indeed other studies have demonstrated that the presence of *SRSF2* mutations negatively affects leukaemia-free survival in MF patients. Recurrent mutations in epigenetic regulators, such as *TET2, ASXL1*, and *IDH1/2*, have also been observed at leukaemic transformation, and *ASXL1* and *IDH1/2* mutations negatively affect leukaemia-free survival. Mutations in the *RAS* signalling pathway have also been observed at the time of leukaemic transformation. Among the most common genomic alterations to occur at the time of transformation are mutations in p*53*, which have been reported to occur with an incidence of approximately 27% in two independent studies. Furthermore, the variant allele frequency of p*53* mutations appears to increase at the time of leukaemic transformation, suggesting that this mutation plays a role in the process of transformation. It is notable that spectrum and frequency of mutations which occur at the time of leukaemic transformation appear to differ from those observed in *de novo* AML. As an example, mutations in genes such as *FLT3, DNMT3a*, and *NMP1* are among the most frequently observed in *de novo* AML, yet these mutations are infrequently observed in post-MPN AML. This suggests the possibility of divergent mechanisms of leukemogenesis, and may have implications for treatment strategies. Table 14.2 depicts a comparative assessment of the somatic mutations in MF and MPN transformed to AML, compared with PV and ET.

While it is clear that the accumulation of new genomic alterations contributes to the process of leukaemic transformation, it is likely that strict temporal acquisition of mutations is but only one process that facilitates transformation. Evidence for this comes from the observation that the *JAK2V617F* mutation is not always retained at the time of evolution to acute leukaemia. Further *TET2* mutations may be acquired at the time of leukaemic transformation or occur before the acquisition of *TET2* mutations, but *ASXL1* mutations are often present in both the leukaemic-phase and chronic-phase MPN. These observations indicate that multiple paths for the development of leukaemic transformation exist, such as acquisition of

Table 14.2 Recurrent somatic mutations enriched in MF and MPN transformed to AML compared with PV and ET

Disease	Somatic mutations						
	TET2	ASXL1	IDH1/2	LNK	EZH2	DNMT3a	TP53
PV	9.8–16%	2.5%	1.9%	Rare VF-patients	–	–	–
ET	4.4–5%	5.6%	0.8%	3–6%	–	–	–
PMF, post-PV/ET MF	7.7–17%	13–23%	3.4%	3–6%	13%	6.5%	3.1%
MPN transformed to AML	18%	18%	21.6–31%	–	0%	0%	27.3%

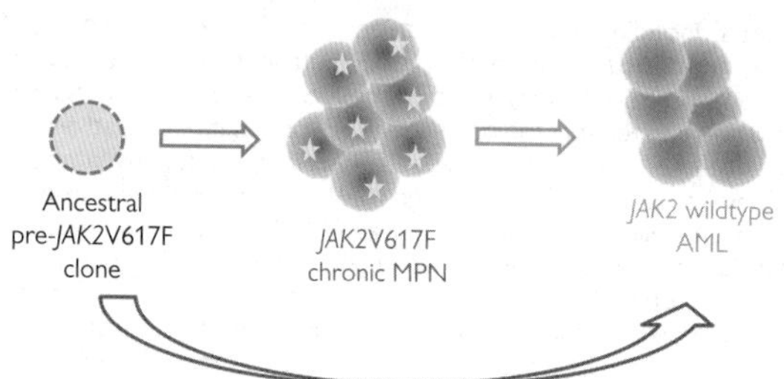

Figure 14.3 Leukaemic transformation of chronic myeloproliferative neoplasms (MPN) may occur from a common precursor clone or distinct precursor. A proportion of patients with leukaemic transformation of JAK2V617F-mutant MPN may develop JAK2 wild-type acute myeloid leukaemia (AML). This finding suggests that leukaemic transformation may occur from a distinct precursor cell than that which give rise to the MPN and/or that the JAK2-mutation is not essential for leukaemic transformation.

additional mutational events in an MPN clone, development of an AML and MPN from a common precursor clone, or development of an MPN and AML from distinct precursor clones (Figure 14.3). Evaluation of clonal evolution using paired MPN and AML samples is required for further understanding of this process.

The use of the genomic data described here to better understand the pathobiology of leukaemic transformation and ultimately to convert such understanding into therapeutic gains requires the development of accurate preclinical models of disease. Towards this end, a murine model of leukaemic transformation in which loss of p*53* cooperates with *JAK2*V617F to promote AML has been developed, thus validating human genetic observations. Given the breadth of genomic alterations observed in post-MPN AML, new models will need to be developed to further understand the biology of transformation, as well as to identify targets for therapeutic intervention.

In MDS/MPN, cytogenetic progression, often involving abnormalities in chromosomes 7 (target genes *EZH2, IKZF1*), 8 (*MYC*), 17p (*TP53*), 21 (*ERG, RUNX1*), and 12 (*ETV6*) is observed at transformation. MDS/MPN with an i(17q) (leading to *TP53* haploinsufficiency) may be a distinct disease entity with further increased risk of AML progression. Patients with chronic neutrophilic leukaemia, who typically have the CSF3R mutation at diagnosis, often develop additional spliceosome gene mutations, in particular involving *SRSF2, SETBP1, NRAS*, and *CBL*, at time of progression to myeloid BC.

Clinical features

Most patients who transform to acute leukaemia present with signs and symptoms which are indistinguishable from those of *de novo* acute

Box 14.1 Highlights of MPN transformed to AML

- Clinical and laboratory features help identify patients with MPN who are at risk of transforming to AML.
- The prognosis of secondary AML remains poor, with few responses to conventional AML therapies.
- Genomic landscape is helping establish somatic mutations, such as in ASXL1, EZH2, IDH1/2, SRSF2, which appear to be predictive of an increased risk of leukaemic transformation in MPN.
- JAK2V617F + TP53 is a common mutational combination in post-MPN AML, and is sufficient to induce AML *in vivo*.
- Best treatment options at present are participating in suitable clinical trials.

leukaemia. They tend to present fatigue, bleeding, and an increased risk of infections; many exhibit weight loss, bone pain, fever, night sweats, and enlarging splenomegaly. The laboratory features include at least 20% blasts in the blood or bone marrow (WHO definition of BC), anaemia and thrombocytopenia, and ACA. Interestingly, there is often a discrepancy in the blast count between blood and bone marrow, which can often be complicated further by the fact that an aspirate is often unobtainable in patients with advanced phases of MPN with its associated fibrosis, particularly in *BCR-ABL1*-negative MPN. Transformation may also arise in regions of extramedullary haematopoiesis and present as extramedullary disease.

AML which emerges from MPN is not restricted to one particular subtype (Box 14.1). Rather, almost all AML morphologic subtypes (excluding acute promyelocytic leukaemia) have been reported in post-MPN AML. Interestingly, acute erythroid leukaemia and acute megakaryocytic leukaemia appear to occur relatively more often in post-MPN AML. As well, although AML is by far the most frequent type of acute leukaemia to occur following an antecedent MPN, cases of lymphoblastic transformation have been reported.

Treatment

The management of most, if not all, MPN patients who transform to acute leukaemia remains unsatisfactory, unlike those in AP, whose outcome is considerably better. Most patients tend to receive conventional acute leukaemia (*de novo*) treatments with little success and often substantial toxicity. In the case of myeloid transformation, it may be in part attributable to the divergent genetic background observed in *de novo* AML and post-MPN AML. In one series, the reported median overall survival of patients with leukaemic transformation was 2.6 months. For patients treated with AML-like induction therapy, survival was lengthened to 3.9 months, with no reported complete remissions. A proportion of patients reverted to chronic-phase disease, with, however, reported median survival of only 6.2 months. Another study demonstrated a complete remission rate (with or without count recovery) of 46%. However, responses were not durable, with median progression-free survival of 5 months.

Treatment of post-MPN AML with the hypomethylating agents azacytidine and decitabine has demonstrated activity in post-MPN AML. The use of azacytidine in a group of MPN patient who had progressed to AML or MDS demonstrated an overall response rate of 52%, including a 24% complete remission rate. A report from a single institution utilizing decitabine in a series of patients with blast-phase MPN demonstrated a median survival beyond 9 months, as well as some spleen and symptom responses. Ruxolitinib, a JAK1/2 inhibitor currently licensed for selected patients with MF and PV refractory/resistant to hydroxyurea (hydroxycarbamide), has demonstrated some activity in a phase II study of refractory AML patients, which included 18 patients with post-MPN AML. Three of these 18 patients demonstrated a response to therapy, including two complete remissions and one complete remission with insufficient recovery of blood counts. The potential role of *FLT3* inhibitors in secondary AML is unclear, though there is a paucity of data. Table 14.3 depicts some of the investigational approaches in clinical trials for both *BCR-ABL1*-positive and negative MPN.

In the case of CML-BC patients who are TKI-naïve, many do respond to treatment with high-dose imatinib, dasatinib, or nilotinib, either alone or in combination with conventional acute leukaemia drugs, but most patients relapse within a few months of achieving apparently complete responses. Dasatinib, with its additional activities on SRC pathway, appears to be the preferred TKI but this requires confirmation. Investigational strategies include combinations of TKI supplemented by other agents, such as antioxidants to abrogate genomic instability caused by overproduction of ROS, downstream signal transduction inhibitors, such as farnesyl

Table 14.3 Treatment strategies for MPN transforming to AML

Treatment strategy	Comment
Induction chemotherapy	CR/CRi 30–50%; minimal impact on survival
Non-induction chemotherapy	Minimal impact on survival compared to BSC
Azacitidine	Median OS 8 months
Decitabine	67% of patients alive at 9 months
Stem cell transplant without prior chemotherapy	Complete responses reported in small number of patients
Induction therapy followed by stem cell transplant	In patients achieving a response to induction, improves survival compared with non-transplant approaches
Ruxolitinib	3/18 patients achieved CR/CRi
Combination ruxolitinib plus hypomethylating agents	Ongoing clinical trials

CR, complete remission; Cri, complete response with incomplete blood count recovery; BSC, best supportive care; OS: overall survival.

transferase inhibitors or mTOR inhibitors, activators of PP2A, such as FTY720 or Forskolin and its derivatives, or Janus kinase (JAK) inhibitors, such as ruxolitinib or pacritinib. Other candidate investigational agents include Bcl-2 inhibitors, such as ABT-199, β-catenin pathway inhibitors, and eigentic modifiers.

In patients who are able to achieve a second indolent or CP, the best current approach appears to be an allogeneic stem cell transplant, provided a suitable donor is available. For patients with BC-CML, who have achieved a second CP, it is useful to place them on 'maintenance' TKI treatment. Several studies have examined the role and efficacy of allogeneic transplant in treating patients with blast-phase MPN or post-MPN AML, with data indicating a potential for prolonged progression-free survival as compared with antileukaemic chemotherapy alone. One study examined patients with post-MPN AML who were treated with induction chemotherapy, following which those who achieved a complete response or reverted back to a chronic-phase MPN were able to proceed to allogeneic stem cell transplant. A total of 38 patients received induction chemotherapy, with 18 patients achieving a complete response or complete response with incomplete count recovery; 11 patients reverted to CP of MPN, while 17 patients received an allogeneic stem cell transplant. The group of patients who received a transplant demonstrated a 2-year overall survival rate (OS) of 47%. In comparison, the group of patients who received induction therapy, and achieved a response, but did not go on to allogeneic stem cell transplant displayed a 2-year OS of 15%. Thus, patients who are able to tolerate and respond to induction chemotherapy, and proceed to transplant, appear to have a relatively improved prognosis.

Conclusion

Though there has been substantial improvement in our understanding of the biology of MPN transformation to advanced phases, much work remains. Recent research highlights potential cooperating mutations, such as DNMT3A and IDH2, which inturn may impact on future treatment options. The treatment in general is unsatisfactory and the optimal goal is prevention. Failing this, it best to consider patients for a suitable clinical trial assessing one of the newer drugs and then consider allogeneic stem cell transplant if a second CP is achieved. The overall prognosis is generally dismal for those who have already transformed to BC. Clearly, this is an area which is evolving rapidly, so it is difficult to make firm treatment recommendations at present.

Further reading

Alvarez-Larran A, Senin A, Fernandez-Rodriguez C, et al. Impact of genotype on leukemic transformation in polycythemia vera and essential thrombocythaemia. *Br J Haem*. 2017;178(5):764–71.

Campbell PJ, Baxter EJ, Beer PA, et al. Mutation of JAK2 in the myeloproliferative disorders: timing, clonality studies, cytogenetic association, and role in leukemic transformation. *Blood*. 2006;108:3548–55.

Eghtedar A, Verstovsek S, Estrov Z, et al. Phase 2 study of the JAK kinase inhibitor ruxolitinib in patients with refractory leukemias, including postmyeloproliferative neoplasm acute myeloid leukemia. *Blood*. 2012;119:4614–18.
Finazzi G, Caruso V, Marchioli R, et al. Acute leukemia in polycythemia vera: an analysis of 1638 patients enrolled in a prospective observational study. *Blood*. 2005;105:2664–70.
Green A, Beer P. Somatic mutations of IDH1 and IDH2 in the leukemic transformation of myeloproliferative neoplasms. *N Engl J Med*. 2010;362(4):369–70.
Haaβ W, Kleiner H, Wieβ C, et al. Clonal evolution and blast crisis correlate with enhanced proteolytic activity of separase in BCR-ABL b3a2 fusion type CML under imatinib therapy. *PLoS One*. 2015;10(6):e129648.
Harutyunyan A, Klampfl T, Cazzola M, Kralovics R. p53 lesions in leukemic transformation. *N Engl J Med*. 2011;364:488–90.
Hehlmann R. How I treat CML blast crisis. *Blood*. 2012;120(4):737–47.
Hiwase DK, Hughes TP. Sudden blast crisis in chronic myeloid leukemia treated with tyrsoine kinase inhibitors. *Leuk Lymphoma*. 2012;53(7):1251–2.
Jamieson CH, Ailles LE, Dylla SJ, et al. Granulocyte-macrophage progenitors as candidate leukemic stem cells in blast-crisis CML. *N Engl J Med*. 2004;351(7):657–67.
Jiang Q, Crews LA, Barrett CL, et al. ADAR1 promotes malignant progenitor programming in chronic myeloid leikemia. *PNAS*. 2013;110(3):1041–6.
Kennedy JA, Atenafu EG, Messner HA, et al. Treatment outcomes following leukemic transformation in Philadelphia-negative myeloproliferative neoplasms. *Blood*. 2013;121:2725–33.
Khan M, Siddiqui R, Gangat N. Therapeutic options for leukemia transformation in patients with myeloproliferative neoplasms. *Leuk Res*. 2017;63:78–84.
Koptyra M, Cramer K, Slupianek A, Richardson C, Skorski T. BCR/ABL promotes accumulation of chromosomal aberrations induced by oxidative and genotoxic stress. *Leukemia*. 2008;22(10):1969–72.
Mughal TI, Goldman JM. A perspective on the molecular evolution of chronic myeloid leukemia from chronic phase to blast transformation. *Clin Leuk*. 2006;1:101–8.
Mughal TI, Goldman JM. Chronic myeloid leukemia: why does it evolve from chronic phase to blast transformation? *Front Biosci*. 2006;11:198–208.
Ortman CA, Kent DG, Nangalia J, et al. Effect of mutation order on myeloproliferative neoplasms. *N Engl J Med*. 2015;372:601–12.
Perrotti D, Cesi, Trotta R, et al. BCR-ABL suppresses C/EBPalpha expression through inhibitory action of hnRNP E2. *Nat Genet*. 2002;30(1):48–58.
Perrotti D, Neviani P. From mRNA metabolism to cancer therapy: chronic myelogenous leukemia shows the way. *Clin Cancer Res*. 2007;13(6):1638–42.
Perrotti D, Neviani P. Protein phosphatase 2A (PP2A), a drugable tumor suppressor in Ph1(+) leukemias. *Cancer Metastasis Rev*. 2008;27(2):159–68.
Quintas-Cardama A, Kantarjian H, Pierce S, Cortes J, Verstovsek S. Prognostic model to identify patients with myelofibrosis at the highest risk of transformation to acute myeloid leukemia. *Clin Lymphoma Myeloma Leuk*. 2013;13:315–18.e2.
Radich JP, Dai H, Mao M, et al. Gene expression changes associated with progression and response in chronic myeloid leukemia. *Proc Natl Acad Sci U S A*. 2006;103(8):2794–9.
Rampal R, Aln J, Abdel-Wahab O, et al. Genomic and functional analysis of leukemic transformation of myeloproliferative neoplasms. *PNAS*. 2014;111:E5401–10.
Sauβelle S, Silver RT. Management of chronic myeloid leukemia in blast crisis. *Ann Hematol*. 2015;94(Suppl2):S159–65.
Tam CS, Nussenzveig RM, Popat U, et al. The natural history and treatment outcome of blast phase BCR-ABL-myeloproliferative neoplasms. *Blood*. 2008;112:1628–37.
Tefferi A, Guiglielmeli P, Larson DR, et al. Long-term survival and blast transformation in molecularly annotated essential thrombocythemia, polycythemia vera, and myelofibrosis. *Blood*. 2014;124:2507–13.
Theocharides A, Boissinot M, Girodon F, et al. Leukemic blasts in transformed JAK2-V617F-positive myeloproliferative disorders are frequently negative for the JAK2-V617F mutation. *Blood*. 2007;110:375–9.
Vannucchi AM, Lasho TL, Guiglielmeli P, et al. Mutations and prognosis in primary myelofibrosis. *Leukemia*. 2013;27:1861–9.
Wang L, Clark RE. Ikaros transcripts Ik6/10 and levels of full-length transcript are critical for chronic myeloid leukemia blast crisis transformation. *Leukemia*. 2014;28(8):1745–7.

Yogarajah M, Tefferi A. Leukemic transformation in myeloproliferative neoplasms: a literature review on risk, characteristics, and outcome. *Mayo Clin Proc*. 2017;7:1118–28.

Zhang SJ, Rampal R, Manshouri T, et al. Genetic analysis of patients with leukemic transformation of myeloproliferative neoplasms shows recurrent SRSF2 mutations that are associated with adverse outcome. *Blood*. 2012;119:4480–5.

Zhou H, Mak PY, Mu H, et al. Combined inhibition of β-catenin and Bcr-Abl synergistically targets tyrosine kinase inhibitor-resistant blast crisis chronic myeloid leukemia invitro and invivo. *Leukemia*. 2017;31:2065–74.

Zoi K, Cross NCP. Genomics of myeloproliferative neoplasms. *J Clin Oncol*. 2017;35:947–54.

Zhang X, Wang X, Wang XQD, et al. Dnmt3a loss and idh2 neomorphic mutations mutually potentiate malignant hematopoiesis. *Blood*. 2020;135:845–856.

Chapter 15

Monitoring efforts in myeloproliferative neoplasms

Daniel Egan and Jerald P. Radich

Introduction *235*

The Philadelphia chromosome and *BCR-ABL1* transcript: The basis of monitoring in CML *235*

Clinical applications of *BCR-ABL1* testing in CML *238*

The definitions of response to therapy in CML *238*

JAK2 in Ph-negative classic MPN *241*

Other relevant diagnostic tests in MPN *244*

Emerging technologies for monitoring MPN *245*

Next major hurdle of monitoring and care in CML *246*

Introduction

Targeted therapy with tyrosine kinase inhibitors (TKI) has transformed the therapy of chronic myeloid leukaemia (CML), and is increasingly playing a role in the management of the myeloproliferative neoplasms (MPN), as a whole. In CML, the BCR-ABL genomic translocation (manifested as the Philadelphia chromosome) drives the pathophysiology of the disease, and is the target of both therapy and monitoring. The relatively recent discovery of the JAK2 V617F mutation and its detection in the majority of patients with essential thrombocytosis (ET), polycythaemia vera (PV), and primary myelofibrosis (PMF) has revolutionized our understanding of these MPN. Assays to detect JAK2 V617F have become incorporated into everyday practice by haematologists, and various inhibitors of the Janus kinase (JAK) tyrosine kinase are similarly being pursued for therapeutic application.

As CML has nearly a decade 'head start' of targeted therapy compared to MPN, the vast bulk of data on the merits of monitoring discussed in this review will be lessons from CML. However, we expect as more of the molecular biology of MPN is understood, and with the development of more active JAK inhibitors or similar targeted therapies, we suspect the lessons learned in CML will be highly relevant to monitoring in MPN. Furthermore, the recent identification of recurrent mutations in calreticulin and colony stimulating factor 3 receptor (CSF3R) have advanced our understanding of the pathophysiology of MPN, as a whole.

The Philadelphia chromosome and *BCR-ABL1* transcript: The basis of monitoring in CML

First recognized by Nowell and Hungerford in 1960 as a recurrent chromosomal abnormality in patients with CML, the Philadelphia chromosome (Ph) was further characterized by Janet. Rowley in 1973 as a reciprocal translocation involving chromosomes 9 and 22 (see Chapter 1). While the specific chromosomal breakpoint regions may differ between patients, the net result in all is fusion of some number of exons of the breakpoint cluster region (*BCR*) gene on chromosome 22 with the tyrosine kinase domain (exons 2–11) of the Abelson (*ABL*) gene on chromosome 9. The resultant *BCR-ABL* fusion ribonucleic acid (RNA) transcript encodes a constitutively active, oncogenic tyrosine kinase that is central to the pathogenesis of disease. Furthermore, because the Ph is found in all cells derived from the abnormal CML clone, but not in normal haematopoietic cells, detectable changes in the frequency of cells harbouring t(9;22) allows for monitoring of response, or loss of response, to therapy. There are three primary methods commonly used in the diagnosis and monitoring of CML: cytogenetics, fluorescence *in situ* hybridization, and molecular testing (PCR-based techniques).

With conventional metaphase *cytogenetics*, the number and appearance of all 46 chromosomes is assessed and, in this manner, the Ph itself may be detected. Cytogenetics has the advantage of allowing for the detection of other chromosomal changes that may be present in advanced phase disease. Disadvantages include the fact that cytogenetic analysis can generally only be performed on bone marrow, cells in metaphase must be captured for analysis, and the procedure itself takes up to two weeks. Because 20 metaphase preparations are often evaluated, the limit of detection is only 1 in 20 cells, or 5%. If less than 20 metaphases are available for review, the sensitivity of the test is significantly limited.

Fluorescence *in situ* hybridization

Fluorescence in situ hybridization (FISH) is a technique in which fluorescently labelled probes are used to identify the spatial locations of desired DNA sequences on chromosomes. In selecting probes specific for corresponding target sequences in *BCR* and *ABL*, rearrangements that result in *BCR-ABL* may then be detected. FISH is considerably more sensitive than cytogenetics in detecting the *BCR-ABL* fusion, with a typical assay demonstrating a limit of detection of roughly 1 in 200 cells, or 0.5%. The test can be performed on either bone marrow or peripheral blood specimens, and turnaround time is often within 1–2 days. However, FISH cannot detect additional chromosomal changes unless those changes are anticipated and screened with specific probes.

Reverse transcription (RT)-PCR

Reverse transcription (RT)-PCR of the chimeric *BCR-ABL* mRNA is the most sensitive assay for detecting CML, and can detect one CML cell in approximately 100 000 cells. The terms 'real-time' or 'quantitative') PCR refer to the measurement of nucleic acid-dependent fluorescence during the exponential phase of the PCR reaction, which is a function of the quantity of starting template. With PCR testing, most of the outcome data in CML is based on peripheral blood specimens, making it both the most convenient and sensitive test available for monitoring. The assay has well documented pitfalls, mostly revolving around the complexity of the assay, and the fact that there is suboptimal standardization across academic and commercial labs.

In CML, two isoforms account for the vast majority of *BCR-ABL* fusion transcripts observed in this population. In the first, commonly referred to as 'e13a2' or 'b2a2', the first 13 exons of *BCR* are fused with exons 2–11 of *ABL* (Figure 15.1). In the second, commonly referred to as 'e14a2' or 'b3a2' the first 14 exons of *BCR* are fused with the same exons 2–11 of *ABL*. Both result in a 210 kDa product, and therefore both are somewhat confusingly referred to as the 'p210' transcript. By contrast, the major isoform detected in Ph+ acute lymphoblastic leukaemia is a 'p190' transcript involving only the first exon of BCR fused with the same exons 2–11 of ABL, and resulting in a 190 kDa product. Less commonly, some patients exhibit a 'p230' BCR-ABL transcript comprised of BCR exons 1–19 fused with ABL exons 2–11 that result in a 230 kDa product. Through appropriate placement of PCR primers, specific approaches for the detection of the p190, p210, or p230 transcripts can be developed. Given that the overwhelming majority of CML and Ph+ ALL patients exhibit p210 or p190 transcripts, respectively, most clinical laboratories have assays for both, though one must typically specify to the lab the particular transcript of interest. Some patients with clinical evidence for CML may be Ph negative, but nonetheless have

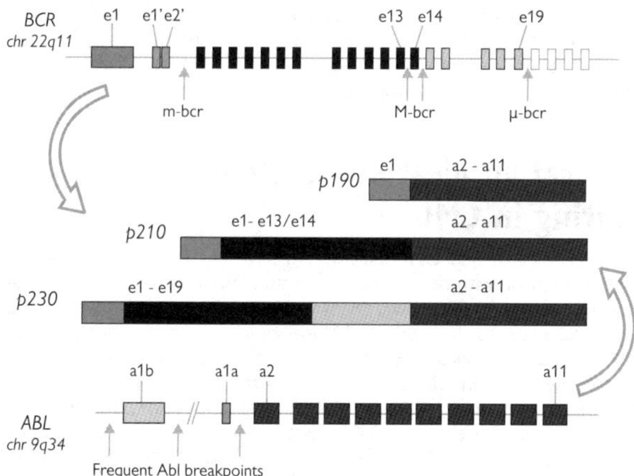

Figure 15.1 Location of breakpoints in BCR gene (on chromosome 22) and ABL gene (on chromosome 9), and resulting BCR-ABL fusion proteins of different sizes. The BCR gene contains three primary breakpoint regions (denoted 'minor breakpoint cluster', m-bcr; 'major breakpoint cluster', M-bcr; and 'micro breakpoint cluster', μ-bcr). Gene rearrangement at m-bcr site results in the p190 fusion protein, composed of BCR exon 1 (e1) (medium grey) fused to ABL exons 2–11 (a2–a11) (dark grey). Gene rearrangement at M-bcr site results in either of two p210 fusion proteins, composed of BCR exons 1–13 or exons 1–14 (medium grey and black) fused to ABL exons 2–11 (dark grey). Gene rearrangement at μ-bcr site results in the p230 fusion protein, composed of BCR exons 1–19 (medium grey, black, and light grey) fused to ABL exons 2–11 (dark grey). Note that BCR e1' and e2' are included in the fusion gene, but splicing events result in loss of corresponding RNA from the BCR-ABL transcript. Fusion transcripts may additionally include ABL exons 1a or 1a/1b with exons 2–11, depending on the ABL breakpoint region. Schematic is not to scale.

detectable BCR-ABL transcripts, a result of alternative chromosomal rearrangements that still result in fusion of the two genes.

The measurement of BCR-ABL mRNA transcript levels using qRT-PCR in a highly accurate manner is crucial for medical decision-making. However, due to the variation in laboratory methods and inconsistent results across laboratories, a standardized approach to measuring and reporting BCR-ABL transcripts has been engineered. Consensus guidelines developed at a 2005 National Institute of Health conference led to the development of what is referred to as the International Scale (IS). The baseline of the IS, set at 100%, correlates with the median BCR-ABL transcript level measured in 30 untreated, chronic phase patients enrolled in the IRIS study. A 1-log reduction in BCR-ABL from that reference level would, thus, be equal to 10% on the IS. In this manner, a 3-log reduction from the baseline would be equal to 0.1%. The original specimen pool used to determine 100% (IS) has since been depleted, but the use of standards from IS reference laboratories, allows for any given laboratory to calculate a site-specific conversion factor (to correct for reagents, etc.). Multiplication of a laboratory's *BCR-ABL* result by the assigned conversion factor results in a standardized value expressed as a percentage on the IS.

Clinical applications of *BCR-ABL1* testing in CML

In a newly diagnosed CML patient, TKI have become standard first-line therapy in those with chronic and accelerated phase disease. TKI are pharmaceuticals with inhibitory activity against the constitutively active *BCR-ABL* tyrosine kinase, so that abnormal clonal CML cells are susceptible to the drug whereas normal cells remain largely unaffected. In reality, TKI are only partially selective and, in fact, each have a range of tyrosine kinases that may be inhibited, in addition to *BCR-ABL* (e.g. c-KIT, PDGFR). Imatinib is well known as the exemplar TKI which initially demonstrated efficacy in newly chronic phase CML patients in the landmark IRIS trial. Since then, multiple new TKI agents have been developed with activity against *BCR-ABL*. The use of a TKI progressively reduces the disease burden in most patients. Therefore, as the number of leukaemia cells decrease, the sensitivity of the techniques used to effectively monitor the disease must increase accordingly.

The definitions of response to therapy in CML

The assessment of response to therapy historically consisted solely of clinical and haematologic measures, such as peripheral blood counts or assessment for any reduction in spleen size. A complete haematologic response, for example, is defined as a normalization in peripheral blood counts, including total leukocyte count of less than 10×10^9/L, platelet count of less than 450×10^9/L, absence of palpable splenomegaly, and absence of immature myeloid cells in the peripheral blood. More recently, cytogenetic and molecular testing has become integrated into standard clinical practice. Monitoring for cytogenetic or molecular response (or failure) not only offers prognostic information, but also allows for early identification of patients with a loss of response or primary treatment failure. In this way, patients at risk for disease progression can be switched to alternative therapy. The National Comprehensive Cancer Network (NCCN), and the European LeukemiaNet (ELN) have defined similar, albeit slightly different, response criteria for CML that are summarized in Table 15.1.

The degree of treatment response, as determined by cytogenetic analysis, is the standard approach to monitoring in CML. A minor cytogenetic response (mCyR) is defined as a reduction in Ph to between 36% and 65%, or between 8 and 13 out of 20 metaphases. A partial cytogenetic response (PCyR) is defined as a reduction in Ph to between 1% and 35%, or up to 7

Table 15.1 Comparison of optimal response and treatment failure definitions, as per 2015 NCCN and 2013 ELN Guidelines

	NCCN Guidelines version 1.2015		2013 European LeukemiaNet Guidelines		
	Optimal	Failure (change of therapy advised)	Optimal	Warning	Failure (change of therapy advised)
3 months	BCR-ABL ≤10% (IS) or PCyR	BCR-ABL >10% (IS); or lack of PCyR	BCR-ABL ≤10% (IS); or PCyR	BCR-ABL >10% (IS); or Ph+ 65–95%	Lack CHR; or Ph+ >95% or new mutations
6 months	BCR-ABL ≤10% (IS); or PCyR	BCR-ABL >10% (IS); or lack of PCyR	BCR-ABL ≤10% (IS); or PCyR	Ph+ 35–65%	BCR-ABL >10% (IS); or Ph+ >65% or new mutations
12 months	CCyR	PCyr (continuation of current TKI/dose may be considered)	BCR-ABL <1% (IS); and/or CCyR	BCR-ABL 1–10% and/or PCyR	BCR-ABL >10% (IS); or Ph+ >35% or new mutations
		Minor or no cytogenetic response; or cytogenetic relapse			
18 months	CCyR	Less than CCyR or cytogenetic relapse	BCR-ABL ≤0.1% (IS)	CCA (−7 or 7q−) in Ph- cells; or BCR-ABL >0.1%	Loss of CHR, or loss of CCyR/PCyR; or new mutations; or loss of MMR; or CCA in Ph+ cells

PCyR, partial cytogenetic response; IS, International Scale; CHR, complete haematologic response; Ph+ Philadelphia chromosome (by cytogenetic analysis); TKI, tyrosine kinase inhibitor; CCA, clonal cytogenetic abnormalities; NCCN, National Comprehensive Cancer Network; ELN, European LeukemiaNet.

Adapted with permission from National Comprehensive Cancer Network (NCCN) Clinical Practice Guidelines in Oncology. (2019). *Chronic Myelogenous Leukemia (Version 1)*. Copyright © National Comprehensive Cancer Network, All Rights Reserved. https://www.nccn.org/professionals/physician_gls/default.aspx; and Baccarani M, et al. (2013). European LeukemiaNet recommendations for the management of chronic myeloid leukemia: 2013. *Blood*. 12(6):872–84. Reprinted with permission from the American Society of Hematology. Copyright © 2013 by The American Society of Hematology. No other use of this material may be made or reprinted without permission. All rights reserved.

out of 20, metaphases. A complete cytogenetic response (CCyR), on the other hand, indicates the absence of detectable Ph. Specific cytogenetic milestones have been shown to correlate extremely well with outcomes. For example, in the IRIS trial, in which newly diagnosed chronic phase patients received interferon or imatinib, the progression-free survival (PFS) was better in patients who either demonstrated any cytogenetic response at 6 months or at least a PCyR at 12 months (compared to those who did not). A more recent update of IRIS trial data also showed that patients achieving CCyR at 18 months were likely to remain in cytogenetic remission for the long-term. The attainment of CCyR correlates with PFS and overall survival regardless of the TKI that is used, and also holds prognostic significance in those who fail first-line therapy and are treated with a second-line TKI. Notably, endpoints in CML have not been defined using FISH, although Testoni et al. demonstrated that in patients with insufficient cells for cytogenetic analysis, FISH <1% could be used as a surrogate for CCyR.

Beyond cytogenetic remission, the additional use of PCR to measure the degree of reduction in BCR-ABL mRNA can further risk-stratify patients. A decrease in BCR-ABL transcripts to 0.1% on the IS, or a 3-log reduction from the untreated, chronic phase IRIS baseline level, has been termed a major molecular response (MMR). In the IRIS trial, considering only those patients with a CCyR, there was a 97% PFS at 54 months in the subset with MMR, at 12 months, as opposed to an 89% PFS in the subset with less than a MMR at 12 months. Multiple studies have confirmed a longer duration of CCyR and higher rates of PFS in those that achieve MMR at either 12 or 18 months. Furthermore, as evidence that molecular monitoring may be useful in identifying patients who may require alternative therapy, Press et al. showed a significant association between loss of MMR and an increased risk of disease relapse. There is further evidence that the degree of molecular response by 3–6 months after starting treatment may be predictive of long-term outcomes. For example, in a study of patients receiving imatinib, the proportion of patients alive at 7 years was 97% if BCR-ABL/ABL was measured at less than 10% at 3 months, compared to only 54% if BCR-ABL/ABL was more than 10% at 3 months. A similar improvement in event-free survival at 3 years was seen in patients taking imatinib or second-generation TKIs.

It is important to point out that the concept of a 'complete molecular remission' (CMR), as defined by the absence of detectable *BCR-ABL*, may not necessarily mean that disease has been completely eradicated, and in fact is somewhat of a moving target as laboratory methods become increasingly sensitive. Inadequate sampling and limitations in assay sensitivity complicate the matter. The comparative inclusion of a 'housekeeping' control gene helps to validate the integrity of the mRNA, and positive control standards can inform as to the relative sensitivity. The term '$CMR^{4.5}$' conveys a lack of detectable BCR-ABL at the level of a 4.5-log reduction from baseline level (equivalent to 0.0032%IS). Clinical studies exploring the possibility of TKI discontinuation in selected patients show that 60% of patients attaining CMR4.5 will relapse after stopping the TKI, illustrating the concept of disease persistence below the lower limit of molecular detection.

qRT-PCR should be performed at the time of diagnosis, in order to establish a baseline, and then every 3 months while on TKI therapy. In this manner, those at greater risk of disease progression can be identified early, with failure to achieve MMR or increase in BCR-ABL level serving as red flags. Even a half-log increase in the quantitative *BCR-ABL* level is associated with decreased relapse-free survival. However, recent surveys suggest that clinicians are actually monitoring patients far less frequently. A retrospective analysis of nearly 300 patients cared for 29 community practitioners found that testing guidelines were followed only 39% of the time, while in another study less than half of patients had two or more PCR tests performed in the preceding 12 months. This poor compliance may be due to inadequate understanding of testing guidelines, access to an appropriate laboratory, or cost.

Mutation testing

Patients may demonstrate primary refractoriness to TKI therapy, or may develop secondary resistance after an initial response. Resistance is commonly due to the emergence of point mutations in the ABL kinase domain, with such mutations detectable in roughly 50% of patients with imatinib resistance. Specific mutations have been established as causing resistance to one or more TKIs, and therefore this knowledge may be used in to inform the selection of an alternative agent. To screen for mutations, direct Sanger sequencing of the BCR-ABL transcript is employed. Importantly, the sensitivity of Sanger sequencing for detection of mutant alleles is estimated to be approximately 20%. Therefore, this testing may be falsely negative if a resistance mutation is present in only a minority of leukaemic cells. There are more sensitive screening methods for ABL mutations, however, it is unclear how such ultra-sensitive mutation analysis should be interpreted in regard to clinical decision-making. It is generally recommended that mutation analysis be performed in patients with accelerated phase or blast crisis, primary failure, or suboptimal response to TKIs, or haematologic or cytogenetic relapse. It is reasonable to perform mutation analysis in those with loss of MMR, as this has correlated with an increased risk of future relapse.

JAK2 in Ph-negative classic MPN

The discovery of *BCR-ABL1* as a disease marker and therapeutic target for CML led to the optimistic expectation that a panel of analogous genetic aberrancies would similarly be identified in other MPN lacking the Philadelphia chromosome. Unfortunately, the successful application of *BCR-ABL1* as a pathognomonic and targetable fusion transcript has in some ways proven to be the exception, rather than the rule. However, mutations have been identified in Janus kinase 2 gene (*JAK2*) in most patients with PV, and roughly half of patients with ET and primary myelofibrosis (PMF), and therefore JAK2 testing is becoming increasingly incorporated into the diagnosis of these disorders.

The Janus kinase (JAK) family consists of related group of signalling kinases that bind to growth factor receptors (e.g. erythropoietin receptor, EpoR) and mediate the effects of haematopoietic growth factors via activation of signal transducer and activator of transcription (STAT) transcription factors. In 2005, multiple groups discovered that a specific mutation in exon

14 of *JAK2* was frequently found in patients with PV, ET, and PMF, resulting in a valine to phenylalanine substitution in the pseudokinase domain (V617F). This results in a gain-of-function that conveys cytokine hypersensitivity and proliferation in affected myeloid cells. The incidence of JAK2 V617F is roughly 65–95% in PV, and approximately 50% in both ET and PMF.

Interestingly, the JAK2 mutant allele burden, or allele frequency, (percentage of myeloid cells carrying the mutation) differs across the spectrum of these disorders, as well. The allele burden may yield important pieces of clinical information. There is evidence to suggest that in each of the three diseases described, JAK2 V617F allele burden may correlate with such clinical characteristics as pruritis, thrombosis, splenomegaly, peripheral cell counts and, most importantly, prognosis. However, the interpretation of the allelic burden is complicated by the biology of the JAK2 mutation. In some cases, JAK2 mutations are heterozygous (that is, present along with a wild-type allele), while in other cases, the mutation is homozygous, with no wild-type component (through the process of acquired uniparental disomy. The situation is further complicated by the fact that JAK2V617F are often homozygous in PV cases, while heterozygous in ET patients. Thus, the allelic ratio is based on the amount of disease (with normal cells contributing two wild-type JAK2 alleles), and whether the JAK2 mutation is heterozygous or homozygous. Thus, it is perhaps not surprising that the significance of allelic burden, and documenting its change with therapy, remains an enigma.

In general, treatment strategies in PV are centred on the reductions in haematocrit, splenomegaly, and risk of thrombosis. Conventional strategies include therapeutic phlebotomy and low-dose aspirin, as well as hydroxyurea for cytoreduction. Because of its antiproliferative effects on haematopoietic cells, interferon-a has been employed as a treatment for PV. While its utility is often limited by adverse effects (e.g. flu-like symptoms), patients receiving interferon often demonstrate a reduction in JAK2 V617F allele burden, with many achieving a CMR, as defined by an undetectable JAK2 mutation. Because of the high frequency of JAK2 mutations in PV, one might naturally predict a great role for JAK inhibition (such as with ruxolitinib), though it has mainly been studied in PV patients intolerant of hydroxyurea. Indeed, ruxolitinib has shown reduction in haematocrit, spleen size, and constitutional symptoms in this population. It is also tempting to assume that use of a ruxolitinib would have an impact on JAK2 allele burden similar to that of interferon, but perhaps surprisingly only modest reductions have been observed. However, it is important to note that while there is a clear correlation between BCR-ABL expression and clinical outcome, the impact of JAK2 V617F reduction on outcomes in PV is unclear, and it's possible that it might not be essential for a clinical response.

In PMF, treatment goals have largely been focused on symptomatic relief from constitutional symptoms and splenomegaly, or haematopoietic stem cell transplantation in selected patients deemed to be at high risk of death or leukaemic transformation. With the discovery of the JAK2 V617F mutation and development of JAK inhibitors, studies of the therapeutic impact of JAK2 inhibition have been performed and more are ongoing. The landmark COMFORT-I and COMFORT-II randomized controlled trials have clearly demonstrated an improvement in splenomegaly and PMF-related constitutional symptoms with ruxolitinib. Furthermore, follow-up analysis has demonstrated a survival benefit in the population receiving ruxolitinib. Intriguingly, responses and survival benefit appear to be independent of JAK2 mutation status. This may be due to the non-selective inhibition of both JAK1 and JAK2 by ruxolitinib, and the fact that JAK1-mediated cytokine effects are likely central to disease pathogenesis in PMF. As with PV, the correlation of JAK2 V617F burden with outcome is not well established in PMF. Therefore, while quantitative assessments of JAK2 V617F allele burden are often performed, interpretation of these results is somewhat limited at present, and additional clinical investigations are required to sort this matter out.

That being said, a reduction of the JAK2 V617F allele burden is a response criterion in MPN according to the ELN and International Working Group-Myeloproliferative Neoplasms Research (IWG-MRT) guidelines. In addition, there is some evidence that monitoring for V617F mutation in the post-stem cell transplant setting may be predictive of disease relapse. Thus, it is important to have reliable quantitative laboratory techniques for accurately measuring the allele frequency of *JAK2* V617F. The presence or absence of the *JAK2* point mutation is often determined by DNA-based laboratory assays, most often through Sanger sequencing, at an estimated sensitivity of 10–20%. For quantitative detection, however, the most common laboratory techniques include qPCR or pyrosequencing, the latter of which involves the sequential determination of incorporated nucleotides and the quantitative measurement of pyrophosphate that is released upon nucleotide incorporation into the growing strand. In both, patient DNA (typically obtained from peripheral blood granulocytes) is referenced against a standard curve generated from dilutions of mutant-to-wild-type DNA or other known reference standards. In quantitative detection of a point mutation, such as V617F, the design of the PCR assay can be optimized to select for mutant or wild-type amplicons of different sizes using multiple forward or reverse primers that are designed to match or mismatch with the nucleotide of interest. This technique is referred to as allele-specific PCR (AS-PCR). Endonuclease digestion (or restriction enzyme digestion) involves the selective digestion of PCR amplicons with sequence-specific enzymatic reagents, so that PCR products are left intact or digested into smaller fragments of known size that may then be separated by electrophoresis or other means and then quantified.

Direct comparisons between the various techniques are somewhat limited, though Lippert et al compared the overall concordance of unknown samples in 16 centres that performed quantitative JAK2 testing through AS-PCR, qPCR, and pyrosequencing. Overall, a coefficient of variation (CV) of 31% was observed, indicating considerable variability in allele quantification between centres. The CV did improve to 21% after references were standardized among all of the centres, illustrating the importance of universal standards in quantitative clinical assays.

Other relevant diagnostic tests in MPN

In those patients with PV, ET, or PMF who do not harbour an identifiable V617F mutation, other (mutually exclusive) mutations in *JAK2* (e.g. exon 12), *MPL*, or calreticulin gene may be implicated. Detection of all can be accomplished through standard sequencing techniques. Curiously, JAK2 exon 12 mutations seem to result in a PV-like phenotype with erythroid hyperplasia and erythrocytosis, there is still considerable phenotypic overlap with V617F-mutant positive patients. It is estimated that point mutations in *MPL*, the gene encoding the thrombopoietin receptor and which signals through JAK-STAT pathway, are found in 5% of patients with ET and PMF. Most often, a point mutation in codon 515 is implicated, resulting in constitutive JAK-STAT signalling. Clinical assays for detection of MPL are, therefore, based on detection of the W515L or W515L mutations for diagnostic purposes. The calreticulin gene (*CALR*) encodes a 46 kDa protein, calreticulin, that is highly conserved and is present in all cells except erythrocytes. Its C terminal domain is thought to be involved in calcium binding, and a specific 'KDEL' amino acid functions to route proteins from the Golgi apparatus to the endoplasmic reticulum. Two groups reported the frequency of *CALR* mutations in roughly half of JAK2-negative cases of PMF (~25% overall). At this time, the mechanism by which *CALR* mutations result in a myelofibrotic phenotype are unknown, though the pathophysiology appears to be dependent on STAT signalling. A variety of different CALR mutations appear to consist of insertion and deletions in exon 9 that all result in a truncated protein with loss of the KDEL retrieval signal. There appear to be important clinical differences between CALR-mutant PMF and JAK2-mutant PMF, with the former associated with younger age and improved survival. At this point in time, there is no role for serial monitoring of MPL or CALR mutations, and standard sequencing approaches are used for detection. A comparison of different methods to detect CALR deletion mutations found that fragment analysis and high resolution melt analysis were superior at detecting low levels (5–10%) of mutant, compared to Sanger sequencing (10–25%), with targeted next-generation demonstrating the lowest limit of detection at 1% allele burden.

In 2013, Maxson et al reported on the frequency of mutations in *CSF3R*, the gene encoding the receptor for colony stimulating factor 3, in patients with chronic neutrophilic leukaemia (CNL) and 'atypical' CML, two disorders on the myeloproliferative spectrum that are both characterized by increased numbers of circulating neutrophils. In fact, 59% of patients with CNL and atypical CML were found to harbour such mutations, whereas no disease-specific genetic markers had previously been identified. A subsequent study confirmed the presence of CSF3R mutations in CNL, but not atypical CML. The CSF3 receptor is fundamentally involved in the regulation of process of granulocyte production, with downstream signalling via the JAK-STAT pathway and other kinases. Notably, mutations have been detected primarily in two distinct regions, each with potentially different effects in downstream signalling. Patients with mutations in the proximal membrane region (e.g. T618I mutation) were shown to activate JAK-STAT, and there is at least some evidence that JAK inhibition with ruxolitinib may be of therapeutic value in this case. Other mutations were identified in the cytoplasmic tail region (e.g. S783fs), correlating with activation of SRC family and signalling via TNK2 kinase. *In vitro* studies suggested sensitivity to dasatinib for such cases. It is expected that the presence of mutations in CSF3R will be incorporated into diagnostic criteria for both conditions, and it is reasonable to suspect that additional cooperating genetic factors will be identified that contribute to either a CNL or atypical CML phenotype. Because the recurrent mutations are localized, a Sanger sequencing or other targeted sequencing assay may be used for diagnostic purposes. At this point, there is no evidence to suggest any utility to serial testing.

Emerging technologies for monitoring MPN

While qPCR techniques remain the standard approach for detecting and monitoring BCR-ABL, increasingly sensitive methods are being developed. In this manner, the concept of a 'complete molecular remission' is entirely dependent upon the context of the sensitivity of the test that is used. As illustrated by the fact that relapse occurs in more than half of patients enrolled on TKI discontinuation trials, there is clearly a need for more sensitive tests that might allow for detection of lower amounts of residual disease. As previously mentioned, differences in laboratory reagents or techniques affects the reproducibility of BCR-ABL testing between labs, and while standardization of references helps to solve this problem, there is the potential that newer, alternative methods may be more precise.

DNA PCR

Detection of BCR-ABL mRNA is the standard monitoring technique in CML, but amplification of the *BCR-ABL* DNA can be done, though time consuming, since multiple primers must be used to identify the exact DNA translocation sequence, then patient specific primers synthesized for use to detect low abundance *BCR-ABL* during therapy (this is analogous to IgH VDJ assays in ALL). Sensitivity can be achieved at a level of sensitivity down to $1{:}10^6$, and DNA sequences can be detected in roughly 50% of cases where BCR-ABL RNA is undetectable.

Digital PCR

Digital PCR is a relatively new method of quantitative detection of rare transcripts. The method involves partitioning the target nucleic acid into myriad separate reactions at a sufficiently low enough target density in each reaction that the target is either there, or not. Thus, each partition yields a binary, or 'digital', result (positive or negative) for which a Poisson distribution can be used to determine the number of mutant or wild-type reads in each partition. These partitioned reactions are either created by a system of pumps, tubes, and well (all, *really* small), or by diluting the target into bubbles (each bubble then becoming the reaction vessel). It has been estimated that digital PCR increases the limit of detection by 1- or 2-logs. The method has the additional advantages of having low technical variation (greater similarity between repeat runs), and calibration curves are not required to yield an absolute numerical value. This technique has been used to detect rare copies of BCR-ABL, as well as single copies of T315I mutated cells.

Mutation detection

Sanger sequencing, currently the most utilized method of mutation testing, has an inherent limit of sensitivity of approximately 10–20%. 'Next-generation sequencing' (NGS) refers to the collective high-throughput methods of sequencing large numbers of RNA or DNA strands in parallel. As with digital PCR, the sequences are digitally tabulated and yield absolute numbers of sequencing reads, thus allowing for detection of low frequency mutations. NGS targeting ABL mutations in CML has revealed the complex world of mutation kinetics that occurs with TKI resistance, with a dynamic mix of compound and polyclonal mutations. However, errors in the polymerase activity during library preparation causes at least 1% or erroneous 'reads', leading to a potential problem with false positives. A new approach to improving upon the error is 'duplex' NGS. In contrast to usual NGS, duplex NGS makes libraries off both DNA strands, and both strands are simultaneously sequenced. 'Mutations' are only declared 'true' is the same base pair in both strands is a mutation, which decreases the potential false positive rate by orders of magnitude. However, it should be noted that the clinical utility of any super-sensitive mutation detection method has not be convincingly demonstrated.

Next major hurdle of monitoring and care in CML

In developed countries we have the luxury of multiple TKIs, sensitive monitoring methods, and healthcare systems largely functional enough to deliver both. For most of the world, this is sadly not the case. Here, we will take the example of CML. TKI therapy has changed the natural history of CML, and now newly diagnose patients enjoy a 10-year survival quite comparable to age-matched controls. However, this therapy costs approximately $80 000 US/year, and thus, the large majority of world-wide cases cannot receive therapy. In addition, the means of diagnosing CML, be it by metaphase cytogenetics, FISH, or BCR-ABL PCR, in unavailable to most of the world's CML patients. To diagnose and monitor patients, physicians in the developing countries have limited options: (1) no diagnostics; (2) send to a nearby lab (but equipment and training of personnel is quite expensive; or (3) send to a referral centre (very costly, especially if this is sent across country borders). The advent of cartridge-based, 'automated' systems (Cepheid) does much to obviate technical training and simplifies the assay, though the system is expensive in low resource areas. Some other options may work, however. First, it may be possible to spot blood on a special filter paper, and ship via 'snail' mail; preliminary works show this technique yields very similar results to samples run fresh (Radich lab, Seattle). In addition, investigators have developed handheld, electricity-free devices to detect

HIV, using the isothermal LAMP assay. This methodology fulfils the WHO 'ASSURED' guidelines for diagnostic devices in low resource settings (A, affordable; S, sensitive; S, specific; U, user-friendly; R, rapid and robust; E, *equipment-free*; D, deliverable to end-users). If similar devices can be developed for BCR-ABL, then the power of diagnosis and monitoring will be placed at the point of care, greatly expanding the potential access of this patients to appropriate CML therapy. We should not settle for anything less.

Further reading

Bartley PA, Ross DM, Latham S, et al. Sensitive detection and quantification of minimal residual disease in chronic myeloid leukaemia using nested quantitative PCR for BCR-ABL DNA. *Int J Lab Hematol*. 2010;32:e222–8.

Harrison C, Kiladjian JJ, Al-Ali HK, et al. JAK inhibition with ruxolitinib versus best available therapy for myelofibrosis. *N Engl J Med*. 2012:366:787–98.

Hochhaus A, Larson RA, Guilhot F, et al. Long-term outcomes of imatinib treatment for chronic myeloid leukemia. *N Engl J Med*. 2017;376:917–27.

Huggett FJ, Cowen S, Foy CA. Considerations for digital PCR as an accurate molecular diagnostic tool. *Clin Chem*. 2015;61:1–10.

Jain P, Kantarjian H, Nazha A, et al. Early responses predict better outcomes in patients with newly diagnosed chronic myeloid leukemia: results with four tyrosine kinase inhibitor modalities. *Blood*. 2013;121:4867–74.

James C, Ugo V, Le Couedic JP, et al. A unique clonal JAK2 mutation leading to constitutive signaling causes polycythaemia vera. *Nature*. 2005;434(7037):1144–8.

Jones AV, Ward D, Lyon M, et al. Evaluation of methods to detect CALR mutations in myeloproliferative neoplasms. *Leuk Res*. 2015;39:82–7.

Khorashad JS, Kelley TW, Szankasi P, et al. BCR-ABL1 compound mutation in tyrosine kinase inhibitor-resistant CML: frequency and clonal relationships. *Blood*. 2013;121:489–98.

Kuriakose E, Vandris K, Wang YL, et al. Decrease in JAK2 V617F allele burden is not a prerequisite to clinical response in patients with polycythemia vera. *Haematologica*. 2012;97:538–42.

LaBarre P, Hawkins KR, Gerlach J, et al. A simple, inexpensive device for nucleic acid amplification without electricity-toward instrument-free molecular diagnostics in low-resource setting. *PLoS One*. 2012;6:e19738.

Lippert E, Girodon F, Hammond E, et al. Concordance of assays designed for the quantification of JAK2V617F: a multicenter study. *Haematologica*. 2009;94:38–45.

Mahon FX, Rea D, Guilhot, et al. Intergroupe Francais des Leucemies Myeloides Chroniques. Discontinuation of imatinib in patients with chronic myeloid leukemia who have maintained complete molecular remission for at least 2 years: the prospective, multicenter Stop Imatinib (STIM) trial. *Lancet Oncol*. 2010;11:1029–35.

Maxson JE, Gotlib J, Polyea DA, et al. Oncogenic CSF3R mutations in chronic neutrophilic leukemia and atypical CML. *N Engl J Med*. 2013;9:1781–90.

Mughal TI, Radich JP, Deininger MW, et al. Chronic myeloid leukemia: reminiscences and dreams. *Haematologica*. 2016;101(5):541–58.

National Comprehensive Cancer Network. NCCN Clinical Practice Guidelines in Oncology. Chronic Myelogenous Leukemia. Version 2019. Available at: https://www.nccn.org/professionals/physician_gls/default.aspx

Nordström T, Ronaghi M, Forsberg L, de Faire U, Morgenstern R, Nyrén P. Direct analysis of single-nucleotide polymorphism on double-stranded DNA by pyrosequencing. *Biotechnol Appl Biochem*. 2000;31:107–12.

Oehler VG, Qin J, Ramakrishnan R, et al. Absolute quantitative detection of ABL tyrosine kinase domain point mutations in chronic myeloid leukemia using a novel nanofluidic platform and mutation-specific PCR. *Leukemia*. 2009;23:396–9.

Quintás-Cardama A, Abdel-Wahab O, Manshouri T, et al. Molecular analysis of patients with polycythemia vera or essential thrombocythemia receiving pegylated interferon-2a. *Blood*. 2013;122:893.

Radich J. The molecular biology of myeloproliferative disorders. *Cancer Cell*. 2010;18:7–8.

Radich JR. Chronic myeloid leukemia: global impact from a local laboratory. *Cancer*. 2017; doi:10.1002/cncr.30776.

Soverini S, De Benedittis C, Polakova KM, et al. Unraveling the complexity of tyrosine kinase inhibitor-resistant populations by ultra-deep sequencing of the BCR-ABL kinase domain. *Blood*. 2013;122:1634–48.

Soverini S, De Benedittis C, Polakova KM, et al. Unraveling the complexity of tyrosine kinase inhibitor-resistant populations by ultra-deep sequencing of the BCR-ABL kinase domain. *Blood*. 2013;122:1634–48.

Testoni N, Marzocchi G, Luatti S, et al. Chronic myeloid leukemia: a prospective comparison of interphase fluorescence *in situ* hybridization and chromosome banding analysis for the definition of complete cytogenetic response: a study of the GIMEMA CML WP. *Blood*. 2009;114:4939–43.

Vannucchi AM, Kiladjian JJ, Griesshammer M, et al. Ruxolitinib versus standard therapy for the treatment of polycythemia vera. *N Engl J Med*. 2015;372:426–35.

Verstovsek S, Mesa RA, Gotlib J, et al. A double-blind, placebo-controlled trial of ruxolitinib for myelofibrosis. *N Engl J Med*. 2012;366:799–807.

Chapter 16

Stem cell transplantation for BCR-ABL1-positive and negative myeloproliferative neoplasms

Alessandro Rambaldi and Nicholas Kröger

Introduction *250*
BCR-ABL1-positive MPN *250*
BCR-ABL1-negative MPN *255*

Introduction

The management of the newly diagnosed patient with chronic myeloid leukaemia (CML) in chronic phase (CP) has changed substantially with the remarkable clinical activity of ABL-tyrosine kinase inhibitors (TKIs). Consequently, allogenic stem cell transplantation (allo-SCT) had a pivotal clinical role in the pre-TKI era, offering long-term remission and probably cure. Allo-SCT, however, remains important for the treatment of patients with CP-resistant to TKI therapy, and many others, including children and those with advanced disease. Additionally, substantial interest progress has been made in the transplant technology optimizing clinical outcomes. For patients with BCR-ABL1-negative myeloproliferative neoplasms (MPN), in particular myelofibrosis (MF), there was a similar initial enthusiasm when the JAK2 inhibitors entered the clinics in 2007. Current clinical experience, however, suggest a qualified impact on the clinical management, with improvements in MF-associated symptoms and splenomegaly but no major effect on the disease process. Allo-SCT is able to accord long-term remission to qualified patients with MF. In efforts to improve eligibility, JAK2 inhibitors are being tested in the peri-transplant period to improve the poor general condition of many candidate patients. In this chapter, we review the scenario pertaining to CML (addressed by AR) and MF (addressed by NK).

BCR-ABL1-positive MPN

Since 1982 when Fefer and colleagues showed the therapeutic activity of allo-SCT performed with identical twin donors, transplantation has been considered the treatment of choice for patients with the BCR-ABL1-postive CML. Younger patients with suitable stem cell donors were offered the option of allo-SCT during the early CP of the disease, possibly within the first year from diagnosis. Following the successful introduction of several TKIs, the therapeutic scenario of CML has dramatically changed. Therefore, for the front-line treatment of CP-CML patients, any of imatinib, nilotinib, or dasatinib is recommended (see Chapter 7). No matter the TKI used, the key objective for first-line treatment is to achieve an 'optimal' response because this endpoint associates with a duration of life comparable with that of the general population. Moreover, when a 'failure' is documented, the patient should receive a different TKI-based treatment to limit the risk of disease progression and death. Following this approach, the probability to achieve a deep haematologic, cytogenetic, or even molecular control of the disease is so good that no one patient should be immediately put at risk of a transplant-related morbidity and mortality. For this reason, starting from the beginning of the new millennium, the number of patients undergoing allogeneic transplant has dramatically diminished (Figure 16.1).

Current indications of allo-SCT for CML in CP

Despite the substantial therapeutic progress achieved by the use of TKIs, allogeneic transplantation remains a curative treatment option and it should be considered and definitely advised under certain circumstances. Human leukocyte antigen (HLA) typing at diagnosis is indicated only in selected

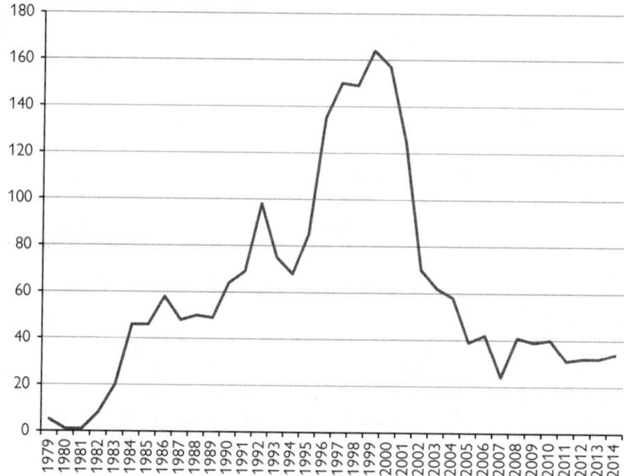

Figure 16.1 Allogeneic transplants performed in Italy in adult CML patients (n = 2215).

Source: data from the Gruppo Italiano Trapianto di Midollo Osseo (GITMO) national registry.

patients with high-risk disease while patients and siblings should be typed when imatinib fails. The search for an unrelated stem cell donor should also be activated if the front-line treatment failure is based on nilotinib or dasatinib, and in any case of a second-line treatment failure. Allo-SCT has to be considered for CP-CML patients who are eligible for the transplant procedure and resistant or intolerant to two lines of treatment including at least one second-generation TKI. In addition, transplant should obviously be considered as a third-line treatment for patients who have failed two different second-generation TKIs and in patients with BCR-ABL-1 kinase domain mutations such as the T315I mutation, which is always associated with resistance to first and second-generation TKIs. For this latter condition, a possible alternative or complementary treatment before transplant is represented by the use of the third-generation TKI, ponatinib, which shows remarkable efficacy in such patients, but also risk of significant cardiovascular toxicity, which remains to be elucidated fully. All in all, for CP-CML patients failing to achieve a durable response with any TKI (less than 20%) allogeneic transplantation remains and effective treatment strategy to eradicate the malignant clone and to achieve a definitive cure in this group of high-risk patients. For patients presenting with or evolving into accelerated phase (AP)/BC the clinical outcome with medical therapy is significantly poorer. Patients with AP or blast phase (BP)-CML at disease onset may receive initial therapy with second-generation TKIs (like nilotinib or dasatinib) which should be selected over imatinib to reduce the CML burden, and to achieve a better haematologic and molecular response. For blast crisis CML, the addition of chemotherapy to TKIs may also improve the rate of response and the survival time. In summary, every effort should be done to achieve at least a good haematologic response in these patients and transplant should be always considered as an early treatment opportunity.

Prognostic factors for outcomes and recent results

The risk assessment before transplant remains a key point to advise CML patients for the transplant procedure. In this regard, in 1998 the European Group for Blood and Marrow Transplantation (EBMT) developed a robust, CML specific, five variables-based, risk score for transplant-related mortality (TRM) and overall survival (OS). The five variables were patient age, disease phase at time of allo-SCT, disease duration, degree of histocompatibility between donor and recipient, and gender of donor. This score was independently validated by the Center for International Blood and Marrow Transplant Research (CIBMTR) and remains a valid tool today, despite having been developed in the pre-TKI era. The EBMT risk score observed a stepwise increase in TRM and a decrease in OS with increasing risk score. More recently, the haematopoietic cell transplantation comorbidity Index (HSCT-CI) has been implemented to better define the non-relapse mortality and OS of different haematologic malignancies and also validated in CML patients mostly treated with TKIs. The clinical outcome of allo-SCT in CML patients has progressively improved over time. The EBMT registry data show that the 2 years survival of patients who underwent transplantation during the first CP of their disease progressively improved from 60% during the 1980s up to 70%, in the early 2000s. A recent survey performed by the Gruppo Italiano Trapianto di Midollo Osseo (GITMO) showed that first CP-CML patients receiving an allogeneic transplant between year 2005–2012 (all being previously treated with TKIs) had a 75% 2-year OS, no matter if the stem cell source was from a matched sibling or unrelated donor (Figure 16.2). On the contrary, the improvement of transplant outcome for patients in advanced phase of the disease is modest, if any. Nonetheless, although the overall rates of cure for AP and BP-CML remains below 40% and 20%, respectively, it is likely that allo-SCT remains at present the most effective curative therapy for these high-risk patients.

Such experiences helped identify transplant toxicity, chronic graft-versus-host disease (cGvHD) and disease relapse as the principal causes of all-SCT failure. The effect of prior medical therapy in the outcome of a subsequent allogeneic transplant remains matter of scientific debate. Current data, however, suggest that prior treatment with any TKI might not increase the probability of TRM, but clearly longer-term follow-up is required, in particular with the newer TKIs. Historical studies have assessed prior cytoreductive therapies and interferon-alfa (IFN), with no major concerns identified. In the case of IFN, patients appear to fare just as well, provided the drug was discontinued approximately 90 days before allo-SCT. A major CIBMTR report on 409 subjects treated with imatinib before transplant and 900 subjects who did not receive imatinib revealed better OS for the imatinib-treated patients, but no statistically significant differences in TRM, disease relapse, or leukaemia-free survival (LFS). No determinantal observations were noted in patients transplanted with advanced CML who had prior imatinib. Interesting, a multivariate analysis confirmed older age to

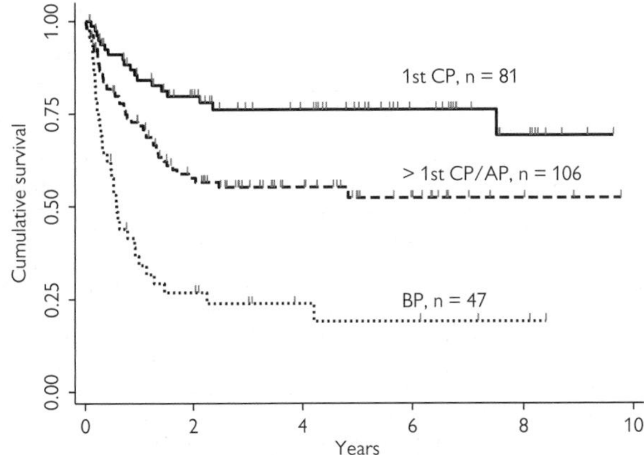

Figure 16.2 Overall survival in adult CML patients after allogeneic stem cell transplantation performed in Italy between 2005 and 2012.

Source: data from the Gruppo Italiano Trapianto di Midollo Osseo (GITMO) national registry.

be a significant prognostic factor for higher TRM. Additionally, major molecular response or complete molecular response (CMR) at 1 month and 3 months, following an allograft, were important predictors of favourable long-term outcomes. Moreover, current experience suggests that with the improving allo-SCT technology, such as reduced intensity conditioning and improved donor availability, the clinical outcomes continue to improve. As illustration, a 3-year OS of 56 imatinib-failure, low EBMT risk CML-CP patients who underwent transplantation was 91%, with a TRM of 8% in a German multicentre study. Such results underscore the importance of allografting patients who probably have biologically more aggressive disease, having failed TKI therapy.

Impact of different types of conditioning regimens donors and stem cells sources

When allo-SCT was the treatment of choice, the combinations of cyclophosphamide (CTX) with total body irradiation (TBI) or Bu were considered the most effective and appropriate options for any young CML patient with a suitable donor. More recently, the combination of intravenous Bu with CTX is considered equally effective and less toxic than CTX-TBI. In addition, the use of reduced intensity or reduced toxicity programmes have shown remarkable tolerability and potent antileukemic activity even in elderly or unfit patients. Many studies have now assessed the usefulness of such pretransplant strategies, which focus on being immunosuppressive, rather than myeloablative, and maximize the graft-versus-leukaemia effect, which is generally considered to play a major role in eradicating CML after transplant.

A retrospective CIBMTR analysis comparing outcomes in adults allografted for CML in first CP observed an i.v. Bu myeloablative conditioning to result in fewer relapses, compared with than TBI or oral Bu and the LFS is better after i.v. or oral Bu compared with TBI. In another retrospective study performed by CIBMTR, the post-allo-SCT outcomes of 306 patients with CML in CP, aged 40 to 75 years, underwent a reduced intensity or a non-myeloablative conditioning from 2001 to 2007; 74% of the study cohort had prior imatinib therapy. Transplant proved to be relatively safe in older CML patients with similar TRM (range 19–29%) across age groups and OS across age cohorts. OS at 3 years ranged from 54% for patients with an age between 40 and 49 years, to 41% for patients older than 60 years. Nonetheless, the incidence of relapse increased with age being at 3 years, 66% in the 60-year age group compared with 36% in the group aged 40 to 49 years. Interestingly, OS after allo-SCT was superior for patients who received imatinib pre-allo-SCT (56% vs. 37% at 2 years). Importantly, the intensity of the conditioning regimens significantly affected relapse and LFS; multivariate analysis demonstrated an inferior outcome for patients receiving a non-myeloablative compared with reduced intensity conditioning.

In a recent study the CIBMTR reported the outcome of more than 1000 patients with CML in CP, aged 40 to 60 years, who received a reduced intensity or myeloablative allo-SCT between 2007 and 2014. Reduced intensity conditioning was associated to a similar survival as myeloablative, albeit with higher early relapse. The efficacy of an allo-SCT using haematopoietic stem cells from unrelated donors has been documented since the early experience and confirmed over the years. The possibility to perform a transplant from alternative donors has also become a feasible option. A haploidentical donor is another option. Recent results confirm that patients with advanced CML receiving a cord blood transplant had a lower relapse rate, a slightly better long-term survival, but a higher early TRM than those receiving HLA-matched related allo-SCT using peripheral blood, compared to bone marrow-derived stem cells. In addition, both in children and adults the development of more effective *in vitro* and *in vivo* manipulations of the graft or the use of post-transplant CTX as graft-versus-host disease (GvHD) prophylaxis has gained a remarkable improvement of the outcome after haploidentical transplantation.

Role of molecular monitoring for minimal (measurable) residual disease following allo-SCT

After allo-SCT, a significant proportion of patients show evidence of haematologic or cytogenetic or molecular recurrence of the underlying CML. The presence of the *BCR-ABL1* transcripts offers a unique opportunity to monitor the presence of the leukaemic clone before and after transplantation. The use of quantitative polymerase chain reaction (PCR) has greatly increased the clinical value of monitoring measurable residual disease (MRD) and several studies have documented that intervention prior to florid relapse improves the outcome of CML. Indeed, while low or absent residual *BCR-ABL1* transcripts are associated with a very low risk of relapse (1%), increasing or persistently high transcript levels are almost invariably associated to relapse. The crucial role of an accurate, quantitative monitoring of minimal residual disease is further emphasized by the therapeutic options that can be taken to correct the kinetic of the leukaemic clone after transplantation. The use of donor lymphocyte infusions (DLI) to restore a remission is well known in CML patients relapsing after allo-SCT. By and large, the amazing ability of donor lymphocytes to induce a complete remission, represents the best evidence of the key role played by the donor immune system in eradicating the patient's leukaemic clone. However, DLI may also induce or precipitate GvHD and this may in turn severely compromise the quality of life of allografted patients. The use of post-transplant TKIs alone or in combination with DLI appears to induce a rapid and durable remission even in patients with AP-CML relapsing after allo-SCT. In addition, it has been examined whether imatinib alone can delay relapse and postpone the requirement for DLI in CML patients allografted using a reduced intensity regimen. In this latter setting, imatinib was commenced on day +35 and continued until 1 year after transplantation. Post-transplantation imatinib was well tolerated and abolished the risk of relapse during this period. For patients who relapsed after imatinib discontinuation, DLI remained highly effective in inducing a molecular remission. More recently, Shimoni and coworkers explored the use of nilotinib for the prevention of relapse after SCT in advanced-phase CML and Ph+ ALL. Patients received prophylactic nilotinib maintenance, starting at a median of 38 days after transplantation. Some patients stopped the treatment because of toxicities (mostly gastrointestinal and hepatic) but after nilotinib maintenance, most patients achieved or maintained a CMR, and only one of them later relapsed. With a median follow-up of 46 months patients on nilotinib maintenance had a 2-year OS and progression-free survival (PFS) of 69% and 56%.

BCR-ABL1-positive MPN summary

TKI-therapies substantially reduces the number of CML cells and confer a survival benefit. However, most patients will relapse, which makes it probable that leukaemia stem cells persist. However, a distinct group of CML patients still require transplant that remains a curable treatment options for an otherwise incurable disease. Most recent results suggest that the outcome after transplantation is improving particularly for patients who remain in a CP of their disease despite a modest or poor response to TKIs. Another key issue remains related to the economic sustainability of long-term treatment with TKIs particularly in low income countries in which the transplant option may be considered a competitive treatment strategy compared to such expensive medical treatments.

BCR-ABL1-negative MPN

The term *BCR-ABL1*-negative MPN includes the classic MPN, primary myelofibrosis (PMF), essential thrombocythaemia (ET), and polycythaemia vera (PV). The majority of allo-SCT are restricted to patients with myelofibrosis (MF), which encompasses three biologically distinct subtypes, PMF, post-ET MF, and post-PV MF. All three subtypes are characterized by worst survival among patients with *BCR-ABL1*-negative MPN, and have significant impact on quality of life. The natural course of the disease is variable and about 25–30% of the patients will transform to acute myeloid leukaemia. Allogeneic haematopoietic stem cell transplantation is a curative treatment option but is associated with therapy-related morbidity and non-relapse mortality, which makes the procedure not applicable to all patients. However, in more recent years transplantation outcome has improved due to the introduction of less toxic conditioning regimens and improved monitoring of minimal residual disease, which allows early strategies (such as reduction of immunosuppression or DLI) to prevent clinical relapse. In addition, the approval of JAK2 inhibitors can be used prior to the transplant in order to reduce spleen size and constitutional symptoms. Despite lacking prospective randomized trials according to the published recommendations of the European LeukemiaNet (ELN), autologous stem cell transplant (ASCT) should be considered in transplant-eligible patients with PMF whose median survival is expected to be less than 5 years, which are patients with intermediate-2 and high risk according to International Prognostic Scoring System (IPSS) or Dynamic International Prognostic Scoring System (DIPSS), respectively. In a recent expert consensus paper, there was a recommendation to consider allogeneic SCT in intermediate-1 patients if other high-risk features such as *ASXL1* mutation, more than 2% peripheral blasts, refractory transfusion-dependent anaemia, or adverse cytogenetics according to DIPSS plus are present.

To properly balance the risk and benefit for the patient, the transplant- and patient-specific risk factor should also be taken into account, as recently proposed by the transplant-specific risk score for myelofibrosis patients.

Results of allogeneic stem cell transplantation for myelofibrosis

The published experience in allo-SCT for MF is growing and has been summarized recently. In the late 1980s and the early 1990s the feasibility of allo-SCT for MF could be shown in small reports. One multicentre international study published in 1999 described a retrospective study with larger cohort in which allo-SCT was performed using myeloablative conditioning (MAC) in patients with a median age of 42 years. Non-relapse mortality (NRM) was 27% and the incidence of graft failure was 9%. The median OS and PFS reached 47% and 39% at 5 years. Another important updated United States study reported on 104 patients who received ASCT after MAC. In this study, NRM at 5 years of 34% and OS at 7 years of 61% were reported. A TBI-based study resulted in a high risk of NRM of 48% and a 2-year OS of 41%.

Myelofibrosis is a disease of the elderly, and reduced intensity regimens were introduced to enable older patients to be considered eligible for allogeneic stem cell transplantation. The evidence of graft vs. leukaemia effect in myelofibrosis could be shown by documented responses to DLI in relapsed patients. This allowed the use of reduced intensity conditioning (RIC) in the setting of ASCT for MF. Smaller studies reported that RIC can reduce toxicity as well as mortality without jeopardizing engraftment. Larger clinical trials were published thereafter but only two prospective studies with a large sample size were reported so far. The EBMT published in 2009 after including 103 patients who received a Bu/fludarabine-based RIC regimen followed by related or unrelated stem cell transplantation. The median age was 55 years and the NRM at 1 year was 16%. Cumulative incidence of relapse was 22% at 3 years. PFS and OS at 5 years were 51% and 67%, respectively. Advanced age and HLA-mismatched donor were independent predictive factors for reduced OS. A recent update of the study after a median follow-up of 60 months confirmed curative potential with an 8-year OS of 65%. A 5-year disease-free survival of 40% and a 5-year cumulative incidence of relapse/progression and NRM of s 28% and 21%, respectively.

The Myeloproliferative Disorders Research Consortium investigated melphalan/fludarabine as conditioning regimen in a prospective phase II trial in 66 myelofibrosis patients. The reported OS was 75% in the sibling group but only 32% in the unrelated group due to a higher NRM (59% vs. 22%). Other studies provided further evidence of the curative effect of allogeneic stem cell transplantation irrespectively of MAC or RIC as condition regimen. In Table 16.1 selected studies of allo-SCT for MF are shown.

Role of conditioning regimen

Registry data from the European Society of Blood and Bone Marrow Transplantation (EBMT) show that nearly 699 allogeneic stem cell procedure are yearly performed in Europe for myelofibrosis. The majority of patients received a RIC regimen (76%) (Figure 16.3). There is a concern that reduction of NRM achieved by using RIC regimens may be offset by the theoretical increased risk of relapse, but retrospective comparisons could not show difference in outcome or relapse incidence. So far no prospective randomized comparison between MAC and RIC in myelofibrosis has been conducted.

Molecular markers and minimal residual disease

The driver mutations *JAK2*^{V617F}, calreticulin, and *MPL* in MF patients enable detection of minimal measurable disease after stem cell transplantation. Highly sensitive PCR methods to monitor *JAK2*^{V617F} or *MPL*$^{W515L/K}$ as well as *CALR* mutations have been developed. These markers are useful to detect minimal residual disease and to guide reduction of the immunosuppressive therapy including donor T-cell mediated adoptive immunotherapy to prevent clinical relapse. Small studies suggest that molecular relapse or residual molecular disease can be treated successfully using escalating DLIs with lower risk of severe GvHD. Other non-driver mutations such as *TET2*, *ASXL1*, *IDH*, or *EHZ2* and *CALR* are also potential marker for detection of MRD, but have not been investigated so far, but since some of them may influence outcome as ASXL-1, these markers may be used to select patient for stem cell transplantation. An older study showed better outcome for JAK2 positive patients in comparison to Janus kinase (JAK) wild-type patients, but more recently CALR and MPL mutated patients had better outcome after allo-SCT compared to *JAK2*^{V617F} and 'triple negative' patients.

Bone marrow fibrosis regression

Beside splenomegaly bone marrow fibrosis is a hallmark of myelofibrosis. The fibrogenesis is only poorly understood and investigators proposed clonal megakaryocytes or monocytes secrete cytokines, such as platelet-derived growth factor (*PDGF*), beta-fibroblast-derived growth factor (βFGF), or/transforming growth factor β (TGF-β). The possibility of bone

Table 16.1 Selected trials of allogeneic stem cell transplantation in myelofibrosis

Author	No. of patients	Conditioning regimen	Median age	Transplant-related mortality at one year	Overall survival
MAC conditioning					
Guardiola et al. 1999	55	TBI based (n = 35), various (n = 20)	42	27%	39% (at 5 years)
Deeg et al. 2003	56	Busulfan-based (n = 44), TBI based (n = 12)	43	20%	31% (at 5 years)
Kerbauy et al. 2007	104	TBI based (n = 15), busulfan-based (n = 80), Reduced intensity (n = 9)	49	34% (at 5 y)	61% (at 7 years)
Daly et al. 2003	25	TBI based		48%	41% (at 2 years)
RIC conditioning					
Hessling et al. 2002	3	Busulfan/ fludarabine	51	0%	100% (at 1 year)
Devine et al. 2002	4	Melphalan/ fludarabine	56	0%	100% (at 1 year)
Rondelli et al. 2005	21	Various	54	10%	85% (at 2.5 years)
Kröger et al. 2005	21	Busulfan/ fludarabine	53	16%	84% (at 3 years)
Bacigalupo et al. 2010	46	Thiotepa-based	51	24% (at 5 years)	45% (at 5 years)
Kröger et al. 2009	103	Busulfan/ fludarabine	55	16%	67% (at 5 years)
Gupta et al. 2014	233	Various	55	24% (at 5 years)	47% (at 5 years)

(Continued)

Table 16.1 *(Contd.)*

Author	No. of patients	Conditioning regimen	Median age	Transplant-related mortality at one year	Overall survival
MAC + RIC					
Stewart et al. 2010	51	RIC + MAC	49	32%	45% (at 5 years)
Ballen et al. 2010	170 (sibling)	RIC + MAC	45	18% at day 100	100% (at 16 months)
	117 (MUD)		47	35% at day 100	67% (at 5 years)
	33 (alternative related)		40	19% at day 100	44% (at 3 years)
Robin et al. 2011	147	RIC + MAC	53	16%	37% (5 years)
Patriaca et al. 2008	100	RIC + MAC	49	43% (at 3 years)	425 (at 3 years)
Gupta et al. 2009	46	RIC + MAC	54 (RIC); 47 (MAC)	48% MAC (at 3 yeas)	48% MAC (at 3 years)
Abelsson et al. 2012	92	RIC + MAC	55 (RIC); 46 (MAC)	32% MAC (at 2 years) 24% RIC (at 2 years)	49% MAC (at 5 years) 59% RIC (at 5 years)
Ditschkowsky et al. 2012	76	RIC + MAC	50	36% (at 5 years)	53% (at 5 years)
Nivison-Smith et al. 2012	57	RIC + MAC	n.a.	25% (at 1 years)	58% (at 5 years)
Scott et al. 2012	170	RIC + MAC	51	34% (at 5 years)	57% (at 5 years)

Adapted with permission from Alchalby H and Kröger N (2014). Allogeneic stem cell transplant vs. Janus kinase inhibition in the treatment of primary myelofibrosis or myelofibrosis after essential thrombocythemia or polycythemia vera. *Clin Lymphoma Myeloma Leuk*. Suppl:S36–41. DOI: 10.1016/j.clml.2014.06.012. Source: data from Kröger N and Mesa RA (2008). Choosing between stem cell therapy and drugs in myelofibrosis. *Leukemia*. 22(3):474–86. DOI: 10.1038/sj.leu.2405080.

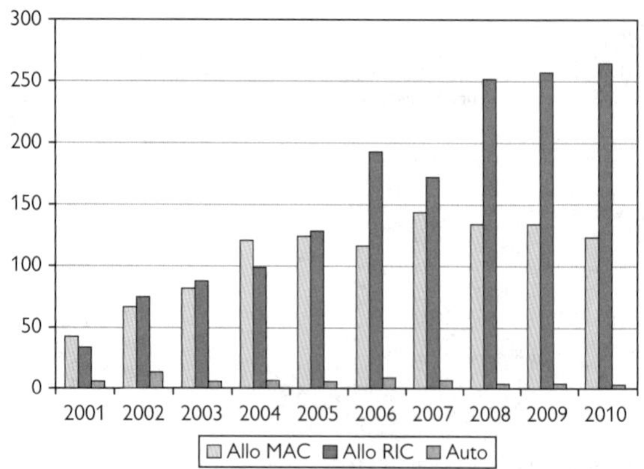

Figure 16.3 Development of allogeneic stem cell transplantation for myelofibrosis in Europe.

Source: data from European Group for Blood and Marrow Transplantation (EBMT). http://www.ebmt.org/.

Table 16.2 Bone marrow fibrosis at transplantation, at day +30, and at day +100 after allogeneic SCT

	MF-0	MF-1	MF-2	MF-3
at SCT (n = 57)			16 (28%)	41 (72%)
day +30 (n = 48)	3 (6%)	7 (15%)	17 (35%)	21 (44%)
day +100 (n = 44)	11 (25%)	13 (29%)	12 (27%)	8 (18%)

Reproduced with permission from Kröger N, et al. (2014). Dynamic of bone marrow fibrosis regression predicts survival after allogeneic stem cell transplantation for myelofibrosis. *Biol Blood Marrow Transplant.* 20(6):812–5. DOI: 10.1016/j.bbmt.2014.02.019.

marrow fibrosis regression by allogeneic stem cell transplantation has been reported in 22 patients who received a complete or nearly complete regression of bone marrow fibrosis in 59% of the patients at day +100, and in 90% at day +180. Furthermore, a complete or near complete resolution of bone marrow fibrosis at day +100 after allogeneic stem cell transplantation resulted in a more favourable survival and with good correlation graft function and reduced blood cell transfusions (Table 16.2). Other methods of monitoring bone marrow fibrosis regression such as magnetic resonance imaging, or positron emission tomography/computed tomography (PET/CT) have been reported.

Role of donor source

The inferiority of unrelated donor transplantation has been reported by several investigators and is in contrast to reports for acute myeloid leukaemia (AML) and myelodysplastic syndrome (MDS). Cord blood transplantation is associated with high risk of graft failure. A retrospective study on haploidentical stem cell transplantation resulted in an NRM rate of 38% and an OS of 54% at 2 years.

Role of disease specific risk scores and timing of transplantation

While in the past only the Lille score and Cervantes score were used to determine prognosis of myelofibrosis patients, more recently new prognostic scoring systems have been proposed, such as the IPSS for PMF which includes five variables: age >65 years, constitutional symptoms; Hb <100 g/L, leukocyte count > 25 × 10^9/L, and the presence of circulating blasts. Median survival differ between low risk (135 months), intermediate –1 (95 months), intermediate –2 (48 months), and high risk (27 months) the dynamic IPSS (DIPSS) was introduced, which includes the same variables used in IPSS but anaemia as risk factor was higher ranked. Unfavourable cytogenetic (+8, −7/7q-, i(17q), inv(3), −5/5q-, 12p-, or 11q23 rearrangement), low platelet count and transfusion dependency were included in the DIPSS system as DIPSS plus These systems are now more frequently used in PMF patients to determine individual risk and to find proper treatment decision. Also, molecular mutations have been included in a more recent proposed scoring system. The prognostic relevance of mutation profile resulted in a mutation-enhanced system (MIPSS70) in transplant-age PMF patients (70 years or younger) incorporating CALR type-1 mutation, presence of *ASXL1, EZH2, SRSF2*, or *IDH1/2* mutations, as well as the number of high-risk mutations. More recently, another prognostic system for post-ET/PV myelofibrosis has been developed and validated by the MYSEC project (MYelofibrosis SECondary to PV and ET). The prognostic model by MYSEC (MYSEC-PM) included the presence of constitutional symptoms, platelets <150 × 10^9/L, haemoglobin <11 g/dL, circulating blasts ≥3%, age, and a CALR-unmutated genotype resulting in improved prognostic ability compared with the IPSS. Larger retrospective comparison between allogeneic stem cell transplantation and conventional therapy in the pre-ruxolitinib era indicates that PMF patients 65 years of age or younger at diagnosis with intermediate-2 or high-risk disease are likely to benefit from allo-SCT, while for patients with low risk disease non-transplant approaches may be appropriate. Individual counselling is indicated for intermediate-1 risk patients.

Even if some correlation between DIPSS score and outcome after transplantation has also been reported (Figure 16.4), a more transplant-specific score which include also transplant-specific and patient-specific risk factors has been proposed and correlated better with outcome after allogeneic stem cell transplantation than IPSS, DIPSS, DIPSS plus, or MIPOSS 70. However, in all the model the use of JAK inhibitor treatment is not fully addressed and need further studies.

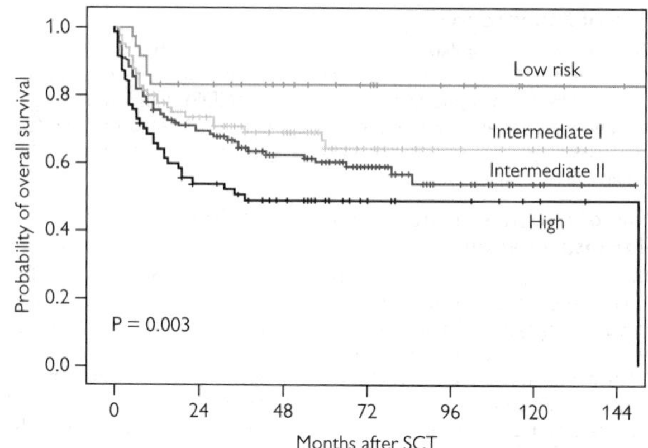

Figure 16.4 Outcome after allogeneic stem cell transplantation according to DIPSS (also see plate section).

Adapted with permission from Kröger N, et al. (2014). Dynamic of bone marrow fibrosis regression predicts survival after allogeneic stem cell transplantation for myelofibrosis. *Biol Blood Marrow Transplant*. 20(6):812–15. DOI: 10.1016/j.bbmt.2014.02.019.

Role of spleen size, splenectomy, and JAK inhibition

A beneficial role of splenectomy before stem cell transplantation for survival has not been detected so far. Some benefit for engraftment of splenectomised patients has been reported but the mortality risk of the procedure has to be taken into account and is reported to be 6–7%. Small series of successful splenectomies after stem cell transplantation have been reported. The approval of JAK inhibitors for the treatment of myelofibrosis resulted in reduction of splenomegaly, improvement of constitutional symptoms, and maybe also to a positive impact on survival. Because reduction of spleen size may positively influence engraftment, graft function, and reduction of constitutional symptoms and therefore could reduce transplant-related morbidity and mortality, the drug may be used to bridge patients with constitutional symptoms and/or splenomegaly to transplantation. Furthermore, the reduction of pro-inflammatory cytokines and the suppressive effect on T cells and NK cells may have some impact on the occurrence of GvHD after allogeneic stem cell transplantation. Studies reporting on use of ruxolitinib before transplantation have shown feasibility and early preliminary results did not negatively affect outcome of transplantation. A small study continued JAK inhibitor treatment during transplantation in myelofibrosis patient and reported 100% engraftment and low incidence of GvHD.

Leukaemic transformation

Transformed AML in MF is generally associated with a dismal outcome (see Chapter 14). In one study for patients with transformed leukaemia did not exceed 4.6 ± 5.5 months independently if patients had PV, ET, or PMF prior to transformation. A retrospective EBMT registry study reported outcome of 47 myelofibrosis patients who received allo-SCT for transformed AML. The OS and PFS at 3 years after allo-SCT were 33% and 26% respectively. Remission status prior to allo-SCT complete remission vs. no complete remission resulted in a better OS (69% vs. 22%). PV which transformed to AML can also be treated successfully by allo-SCT. In another retrospective EBMT study on 57 PV patients who transformed to AML and received allogeneic stem cell transplantation, an NRM of 29% and an OS of 28% were reported.

Treatment and prevention of relapse

The risk of relapse after allogeneic stem cell transplantation is between 10% and 18% after myeloablative and 29% and 43% after RIC. DLI are effective, but the numbers reported so far are limited. In a two-step approach for 30 relapsed patients, first DLI was given to 26 patients and 39% responded; 13 patients did not respond, and 4 patients with primary graft failure received a second allograft with a 2-year relapse-free and OS of 67% and 70%, respectively.

In summary, improvement in the management of allogeneic stem cell transplantation for myelofibrosis has increased the popularity of the procedure, especially in older patients. However, careful donor selection is needed to improve outcome. Harnessing the major effect of JAK inhibitors, such as spleen size reduction and improvement of constitutional symptoms before transplantation, will increase the likelihood that treatment-related complications will reduce. This will ultimately further improve survival.

Further reading

Abelsson J, Merup M, Birgegard G, et al. The outcome of allo-HSCT for 92 patients with myelofibrosis in the Nordic countries. *Bone Marrow Transplant.* 2012;47:380–6.

Baccarani M, Deininger MW, Rosti G, et al. European LeukemiaNet recommendations for the management of chronic myeloid leukemia. *Blood.* 2013;122:872–84.

Bacigalupo A, Soraru M, Dominietto A, et al. Allogeneic hemopoietic SCT for patients with primary myelofibrosis: a predictive transplant score based on transfusion requirement, spleen, and donor type. *Bone Marrow Transplant.* 2010;45:458–63.

Ballen KK, Shrestha A, Sobocinski KA, et al. Outcome of transplantation for myelofibrosis. *Biol Blood Marrow Transplant.* 2010;16:358–67.

Chhabra S, Ahn KW, Hu ZH, et al. Myeloablative vs reduced-intensity conditioning allogeneic hematopoietic cell transplantation for chronic myeloid leukemia. *Blood Adv.* 2018;2(21):2922–36.

Copelan EA, Avalos BR, Ahn KW, et al. Comparison of outcomes of allogeneic transplantation for chronic myeloid leukemia with cyclophosphamide in combination with intravenous busulfan, oral busulfan, or total body irradiation. *Biol Blood Marrow Transplant.* 2015;21(3):552–8.

Copelan EA, Avalos BR, Ahn KW, et al. Comparison of outcomes of allogeneic transplantation for chronic myeloid leukemia with cyclophosphamide in combination with intravenous busulfan, oral busulfan, or total body irradiation. *Biol Blood Marrow Transplant.* 2015;21:552–8.

Daly A, Song K, Nevill T, et al. Stem cell transplantation for myelofibrosis: a report from two Canadian centers. *Bone Marrow Transplant.* 2003;32:35–40.

Deeg HJ, Gooley TA, Flowers ME, et al. Allogeneic hematopoietic stem cell transplantation for myelofibrosis. *Blood.* 2003;102:3912–18.

Derlin T, Alchalby H, Bannas P, et al. Assessment of bone marrow inflammation in patients with myelofibrosis: an (18)F-fluorodeoxyglucose PET/CT study. *Eur J Nucl Med Mol Imaging.* 2015;42:696–705.

Devine SM, Hoffman R, Verma A, et al. Allogeneic blood cell transplantation following reduced-intensity conditioning is effective therapy for older patients with myelofibrosis with myeloid metaplasia. *Blood*. 2002;99:2255–8.

Ditschkowski M, Elmaagacli AH, Trenschel R, et al. Dynamic International Prognostic Scoring System scores, pre-transplant therapy and chronic graft-versus-host disease determine outcome after allogeneic hematopoietic stem cell transplantation for myelofibrosis. *Haematologica*. 2012;97:1574–81.

Fefer A, Cheever MA, Greenberg PD, et al. Treatment of chronic granulocytic leukemia with chemoradiotherapy and transplantation of marrow from identical twins. *N Engl J Med*. 1982;306:63–8.

Gagelmann N, Ditschkowski M, Bogdanov R, et al. Comprehensive clinical-molecular transplant scoring system for myelofibrosis undergoing stem cell transplantation. *Blood*. 2019;133(20):2233–42.

Gratwohl A, Heim D. Current role of stem cell transplantation in chronic myeloid leukaemia. *Best Pract Res Clin Haematol*. 2009;22:431–43.

Gratwohl A, Hermans J, Goldman J, et al. Risk assessment for patients with chronic myeloid leukaemia before allogeneic blood or marrow transplantation. *Lancet*. 1998;352:1087–92.

Guardiola P, Anderson JE, Bandini G, et al. Allogeneic stem cell transplantation for agnogenic myeloid metaplasia: a European Group for Blood and Marrow Transplantation, Société Francaise de Greffe de Moelle, Gruppo Italiano per il Trapianto del Midollo Osseo, and Fred Hutchinson Cancer Research Center Collaborative Study. *Blood*. 1999;93:2831–8.

Guglielmelli P, Lasho TL, Rotunno G, et al. MIPSS70: mutation-enhanced International Prognostic Score System for transplantation-age patients with primary myelofibrosis. *J Clin Oncol*. 2018;36:310–18.

Gupta V, Kröger N, Aschan J, et al. A retrospective comparison of conventional intensity conditioning and reduced-intensity conditioning for allogeneic hematopoietic cell transplantation in myelofibrosis. *Bone Marrow Transplant*. 2009;44:317–20.

Gupta V, Malone AK, Hari PN, et al. Reduced-intensity hematopoietic cell transplantation for patients with primary myelofibrosis: a cohort analysis from the center for international blood and marrow transplant research. *Biol Blood Marrow Transplant*. 2014;20:89–97.

Hessling J, Kröger N, Werner M, et al. Dose-reduced conditioning regimen followed by allogeneic stem cell transplantation in patients with myelofibrosis with myeloid metaplasia. *Br J Haematol*. 2002;119:769–72.

Hochhaus A, Larson RA, Guilhot F, et al. Long-term outcomes of imatinib treatment for chronic myeloid leukemia. *N Engl J Med*. 2017;376:917–27.

Innes AJ, Apperley JF. Chronic myeloid leukemia-transplantation in the tyrosine kinase era. *Hematol Oncol Clin North Am*. 2014;28:1037–53.

Jain T, Temkit M, Partain DK, et al. Comparison of reduced-intensity conditioning regimen used in patients undergoing hematopoietic stem cell transplantation for myelofibrosis. *Bone Marrow Transp*. 2017;23(3):S280–1.

Kerbauy DM, Gooley TA, Sale GE, et al. Hematopoietic cell transplantation as curative therapy for idiopathic myelofibrosis, advanced polycythemia vera, and essential thrombocythemia. *Biol Blood Marrow Transplant*. 2007;13:355–65.

Kolb HJ. Graft-versus-leukemia effects of transplantation and donor lymphocytes. *Blood*. 2008;112:4371–83.

Kröger N, Ditschkowski M, Scott BL, et al. Impact of conditioning regimen, donor source, and DIPSS score on outcome of allogeneic stem cell transplantation for myelofibrosis. *Blood*. 2013;122:712.

Kröger N, Giorgino T, Scott BL, et al. Impact of allogeneic stem cell transplantation on survival of patients less than 65 years with primary myelofibrosis. *Blood*. 2015;125(21):3347–50.

Kröger N, Holler E, Kobbe G, et al. Allogeneic stem cell transplantation after reduced-intensity conditioning in patients with myelofibrosis: a prospective, multicenter study of the Chronic Leukemia Working Party of the European Group for Blood and Marrow Transplantation. *Blood*. 2009;114:5264–70.

Kröger N, Zabelina T, Alchalby H, et al. Dynamic of bone marrow fibrosis regression predicts survival after allogeneic stem cell transplantation for myelofibrosis. *Biol Blood Marrow Transplant*. 2014;20:812–15.

Kröger N, Zabelina T, Schieder H, et al. Pilot study of reduced-intensity conditioning followed by allogeneic stem cell transplantation from related and unrelated donors in patients with myelofibrosis. *Br J Haematol*. 2005;128:690–7.

Kröger NM, Deeg JH, Olavarria E, et al. Indication and management of allogeneic stem cell transplantation in primary myelofibrosis: a consensus process by an EBMT/ELN international working group. *Leukemia*. 2015;29:2126–33.

Kröger N, Shahnaz Syed Abd Kadir S, Zabelina T, et al. Peritransplantation ruxolitinib prevents acute graft-versus-host disease in patients with myelofibrosis undergoing allogenic stem cell transplantation. *Biol Blood Marrow Transplant*. 2018;24(10):2152–6.

Lee SE, Choi SY, Kim SH, et al. Prognostic factors for outcomes of allogeneic stem cell transplantation in chronic phase chronic myeloid leukemia in the era of tyrosine kinase inhibitors. *Hematology*. 2014;19:63–72.

Lee SJ, Kukreja M, Wang T, et al. Impact of prior imatinib mesylate on the outcome of hematopoietic cell transplantation for chronic myeloid leukemia. *Blood*. 2008;112:3500–7.

Lussana F, Rambaldi A, Finazzi MC, et al. Allogeneic hematopoietic stem cell transplantation in patients with polycythemia vera or essential thrombocythemia transformed to myelofibrosis or acute myeloid leukemia: a report from the MPN Subcommittee of the Chronic Malignancies Working Party of the European Group for Blood and Marrow Transplantation. *Haematologica*. 2014;99:916–21.

Mughal TI, Radich JP, Deininger MW, et al. Chronic myeloid leukemia: reminiscences and dreams. *Haematologica*. 2016;101:541–58.

Nicolini FE, Basak GW, Kim D-W, et al. Overall survival with ponatinib versus allogeneic stem cell transplantation in Philadelphia chromosome-positive leukemias. *Cancer*. 2017;123(15):2875–80.

Nivison-Smith I, Dodds AJ, Butler J, et al. Allogeneic hematopoietic cell transplantation for chronic myelofibrosis in Australia and New Zealand: older recipients receiving myeloablative conditioning at increased mortality risk. *Biol Blood Marrow Transplantation*. 2012;18(2):302–30.

Panagiota V, Thol F, Markus B, et al. Prognostic effect of calreticulin mutations in patients with myelofibrosis after allogeneic stem cell transplantation. *Leukemia*. 2014;28:1552–5.

Passamonti F, Giorgino T, Mora B, et al. A clinical-molecular prognostic model to predict survival in patients with post polycythemia vera and post essential thrombo-cythemia myelofibrosis. *Leukemia*. 2017;31:2726–31.

Passweg JR, Baldomero H, Bader P, et al. Impact of drug development on the use of stem cell transplantation: a report from the EBMT. *Bone Marroq Transp*. 2017;52:191–6.

Passweg JR, Walker I, Sobocinski KA, et al. Validation and extension of the EBMT Risk Score for patients with chronic myeloid leukaemia (CML) receiving allogeneic haematopoietic stem cell transplants. *Br J Haematol*. 2004;125:613–20.

Patriarca F, Bacigalupo A, Sperotto A, et al. Allogeneic hematopoietic stem cell transplantation in myelofibrosis: the 20-year experience of the Gruppo Italiano Trapianto di Midollo Osseo (GITMO). *Haematologica*. 2008;93:1514–22.

Pavlu J, Szydlo RM, Goldman JM, Apperley JF. Three decades of transplantation for chronic myeloid leukemia: what have we learned? *Blood*. 2011;117:755–63.

Robin M, Tabrizi R, Mohty M, et al. Allogeneic haematopoietic stem cell transplantation for myelofibrosis: a report of the Société Française de Greffe de Moelle et de Thérapie Cellulaire (SFGM-TC). *Br J Haematol*. 2011;152:331–9.

Rondelli D, Barosi G, Bacigalupo A, et al. Allogeneic hematopoietic stem-cell transplantation with reduced-intensity conditioning in intermediate- or high-risk patients with myelofibrosis with myeloid metaplasia. *Blood*. 2005;105:4115–19.

Saber W, Cutler CS, Nakamura R, et al. Impact of donor source on hematopoietic cell transplantation outcomes for patients with myelodysplastic syndromes (MDS). *Blood*. 2013;122:1974–82.

Saussele S, Lauseker M, Gratwohl A, et al. Allogeneic hematopoietic stem cell transplantation (allo SCT) for chronic myeloid leukemia in the imatinib era: evaluation of its impact within a subgroup of the randomized German CML Study IV. *Blood*. 2010;115:1880–5.

Savani BN, Montero A, Kurlander R, Childs R, Hensel N, Barrett AJ. Imatinib synergizes with donor lymphocyte infusions to achieve rapid molecular remission of CML relapsing after allogeneic stem cell transplantation. *Bone Marrow Transplant*. 2005;36:1009–15.

Scott BL, Gooley TA, Sorror ML, et al. The Dynamic International Prognostic Scoring System for myelofibrosis predicts outcomes after hematopoietic cell transplantation. *Blood*. 2012;119:2657–64.

Shahnaz Syed Abd Kadir S, Christopeit M, et al. Impact of ruxolitinib pretreatment on outcomes after allogeneic stem cell transplantation in patients with myelofibrosis. *Eur J Haematol*. 2018;101(3):305–17.

Stewart WA, Pearce R, Kirkland KE, et al. The role of allogeneic SCT in primary myelofibrosis: a British Society for Blood and Marrow Transplantation study. *Bone Marrow Transplant*. 2010;45:1587–93.

Stübig T, Alchalby H, Ditschkowski M, et al. JAK inhibition with ruxolitinib as pretreatment for allogeneic stem cell transplantation in primary or post-ET/PV myelofibrosis. *Leukemia*. 2014;28:1736–8.

Tamari R, Mughal TI, Rondelli D, et al. Allogeneic stem cell transplantation for myelofibrosis: reversing the chronic phase in the JAK inhibitors' era? *Bone Marrow Transplantation*. 2015;50:628–36.

Warlick E, Ahn KW, Pedersen TL, et al. Reduced intensity conditioning is superior to nonmyeloablative conditioning for older chronic myelogenous leukemia patients undergoing hematopoietic cell transplant during the tyrosine kinase inhibitor era. *Blood*. 2012;119(17):4083–90.

Zheng C, Tang B, Yao W, et al. Comparison of unrelated cord blood transplantation and HLA-matched sibling hematopoietic stem cell transplantation for patients with chronic myeloid leukemia in advanced stage. *Biol Blood Marrow Transplant*. 2013;19:1708–12.

Chapter 17

Assessment of disease burden in patients with myeloproliferative neoplasms

Holly L. Geyer, Deepti Radia, Nicholas Sarlis, and Ruben A. Mesa

Introduction *268*
Spectrum of disease burden *270*
Tools to assess the MPN disorders *272*
Disease burden assessment in MPN *276*
PRO validation for FDA/EMA submission *280*
Patient outcomes as trial endpoints *281*
Conclusion *283*

Introduction

The individual conditions comprising the myeloproliferative neoplasms (MPN) are best understood as a mosaic of phenotypically diverse disorders united by similar genotypic and prognostic characteristics (Table 17.1). Essential thrombocythaemia (ET), polycythaemia vera (PV), and myelofibrosis (MF) have been particularly well studied as a result of their significant symptomatic disease burdens. Each is associated with splenomegaly, profound constitutional symptoms, cytopenias, and heightened risk of transformation. Mortality is typically attributable to disease transformation, infection, anaemia, or thrombotic/bleeding complications. Indeed, MPN-related thrombosis risk is five to sevenfold times that of the general population. Though life expectancy in ET and PV patients frequently nears that of the general population, patients remain at risk for clonal evolution into myelofibrosis with subsequent mortality rates similar to those of patients with primary myelofibrosis (PMF). Advancement to acute myeloid leukaemia is typically fatal within 12 months of diagnosis and occurs in roughly 7.8% of MPN patients.

The disease burden of MF patients is distinguishable from that of ET and PV via its magnified severity and expanded index of symptoms. Independent of arising *de novo* (PMF) or as secondary transformation from ET and PV, MF patients face a reduced life expectancy of 6–10 years which are dominated by considerable morbidity. Blastic transformation occurs in up to 23% of MF patients within 10 years of diagnosis. Median survival is an estimated 2.6 months. MF symptoms are generally more severe than those seen in ET and PV and include fatigue (96%), early satiety (77%), abdominal discomfort (66%), inactivity (74%), concentration problems (69%), night sweats (62%), itching (50%), bone pain (52%), fevers (22%), and weight loss (42%). Up to 42% of MF patients describe clinically deficient quality of life (QoL). Treatments for MF have historically been limited. With the exception of the recently released targeted therapies, few treatments offered any meaningful symptom relief and many paradoxically foster symptom developments.

Systemic mastocytosis (SM) is a rare heterogeneous multisystem disorder resulting from clonal mast cells in the skin and other tissues (see Chapter 11). The World Health Organization classification system for mast cell disease defines two major subgroups: cutaneous mastocytosis (CM, 80%) and systemic mastocytosis (SM, 20%). These are further divided into seven subtypes: indolent (ISM); smouldering (SSM); aggressive (ASM); SM associated with clonal haematological non-mast cell lineage disease (AHNMD); mast cell leukaemia (MCL); mast cell sarcoma; and extracutaneous mastocytosis (EM). Confirmation of SM is commonly performed via bone marrow biopsy or tissue biopsy demonstrating an aberrant mast cell immunophenotype with clonal mast cells expressing mutations in the encoding receptor for stem cell factor KIT with >90% patients harbouring the D816V point mutation and a tryptase level of >20 ng/mL. Although the incidence rate remains opaque, available data estimates it to be between 0.3 and 0.89/10 000 cases per year.

This orphan disease is challenging in its classification and clinical heterogeneity. Patients with SM can range from being completely asymptomatic to having debilitating symptoms. Patients suffer from a variety of clinical

Table 17.1 MPN symptoms by subtype

	Fatigue	Itching	Sweats	Bone pain	Abdominal fullness/ gastrointestinal symptoms	Fever	Undesired weight loss	Anxiety	Sleep disturbance	Intimacy issues	Breathing problems	Allergic/ mediator symptoms
MF	+++	+(+)	+++	++	+++	+(+)	++	+++	++	++	++	–
PV	++	+++	(+)	–	(+)	–	–	+	+	(+)	–	–
ET	+(+)	–	–	–	–	–	–	+	(+)	(+)	(+)	–
CM	++	++(+)	–	+	+(++)	(+)	(+)	++(+)	+	+	(+)	++(+)
SM	++(+)	+(++)	+(+)	+(+)	+(++)	(+)	(+)	++(+)	+	+	(+)	+(++)
MCAS	+++	++	++	(+)	++(+)	+	+(+)	+++	++	+(+)	+(+)	+++
HES	+(+)	+(++)	(+)	(+)	+(++)	(+)	+(+)	+(+)	(+)	(+)	+(++)	+(+)
CEL	+(+)	(+)	+(+)	(+)	(+)	+(+)	+(+)	+	(+)	(+)	+(+)	(+)

CEL, chronic eosinophilic syndrome; CM, cutaneous mastocytosis; ET, essential thrombocythaemia; HES, hypereosinophilic syndrome; MCAS, mast cell activation syndrome; MF, myelofibrosis; PV, polycythaemia vera; SM, systemic mastocytosis.

signs and symptoms as a result of local mast cell infiltration and mast cell mediator release of pro and anti-inflammatory mediators such as proteases (predominantly tryptase) histamine, PGD2, LTC4, LTD4, E4, TNF, IL-1, IL-4, IL-5, IL-8, IL-13, IL-1RA. There is considerable variation in the release of these mediators which likely impacts the heterogeneity of symptoms experienced by patients. Symptoms include pruritus, flushing, fatigue, dizzy spells, anaphylactic reactions, headaches, palpitations, fainting, breathlessness, throat swelling/tightness, indigestion, abdominal pain/discomfort, nausea, vomiting, diarrhoea, memory loss, bone pain, fractures due to osteoporosis, arthralgia, myalgia, alteration in mood, impending sense of doom, and depression. The severity and frequency of these symptoms have intra- and interpatient variability and do not correlate with baseline tryptase levels or clinical classification. Unlike patients with classical MPN who invariably are under the care of a haematologist, those with mast cell disorders may present to various clinicians as a result of the multiple manifestations of their disorder. Medical professionals have historically included dermatologists, immunologists, allergists, gastroenterologists, pulmonologists, and haematologists. The majority of patients with SM (>90%) have indolent SM. Current treatment is based on symptom control with few patients demonstrating symptomatic SM, ASM, MCL, and AHNMD being able to access targeted treatment on a compassionate-use basis or within a clinical trial.

Spectrum of disease burden

The heterogeneity both within and between MPN subtypes has made assessment and treatments of MPN disorders a challenging process. Until this past decade, little focus has been spent on advancing our knowledge of the MPN disease spectrum given the paucity of symptom or prognostic assessment tools. The field evolved dramatically following the 2005 discovery of the JAK2V617F mutation present in variable expression within PV, ET, and MF. Subsequent development of gene-targeted therapies revived interest into the quandary of MPN diversity and its impact on therapeutic response. Exploration of the MPN disease burden was first undertaken through a cross-sectional, internet-based symptom survey of 1179 PV, ET, and MF patients. Outcomes of this study highlighted the reality that most MPN patients struggle with daily fatigue (81%), itching (53%), night sweats (50%), bone pain (44%), fevers (14%), undesired weight loss (13%), and spleen pain (6%). Symptoms furthermore compromised many aspects of daily living. Patients described impairments in social functioning, were unable to achieve independence in daily tasks, and had reduced levels of physical activity and global QoL.

A recent prospective evaluation of 1470 MPN patients aimed to further determine whether the marked heterogeneity demarking MPN subtypes was indeed evidence of subtype subclusters. In a novel heat-map statistical presentation, five distinct subclusters emerged within both PV and ET. These subclusters contrasted by features such as Myeloproliferative Neoplasm Symptom Assessment Form Total Symptom Scores (MPN-SAF TSS), splenic size, bleeding history, spoken language, age, gender, and the presence of laboratory derangements. Interestingly, no correlations were noted between symptomatic burden and MPN risk score. Four subclusters were noted in MF. In contrast to PV and ET, correlations were identified linking higher MPN-SAF TSS scores with increased risk scores (Dynamic International Prognostic Scoring System, DIPSS). The results of this landmark study intimated that previously noted MPN subtype heterogeneity was indeed driven by unique biological and social influences with resultant phenotypic clustering. Furthermore, the study confirmed that disease risk is not an adequate surrogate for MPN symptom burden or patient QoL (as observed in PV and ET). Similarly, within mast cell disorders, correlations fail to exist between the clinical classification and predictable patient symptomatology, likely a reflection of the inherent phenotypic heterogeneity among patients.

Another area of study has focused on evaluating how the MPN patients perceive and cope with their disease burden. In a recent study, MPN patients were surveyed on their disease burden impacts their activities of daily living (ADLs), productivity, and QoL.

The MPN Landmark Survey evaluated 813 MPN patients (MF, 91%; PV, 78%; ET, 74%). Most patients that were surveyed reported feeling 'anxious' or 'worried' about their condition. They furthermore disclosed that MPN symptoms reduced their QoL (MF, 81%; PV, 66%; ET, 57%).

Patients also reported vocational impairments in the form of reduced work hours, increased sick days, voluntary job termination, receipt of medical disability, early retirement, or negative impact on ADLs. Within the previous 30 days prior to administering the survey, almost 35% of low-risk prognostic score patients reported missing >/=1 day of work or cancelling >/=1 day of planned activities. Interest into the potency of individual MPN symptoms as negative QoL drivers has also grown. MPN-related fatigue is routinely reported as the primary driver of the MPN disease burden. Its multifactorial nature (cytopenias, inflammation, pain, etc.) has made full understanding of its impact difficult. However, new research has discovered that associations are present between fatigue severity and patient education level, female gender, the presence of mental health disorders (depression), substance abuse (alcohol, tobacco) and body mass index (BMI). The marked inflammatory burden in MPN was also found to correlate with fatigue in a recent analysis of 309 JAK2-inhibitor treated MF patients. Symptom burden correlated closely with cytokines including TNFRII, VCAM1, TIMP1, B2MICG, and leptin. Gender also plays a key role in MPN symptom manifestation. In general, female MPN patients struggle with more significant MPN symptom burdens than their male counterparts. Fatigue and abdominal complaints appear to be particularly burdensome, and persist in spite of females having lower red blood cell transfusion requirements and being of younger age. Of special interest was the finding that despite more significant symptom burdens, females generally score higher for overall QoL. The interrelationships between symptoms have proven perplexing. Available evidence suggests that symptoms correlate closely with other symptoms, along with functional domains. Studies into these complex relationships are ongoing.

Tools to assess the MPN disorders

MPN-dedicated resources are available to assess patient disease burden. These include patient-reported outcome (PRO) tools to evaluate symptom severity and risk scoring instruments for prognostic evaluation (Table 17.2). These instruments are applicable at the time of initial patient evaluation and through the duration of the disorder. The MPN PRO tools have been a particularly timely resource as the scientific arena has focused on the development of targeted therapies whose scope of impact includes symptoms. Prognostic instruments for ET, PV, and MF continue to be updated as new clinical, cytogenic, and molecular risk factors are uncovered. Next we describe the available MPN symptom burden assessment tools in detail.

Prognostic tools

Essential thrombocythaemia

The International Prognostic Scoring System for Essential Thrombocythemia (IPSET; 2012) criteria are most frequently employed to predict thrombosis risk and median survival. The criteria utilize leukocyte count >/= 11 × 10(9)/L (1 point), age >/= 60 (2 points), and history of thrombosis (1 point). Low risk (survival not predicted), intermediate risk (24.5 year survival), and high risk (13.8 year survival) are denoted by scores of 0 points, 1–2 points, and 3–4 points, respectively.

Polycythaemia vera

The International Working Group for Myeloproliferative Neoplasm Research and Treatment (IWG-MRT) criteria are validated to predict PV survival. Leukocyte count >/= 15 × 10(9)/L (1 point), venous thrombosis (1 point), age 57–66 years (2 points), and age >/= 67 years (5 points) to assign patients as low risk (26 year survival), intermediate risk (15 year survival), and high risk (8.3 year survival) are denoted by scores of 0 points, 1–2 points, and >/=3 points, respectively.

Myelofibrosis

As with PV, numerous prognostic algorithms are available to estimate survival in MF. The International Prognostic Scoring System (IPSS) is available for use in PMF patients at the time of diagnosis. Similarly, the DIPSS may be applied throughout the disease course and is applicable to post-ET and post-PV MF patients as well. DIPSS includes the variables of age >65 (1 point), circulating blasts >/=1% (1 point), leukocyte count >25 × 10(9)/L (1 point), haemoglobin <10 g/dL (2 points), and the presence of constitutional symptoms (1 point) to stratify patients into low risk (0 factors, median survival not reached), intermediate-1 risk (1 to 2 factors, 14.2 year survival), intermediate-2 risk (3 to 4 factors, 4.0 year survival), and high risk (5 to 6 factors, 1.5 year survival). The updated DIPSS-PLUS criteria furthermore incorporate the risk factors of platelet count <100 × 10(9)/L, red cell transfusion need, and unfavourable karyotype.

Table 17.2 MPN-specific patient-reported outcome tools

PRO	Year	Total number of questions	Areas covered	Question content	Languages	Therapies investigated	Validation tools
MF-SAF (Deisseroth A. et al. 2012)	2009	20	• Fatigue • Splenomegaly-related complaints • Catabolic/ proliferative symptoms • Constitutional symptoms • QoL	• Early satiety • Abdominal discomfort • Abdominal pain • Fatigue • Inactivity • Cough • Pruritus • Night sweats • Fever • Bone pain • Quality of life • Weight loss	• English	• Ruxolitinib (Mesa et al. 2011)	• BPI • BFI • MSAS

(Continued)

Table 17.2 *(contd.)*

PRO	Year	Total number of questions	Areas covered	Question content	Languages	Therapies investigated	Validation tools
MPN-SAF (Falcone R. et al. 2012)	2011	27	• Fatigue • Splenomegaly-related complaints • Catabolic/ proliferative symptoms • Constitutional symptoms • QoL • Microvascular Symptoms	• Fatigue • Early satiety • Abdominal pain • Abdominal discomfort • Inactivity • Headache • Concentration problems • Dizziness • Numbness • Insomnia • Sad mood • Sexuality problems • Cough • Night sweats • Itching • Bone pain • Fever • Weight loss • Quality of life	• English • French • German • Spanish • Dutch • Swedish • Italian • Portuguese • Mandarin • Japanese • Hebrew • Czech • Arabic	• Ruxolitinib (Geyer et al. 2014) • Ruxolitinib (Vannucchi et al. 2015) • SAR302503 (Jamieson et al. 2013) • LY2784544 (Verstovsek et al. 2011) • Vorinostat (Andersen et al. 2014) • Pegylated Interferon (NCT01259856)	• BFI • EORTC-QLQC30

MPN-SAF TSS (Valent P et al. 2010)	2013	10	• Fatigue • Splenomegaly-related complaints • Catabolic/ proliferative symptoms • Constitutional symptoms • Microvascular symptoms	• Fatigue • Early satiety • Abdominal discomfort • Inactivity • Concentration problems • Night sweats • Itching • Bone pain • Fever • Weight loss	• English • French • German • Spanish • Dutch • Swedish • Italian • Portuguese • Mandarin • Japanese • Hebrew • Czech • Arabic	• PRM-151 (Verstovsek et al. 2014) • Ruxolitinib (Scherber et al. 2014) • Ruxolitinib (NCT02092324) • Pacritinib (NCT02055781)	• BFI • EORTC QLQ-C30

BFI, Brief Fatigue Inventory; BPI, Brief Pain Inventory; EORTC QLQ-C30, European Organization for Research and Treatment of Cancer Quality of Life Questionnaire; MF-SAF, Myelofibrosis Symptom Assessment Form; MPN-SAF, Myeloproliferative Neoplasm Symptom Assessment Form; MPN-SAF TSS, Myelofibrosis Symptom Assessment Form Total Symptom Score; MSAS, Memorial Symptom Assessment Survey; QoL, quality of life.

Adapted with permission from Radia D and Geyer HL (2015). Management of symptoms in polycythemia vera and essential thrombocythemia patients. *Hematology Am Soc Hematol Educ Program.* 2015:340–8. DOI: 10.1182/asheducation-2015.1.340.

Symptom assessment tools

MF-SAF

The Myelofibrosis Symptom Assessment Form (MF-SAF, 2009) was the first PRO tool developed for MPN symptom assessment. The PRO is comprised of 20 items and designed to capture the most applicable MPN symptoms on 'yes', 'no', or 0 (absent) to 10 (worst imaginable) scale. Initial validation took place against the Memorial Symptom Assessment Scale (MSAS), Brief Pain Inventory (BPI), and Brief Fatigue Inventory (BFI).

MPN-SAF

The Myeloproliferative Neoplasm Symptom Assessment Form (MPN-SAF, 2012) served as an expansion of the MF-SAF and includes symptom assessment for PV and ET patients as well. The study included complaints related to microvasculature such as dizziness, headaches, and numbness/tingling. The form has been validated in a variety of languages and played a valuable role in clinical trials such as COMFORT-1 and RESPONSE investigating JAK-2 inhibitor therapy.

MPN-SAF TSS

The Myeloproliferative Neoplasm Symptom Assessment Form Total Symptom Score (MPN-SAF TSS), also referred to as the MPN-10, is an upgraded version of the MPN-SAF, containing only the most frequent and representative MPN symptoms. Designed to facilitate administration in office and trial environments, this 10-item scoring tool has been employed in MPN clinical trials such as RELIEF. Assessed symptoms include worst fatigue, early satiety, abdominal discomfort, inactivity, itching, concentration problems, night sweats, fever, bone pain, and weight loss.

MPN-SAF TSS mast cell

Collaboration between the Stanford University School of Medicine (US), Guys and St Thomas' Hospitals NHS Foundation Trust (UK), The Mayo Clinic, Scottsdale (US) with patients from the UK Mastocytosis Patient Support Group and the US Mastocytosis Society led to the development of a modified MPN-SAF for patients with mast cell disorders. This tool included a combination of baseline questions from the MPN-SAF TSS and a 12-inventory questionnaire specific to mast cell symptoms. An initial survey to validate this PRO tool was carried out via electronic participation of members of the Mastocytosis Society (US) and the UK Mastocytosis Patient Support Group. This survey is discussed in detail next.

Disease burden assessment in MPN

Repetitive assessment of disease burden in MPN disorders is integral to management as disease advancement commonly involves life-threatening complications and progressive, debilitating symptoms. Prognostic evaluation upon discovery of the MPN and routinely if complications or worsening symptoms be encountered. The phenotypic symptom profile of PV and ET patients is not accurately predicted by prognostic criteria and frequently presents out of proportion to that expected for low- to intermediate-risk patients. As such, in addition to prognostic evaluation, symptom assessment utilizing the MPN-SAF TSS should also be performed at regular intervals, beginning at the time of diagnosis. A recent study (MPN Quartile Study) identified that MPN-10 scores could be divided into quartiles when assessing symptom improvement/worsening (MPN-10 Q1:<8; MPN-10 Q2: 8–17; MPN-10 Q3: 18–31; MPN-10 Q4: >/=32).

Treatment of ET and PV includes three prime objectives: first, avoidance and management of complications; second, the prevention of transformation; and finally, adequate symptom control. All PV and ET should be treated with daily aspirin therapy. PV haematocrit levels should be targeted to <45%. Cytoreductive therapy, beginning with hydroxyurea, is indicated if patients develop high-risk profiles or incur a thrombotic complication. Based on the successful outcomes of the RESPONSE and RELIEF trials, the JAK2 inhibitor, ruxolitinib, was licensed in December 2014 for use in PV patients unresponsive or intolerant to hydroxyurea. For high-risk ET or PV patients with significant symptom burdens, JAK2 inhibitor therapy should be considered.

As with PV and ET, evaluation of the MF disease burden requires estimation of disease risk (DIPSS) and a comprehensive symptom assessment. As reflected in the DIPSS scoring system, MF symptoms positively correlate with disease risk and therefore require diligent supervision. Management of MF involves two objectives: (1) early evaluation for curative options in eligible patients (stem cell transplant); (2) symptom management. For suitable intermediate- to high-risk MF patients, stem cell transplant remains first line therapy regardless of symptom profile. For those not deemed candidates, JAK2 inhibitors remain the most efficacious class of approved therapies for MF symptoms. As revealed in the COMFORT-I/II studies and their subsequent analysis, the JAK2 inhibitor ruxolitinib demonstrates impressive efficacy in reducing splenic size, managing MPN-related symptoms and complications (thromboembolic events, secondary malignancies), altering cytokine profiles, and delaying bone marrow fibrosis. Pooled evaluation studies have further shown up to a 35% reduced risk of death in ruxolitinib-treated patients vs. controls. JAK2 inhibitors have also proven beneficial for low- and intermediate-1 risk MF but are not yet FDA approved for use in this population. Therefore, low-risk, low-symptom burden MF patients may simply be observed. Patients with symptom advancement objectified by symptom quartile changes may benefit from JAK2 inhibitor treatment or interferon trials.

Mastocytosis

There have been a few studies looking at how to assess and measure the symptoms/disability experienced by patients with mastocytosis. A French case-control study investigating patient perceptions of disability in mastocytosis was carried out in 2004 with 363 mastocytosis patients (CM, ISM, and ASM) and 90 controls using an OPA and AFFIRM score. The OPA score was derived from a one-dimensional questionnaire asking patients how they assessed their disability in general on the health status and QoL graded as follows: 0—no disability, 1—light, 2—moderate, 3—severe, and 4—intolerable. AFFIRM was developed by the French network to support patients with mastocytosis. The design of this multidimensional questionnaire was based upon patient interviews to include the most frequently reported symptoms. At total of 38 symptoms are offered in 12 categories (skin, allergy/flush/shock, gastrointestinal, rheumatologic, asthenia, neurology/psychiatry, respiratory, urologic, infection, haemorrhoid inflammation, libido, and sweating difficulties). These were graded 0–4 (none, light, moderate, severe, and intolerable). Each disability was also weighted 1–5 to reflect the impact on overall (QoL) and a composite AFFIRM score calculated for the total results ranging from 0 to 760 (none to most severe disability). Validated questionnaires were also used including the Hamilton score for depression and QLQ-C30 score designed to measure QoL.

The results from this study showed a significant burden of disability in the French patients with mastocytosis compared to the controls and no direct correlation with tryptase levels, presence of D816V mutation, or subclassification of mastocytosis (no statistical difference between symptom reports by patients with CM/ISM and ASM). Symptoms included rash (72%; 23% grade 4), asthenia (82%; 28% grade 4), reduced performance status (52%), difficulty in social interaction (53%), memory loss (66%), headaches (20%), pain (20%), reduced sexual performance (18%), and grade IV bronchospasm (26%). Depression was common with >70% of patients reporting a Hamilton score >10. Two hundred and sixty-two (262) patients completed the QLQ-C30 QoL questionnaire and 32% (124 patients) had a score ≥60. A subgroup of 262 patients were assessed for the presence of life-threatening reactions; 19% had recurrent episodes of life-threatening anaphylactoid reactions, 32% had ≥7 flushes/ week, 12% ≥4 stools/day, 32% ≥8 micturitions/day, 77% had a pruritis score ≥6, 75% had a Hamilton scale ≥10, and 32% had a QLQ C30 score ≥60.

A further survey carried out in 2010 by the Mastocytosis Society, a US-based patient advocacy organization, aimed to identify experiences and perceptions of patients with mastocytosis including patients with mast cell activation syndromes and related disorders. The survey, containing 68 questions developed by the Society in conjunction with clinical advisors with an expertise in mast cells disorders, was administered to 428 patients. Patient populations included CM (100), SM (215), mast cell activation syndrome (MCAS), IA (idiopathic anaphylaxis, 19), and others (34). Most responders were female (62.5%) with a median age of 48. More than 66% of the respondents described itching, flushing, fatigue, and stomach pain. Fifty per cent (50%) of patients also noted these symptoms daily or occasionally with moderate or extreme severity. Fatigue and stomach pain were common complaints, with 21.7% of responders suffering daily extreme fatigue and 14.8% stomach pains. Other commonly reported symptoms included brain fog/cognitive difficulties, diarrhoea, headache, joint pain, rash, or telangiectasia macularis eruptiva perstans eruptions, light-headedness/syncope, abdominal bloating, anxiety, bone pain, and lower abdominal pain. Data regarding allergies was provided by 91.4% of responders. Fifty-eight per cent (58%) of patients declared drug allergies confirmed by positive allergy tests, and 58% also declared allergies to environmental substances/inhalants. More than 95% of patients listed triggers for allergic reactions which included heat, stress, exercise, alcohol, medications, odours, and insect stings. When questioned about overall mast cell disease (MCD) emotional impact on their lives, patients felt it impacted them either extremely (40%), moderately (35.4%), a little bit (15.6%), or none at all (3.4%). Twenty-five per cent (25%) reported that the greatest single distress-causing aspect of living with an MCD was the unpredictability of symptoms. This was followed by gastrointestinal symptoms (17.9%), an inability to work or participate in daily living activities (15.3%), pain (12.9%), anaphylactic episodes (12.1%), fatigue (10.3%), and fear or anxiety (4.2%). Over 60% of respondents were affected either moderately or extremely in regard to their need to cope with the unpredictability of symptoms, gastrointestinal problems, and fatigue.

Moreover, an earlier collaborative project between the same groups resulted in the development of a modified MPN-SAF for patients with mast cell disorders. This tool included a combination of baseline questions from the Myeloproliferative Neoplasm Symptom Assessment Form Total Symptom Score (MPN-SAF TSS) in addition to a 12-inventory questionnaire specific to mast cell symptoms relating to gastrointestinal symptoms, fainting/allergic reactions, and anaphylactic reactions with/without hospitalization. A survey of this PRO tool was carried out via electronic participation by members of the Mastocytosis Society (US) and the UK Masto patient support groups. A total of 285 responders completed the survey (85% female) with a median age of 49 years (range 18–87 years). Self-reported diagnoses were recorded as follows: 102 ISM (37%); 46 CM (17%); 13 SSM (4%); 12 systemic mastocytosis with an associated clonal haematological non-mast cell lineage disease (SM-AHNMD (4%); 74 MCAS; 26%); 13 airway smooth muscle (ASM) disorders (5%); and 20 of unknown diagnosis (7%).

Analysis of the MPN-SAF TSS Mast Cell PRO validation data showed that the mean MPN-SAF TSS scores were higher in the mast cell patient groups than those reported by MF patient cohorts (reported by Scherber et al. (2011)): CM 3.3, ISM 4.1, SSM 4.4, ASM 3.9, SM-AHNMD 3.9, MCAS 4.5 vs. PMF 2.5, PPV MF 2.7, and PET MF 2.7. Total numbers of patients were similar in both groups (285 vs. 284) although numbers in mast cell subgroups were smaller. Almost half of mast cell patients (46%) reported anaphylactic reactions with 21% having been seen in the emergency rooms in the previous 6 months. Sixty per cent (61%) of patients had cutaneous symptoms and the majority of these patients found the cosmetic appearance distressing. The study also identified that mast cell patients have utilized up to 15 different medications to manage symptoms.

In SM/MCD the clinicopathological diagnosis and classification of the disease has evolved greatly over the last decade in response to increased experience, development of multidisciplinary collaborative networks, and cooperative sharing of knowledge and research. In order to better understand the pathophysiology of the disease spectrum and subsequent impact on patient symptoms and QoL, it is imperative that we evaluate patient-reported symptoms with appropriate PRO tools, as well as develop tailored prognostic indictors and evaluate potential new targeted molecules. This is particularly important for mast cell patients with indolent or cutaneous disease, high symptom burden profiles, and those with limited symptomatic response to available therapies.

PRO validation for FDA/EMA submission

Historically, the incorporation PROs into clinical trials and subsequently product labelling was based on assessment tools that were not always disease specific. Such generic instruments may not be suitable for all conditions, especially for even rarer diseases with no precedent to identify appropriate regulatory endpoints. Ruxolitinib, a JAK1/JAK2 inhibitor, is the first agent licensed, by the FDA for the treatment of intermediate or high-risk myelofibrosis (MF), and by the European Medicine Agency (EMA), for disease-related splenomegaly or symptoms in patients with MF. It received a subsequent approval by the FDA for the treatment of patients with PV who have had an inadequate response to or are intolerant of hydroxyurea. The initial approval of ruxolitinib in MF was based in part on its ability to improve MF-related symptoms as measured by a novel, validated PRO instrument developed specifically for this patient population (i.e. 'fit for purpose'). Since the issuance of the FDA draft guidance on the use of PROs to support labelling claims in 2006 (guidance finalized in 2009), ruxolitinib is also the first oncology product to have a PRO incorporated in its US prescribing information.

The decision to pursue inclusion of symptoms in the ruxolitinib label was prompted by initial findings in the phase I/II study (INCB28424-251; NCT00509899). In addition to reductions in splenomegaly, improvements in many of the debilitating symptoms of MF were observed with ruxolitinib treatment. As a result of these findings, the protocol was amended to include a formal assessment of MF-related symptoms and thus better understand the clinical meaningfulness of therapy-related changes over time. Incyte also had several discussions with the FDA regarding a special protocol assessment that included a PRO instrument for the phase III, randomized, double-blind, placebo-controlled COMFORT-I study. During the course of these interactions, the FDA proposed the incorporation of a secondary endpoint based on an early version of the Myelofibrosis Symptom Assessment Form (MF-SAF) published by Mesa et al., a modification of the 19-item MF-SAF incorporated into the phase I/II study. After extensive qualitative patient interviews and cognitive testing, the PRO instrument was ultimately accepted for use in COMFORT-I as the modified MF-SAF version 2.0 (Figure 17.1). This electronic handheld diary included seven symptoms previously identified as common in patients with MF (night sweats, itching, abdominal discomfort, pain under the left rib, early satiety, bone/muscle pain, and inactivity), rated on a scale of 0 (absent) to 10 (worst imaginable). A TSS was calculated daily from the sum of patient ratings of the individual symptoms with the exception of inactivity. The key secondary endpoint in COMFORT-I was the proportion of patients who had at least a 50% improvement in the TSS from baseline to week 24.

Ruxolitinib treatment demonstrated significant benefit on the TSS compared with placebo, with changes in each of the six individual symptoms contributing to this overall benefit. Test-retest reliability coefficients from week 7 to week 8 were 0.98 with ruxolitinib and 0.97 with placebo, and compliance with data entry was ≥95%. Evaluation of the relationship between patient-reported symptom improvement measured with the TSS and responses on the Patient Global Impression of Change (PGIC) provided additional support for the use of the MF-SAF v2.0 as a 'fit for

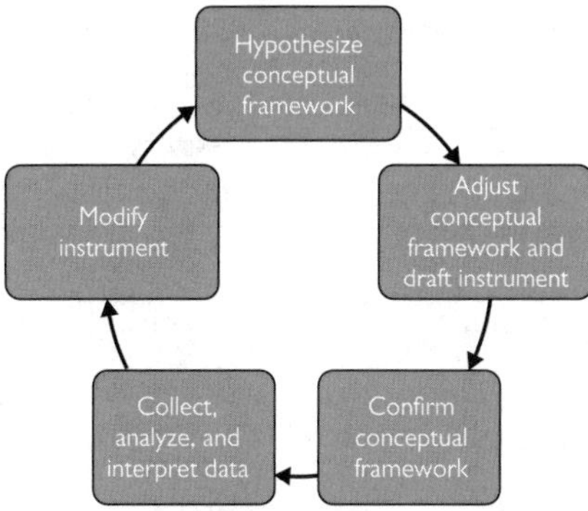

Figure 17.1 Development of the modified MF-SAF v.2.0.

purpose' PRO instrument. The PGIC asked patients to respond to the following item: 'Since the start of the treatment you've received in this study, your MF symptoms are: (1) very much improved; (2) much improved; (3) minimally improved; (4) no change; (5) minimally worse; (6) much worse; (7) very much worse.' Over 90% of ruxolitinib-treated patients who achieved a ≥50% improvement in TSS responded that their condition was 'much improved' or 'very much improved' on the PGIC, suggesting that the improvements measured by the TSS were clinically meaningful. In addition, >70% of placebo-treated patients who achieved <50% improvement in TSS responded that their condition was unchanged or had worsened (Table 17.3).

Patient outcomes as trial endpoints

An understanding of the impact of a given treatment on patient symptoms can facilitate informed decision making by patients, clinicians, manufacturers, regulators, and payers (reimbursement authorities). Such endpoints reflect important aspects of a disease that may not be captured by more objective disease assessments (e.g. laboratory values, MRI of the spleen), but can have a profound influence on a patient's QoL (e.g. severe itching, insomnia, pain). Consequently, such measures can provide valuable information in clinical trials not only to understand this aspect of treatment efficacy, but also the burden of disease from the patient's perspective.

Following the recognition of the importance of PROs, the FDA issued guidance for the use of PROs to support labelling claims. This guidance states: 'Generally, findings measured by a well-defined and reliable PRO instrument in appropriately designed investigations can be used to support a claim in medical product labeling if the claim is consistent with the instrument's documented measurement capability.'[1] As noted in this guidance, demonstration of a 'fit for purpose' instrument requires that it

Table 17.3 Associations between modified MF-SAF v2.0 TSS and PGIC in COMFORT-I

PGIC response, n (%)	Ruxolitinib n = 127		Placebo n = 100	
	≥50% TSS improvement (n = 68)	<50% TSS improvement (n = 59)	≥50% TSS improvement (n = 9)	<50% TSS improvement (n = 91)
Very much improved	35 (51.5)	8 (13.6)	1 (11.1)	0
Much improved	27 (39.7)	19 (32.3)	3 (33.3)	7 (7.7)
Minimally improved	3 (4.4)	22 (37.3)	3 (33.3)	17 (18.7)
No change	0	6 (10.2)	2 (22.2)	30 (33.0)
Minimally worse	2 (2.9)	3 (5.1)	0	19 (20.9)
Much worse	1 (1.5)	0	0	14 (15.4)
Very much worse	0	1 (1.7)	0	4 (4.4)

PGIC, Patient Global Impression of Change; TSS, total symptom score.

Adapted with permission from Mesa RA, et al. (2013). Effect of Ruxolitinib Therapy on Myelofibrosis-Related Symptoms and Other Patient-Reported Outcomes in COMFORT-I: A Randomized, Double-Blind, Placebo-Controlled Trial. *J Clin Oncol.* 31(10):1285–92. DOI: 10.1200/JCO.2012.44.4489.

measures symptoms important to patients, as identified through concept elicitation interviews, and that it contains questions that are interpretable and meaningful to patients, as established through cognitive debriefing interviews. The instrument must demonstrate reliability (internal consistency, test/retest correlations), construct validity (correlations with change in established measures), and ability to detect a meaningful change, and the definition of response must be clinically meaningful to the patient.

Factors to consider when deciding whether or not to include patient outcomes as trial endpoints include the presence of symptoms in the targeted patient population, the ability of the drug to improve a set of given symptoms without making others worse, and the overall toxicity profile of the drug. Study designs should take into account various sources of potential bias. Although placebo-controlled trials are optimal for assessing PROs, other potential elements of bias should be assessed, such as trial design factors (including characteristics of the blinding), as well as signs of efficacy and safety that can be attributed to specific treatment effects. Finally, compliance with the use of the instrument measuring the PRO of interest is an important factor in obtaining useful and meaningful results from the trial, and therefore, instruments that ensure maximal and reliable patient participation (e.g. electronic diaries, electronic reminders to complete) with a low burden to the patient are critical.

In patients with MPN, symptom burden is considerable and negatively impacts QoL. The MF-SAF v2.0 was developed specifically for patients with myelofibrosis; thus, other PRO instruments may need to be developed to evaluate symptomatic improvement with treatment in patients with other MPN.

Conclusion

Over the past decade, the substantial advancements in our understanding of the MPN disease burden have emerged from acknowledging the therapeutic deficiencies offered through standard therapies. Early exploration of aberrant MPN genotypic infrastructures, followed by subsequent development of targeted molecular mediators, has provided researchers an expansive arsenal of targeted therapies whose full potential awaits discovery. Through the dedicated, collaborative efforts of the international MPN research community, we now have tools at our disposal capable of objectively assessing the MPN disease burden. Development and continual revision of MPN prognostic scoring systems offers patients realistic survival timelines and assists in determining the most appropriate therapies. MPN-specific PRO tools have further allowed us to evaluate patient symptoms and subsequent response to therapies and have been of particular interest to the FDA as new therapies are developed. The confinements of subjective estimation that once limited the MPN field have been replaced with validated, objective tools whose usance holds unlimited potential. As we evolve from a decade of 'understanding' to that of 'application', we anticipate tremendous advancements in treatments and symptom management for all patients facing the MPN disease burden.

Reference

1. U.S. Department of Health and Human Services. *Guidance for Industry Patient-Reported Outcome Measures: Use in Medical Product Development to Support Labeling Claims*. Food and Drug Administration, 2019. Available at: https://www.fda.gov/media/77832/download

Further reading

Akin C, Fumo G, Yavuz AS, Lipsky PE, Neckers L, Metcalfe DD. A novel form of mastocytosis associated with a transmembrane c-kit mutation and response to imatinib. *Blood*. 2004;103(8):3222–5.

Andersen CL, Mortensen NB, Klausen TW, Vestergaard H, Bjerrum OW, Hasselbalch HC. A phase II study of vorinostat (MK-0683) in patients with primary myelofibrosis and post-polycythemia vera myelofibrosis. *Haematologica*. 2014;99(1):e5–7.

Barbui T, Barosi G, Birgegard G, et al. Philadelphia-negative classical myeloproliferative neoplasms: critical concepts and management recommendations from European Leukemia Net. *J Clin Oncol*. 2011;29(6):761–70.

Cervantes F, Dupriez B, Pereira A, et al. New prognostic scoring system for primary myelofibrosis based on a study of the International Working Group for Myelofibrosis Research and Treatment. *Blood*. 2009;113(13):2895–901.

Cervantes F, Vannucchi AM, Kiladjian JJ, et al. Three-year efficacy, safety, and survival findings from COMFORT-II, a phase 3 study comparing ruxolitinib with best available therapy for myelofibrosis. *Blood*. 2013;122(25):4047–53.

Deisseroth A, Kaminskas E, Grillo J, et al. U.S. Food and Drug Administration approval: ruxolitinib for the treatment of patients with intermediate and high-risk myelofibrosis. *Clin Cancer Res*. 2012;18(12):3212–17.

Emanuel RM, Dueck AC, Geyer HL, et al. Myeloproliferative neoplasm (MPN) symptom assessment form total symptom score: prospective international assessment of an abbreviated symptom burden scoring system among patients with MPNs. *J Clin Oncol*. 2012;30(33):4098–103.

Falcone R, Levy R. Approval of Jakafi (ruxolitinib) based on a home-grown, patient-reported outcome instrument: a case study. *Regulatory Focus*. 2012. Available at: https://www.raps.org/focus-online/quality-and-compliance/quality-and-compliance-article/article/1854/approval-of-jakafi-ruxolitinib-based-on-a-home-grown-patient-reported-outcome-i.aspx

Gangat N, Caramazza D, Vaidya R, et al. DIPSS plus: a refined dynamic international prognostic scoring system for primary myelofibrosis that incorporates prognostic information from karyotype, platelet count, and transfusion status. *J Clin Oncol*. 2011;29(4):392–7.

Geyer HL, Scherber R, Dueck A, et al. Gender differences and MPN symptom burden: an analysis by the MPN quality of life international study group (MPN-QOL ISG). *European Hematology Association Annual Meeting Abstracts*. 2014; Abstract 1039.

Gotlib J, Kluin-Nelemans HC, George TI, et al. Efficacy and safety of midostaurin in advanced systemic mastocytosis. *N Engl J Med*. 2016;374(26):2530–41.

Gotlib J, Pardanani A, Akin C, et al. International Working Group-Myeloproliferative Neoplasms Research and Treatment (IWG-MRT) & European Competence Network on Mastocytosis (ECNM) consensus response criteria in advanced systemic mastocytosis. *Blood*. 2013;121(13):2393–401.

Gotlib J. A molecular roadmap for midostaurin in mastocytosis. *Blood*. 2017;130:98–100.

Harrison C, Kiladjian JJ, Al-Ali HK, et al. JAK inhibition with ruxolitinib versus best available therapy for myelofibrosis. *N Engl J Med*. 2012;366(9):787–98.

Hermine O, Lortholary O, Leventhal PS, et al. Case-control cohort study of patients' perceptions of disability in mastocytosis. *PloS One*. 2008;3(5):e2266.

Jennings S, Russell N, Jennings B, et al. The Mastocytosis Society survey on mast cell disorders: patient experiences and perceptions. *J Allergy Clin Immunol Pract*. 2014;2(1):70–6.

Kvasnicka HM, Thiele J, Bueso-Ramos CE, et al. Effects of long-term ruxolitinib (RUX) on bone marrow (BM) morphology in patients with myelofibrosis (MF) enrolled in the COMFORT-I Study. *Blood*. 2016;128(22):1949.

Landolfi R, Marchioli R, Kutti J, et al. Efficacy and safety of low-dose aspirin in polycythemia vera. *N Engl J Med*. 2004;350(2):114–24.

Marchioli R, Finazzi G, Specchia G, et al. Cardiovascular events and intensity of treatment in polycythemia vera. *N Engl J Med*. 2013;368(1):22–33.

Mesa RA, Hoffman R, Kosiorek HE, et al. Impact on MPN symptoms and quality of life of front line pegylated interferon alpha-2a Vs. Hydroxyurea in high risk polycythemia vera and essential thrombocythemia: interim analysis results of Myeloproliferative Disorders Research Consortium (MPD-RC) 112 global phase III trial. *Blood*. 2016;128(22):4271.

Mesa RA, Kantarjian H, Tefferi A, et al. Evaluating the serial use of the Myelofibrosis Symptom Assessment Form for measuring symptomatic improvement: performance in 87 myelofibrosis patients on a JAK1 and JAK2 inhibitor (INCB018424) clinical trial. *Cancer*. 2011;117(21):4869–77.

Mesa RA, Li CY, Ketterling RP, Schroeder GS, Knudson RA, Tefferi A. Leukemic transformation in myelofibrosis with myeloid metaplasia: a single-institution experience with 91 cases. *Blood*. 2005;105(3):973–7.

Mesa RA, Niblack J, Wadleigh M, et al. The burden of fatigue and quality of life in myeloproliferative disorders (MPDs): an international Internet-based survey of 1179 MPD patients. *Cancer*. 2007;109(1):68–76.

Mesa RA, Schwager S, Radia D, et al. The Myelofibrosis Symptom Assessment Form (MFSAF): an evidence-based brief inventory to measure quality of life and symptomatic response to treatment in myelofibrosis. *Leuk Res*. 2009;33(9):1199–203.

Pardanani A. Systemic mastocytosis in adults: 2017 update on diagnosis, risk stratification, and management. *Am J Hematol*. 2016;91(11):1146–59.

Pardanini A, Tefferi A, Jamieson C, et al. Updated results from a randomized phase II dose-ranging study of the JAK2-selective inhibitor SAR302503 in patients with myelofibrosis (MF). *J Clin Oncol*. 2013;31:7109.

Passamonti F, Rumi E, Caramella M, et al. A dynamic prognostic model to predict survival in post-polycythemia vera myelofibrosis. *Blood*. 2008;111(7):3383–7.

Passamonti F, Thiele J, Girodon F, et al. A prognostic model to predict survival in 867 World Health Organization-defined essential thrombocythemia at diagnosis: a study by the International Working Group on Myelofibrosis Research and Treatment. *Blood*. 2012;120(6):1197–201.

Reiter A, Gotlib J. Myeloid neoplasms with eosinophilia. *Blood*. 2017;129:704–14.

Scherber R, Dueck AC, Johansson P, et al. The Myeloproliferative Neoplasm Symptom Assessment Form (MPN-SAF): international prospective validation and reliability trial in 402 patients. *Blood*. 2011;118(2):401–8.

Scherber RM, Senyak Z, Dueck AC, et al. High prevalence of mood disorders in MPNs and their possible role in MPN-related fatigue. *Blood*. 2014;124:3173.

Tefferi A, Rumi E, Finazzi G, et al. Survival and prognosis among 1545 patients with contemporary polycythemia vera: an international study. *Leukemia*. 2013;27(9):1874–81.

Valent P, Akin C, Hartmann K, et al. Advances in the classification and treatment of mastocytosis: current status and outlook toward the future. *Cancer Res*. 2017;77(6):1261–70.

Valent P, Sperr WR, Akin C. How I treat patients with advanced systemic mastocytosis. *Blood*. 2010;116(26):5812–17.

Vannucchi AM, Kiladjian JJ, Griesshammer M, et al. Ruxolitinib versus standard therapy for the treatment of polycythemia vera. *N Engl J Med*. 2015;372(5):426–35.

Verstovsek S, Mesa R, Foltz L, et al. Phase 2 trial of PRM-151, an antifibrotic agent, in patients with myelofibrosis: stage 1 results. *J Clin Oncol*. 2014;32(5):7114.

Verstovsek S, Mesa RA, Gotlib J, et al. A double-blind, placebo-controlled trial of ruxolitinib for myelofibrosis. *N Engl J Med*. 2012;366(9):799–807.

Verstovsek S, Mesa RA, Rhoades SK, et al. Phase I study of the JAK2 V617F inhibitor, LY2784544, in patients with myelofibrosis (MF), polycythemia vera (PV), and essential thrombocythemia (ET). *Blood*. 2011;118(21):1213–14.

Chapter 18

Clinical trials in myeloproliferative neoplasms

Giovanni Barosi and Gianni Tognoni

Introduction *287*
Genomic characterization of MPN *288*
Treatment goals of MPN *288*
Clinical trials in MPN measuring overall survival (OS) *290*
Clinical trials in MPN measuring progression-free survival (PFS) *292*
Clinical trials in MPN measuring objective response rate (ORR) *293*
Clinical trials in MPN measuring time-to-vascular-event (TTE) *296*
Clinical trials in MPN measuring patient-reported outcomes (PROs) *297*
Conclusion and future directions *299*

Introduction

The classic *BCR-ABL1*-negative myeloproliferative neoplasms (MPN) are clonal haematopoietic stem cell disorders comprising essential thrombocythaemia (ET), polycythaemia vera (PV), and myelofibrosis (MF), which are defined by unique clinical and laboratory characteristics, natural history, and prognosis. As an illustration, MF, which includes primary myelofibrosis (PMF), and ET and PV which transforms to MF (post-ET-MF and post-PV MF, respectively), is defined by bone marrow fibrosis and represents an advanced phase of MPN with a median survival of about 5 years. In contrast, ET and PV are chronic-phase diseases associated with remarkable long natural history where many patients have a survival that is similar to that of the general population. Such patients, when they develop disease-related symptoms, can be managed well with supportive measures alone. The median survival of patients with ET is essentially normal, and that for patients with PV is 27 years. It is therefore important to stratify the risk of all MPN patients carefully in order to avoid unnecessary treatment and treatment-related side effects. A key priority, therefore, is to develop effective treatments that enable MPN patients to live better and longer.

The gold standard to assess therapeutic efficacy of experimental agents in cancer is either a statistically significant and clinically meaningful improvement in overall survival (OS) and health-related quality of life (HRQoL), or a decrease in disease-related symptoms and adverse events In this chapter we address the current practices in the measurement of clinical outcomes in MPN trials, and discuss the benefits and limitations of trials endpoints in use in MPN clinical research. Our recent effort as part of the working group from the European LeukemiaNet (ELN) and the International Working Group-Myeloproliferative Neoplasm Research and Treatment (IWG-MRT) effort in improving clinical outcomes and endpoints in MPN served as a platform for this initiative.

In patients with MPN, in particular MF, improvements in trial design by incorporating patient-reported outcomes (PROs) beyond disease-related symptoms, and improvements in available endpoints of clinical relevance, has enabled patients, physicians, and other stakeholders to work together over the past decade to help determine good clinical practice approaches. As an illustration, for patients with MF, improvement in OS was a secondary endpoint in three randomized trials, with confounding results related to sample size, trial duration, and treatment choices after progression. Progression-free survival (PFS) was the secondary endpoint in one trial in MF with a greater clinical impact with respect to OS; however, the reflection of its benefit on OS was not demonstrated. Objective response rate (ORR) was widely used in MPN, however, it reflects heterogeneous objective benefits for the patients and biological rationales. In patients with ET and PV, event-free survival documented the capacity of therapies to prevent thrombotic occurrences, reflecting clinically relevant benefit to patients. PROs were secondary endpoints in MF and PV, and their support to change in ORR was the reason of drug approval by regulatory agencies. We know now that selected patients with MF can be treated, with short-term reduction in disease-related symptoms and splenomegaly, but at present most MF patients remain incurable and thus inexorably fatal, with the sole exception of those who receive an allogeneic stem cell transplant (allo-SCT) (Chapter 16).

Genomic characterization of MPN

Compared to *BCR-ABL1*-positive MPN, chronic myeloid leukaemia (CML), the *BCR-ABL1*-negative MPN demonstrate a remarkable genetic complexity, with multiple somatic mutations impacting disease biology, in particular the number of non-driver mutations present, as well as the effect of the order of acquisition of these aberrations on the phenotypic characteristics of MPN and its treatment. The phenotypic driver mutations include *JAK2*^{V617F} (located on chromosome 9p24), *MPL* (located on chromosome 1p34), *JAK2* exon 12, and *CALR* (located on chromosome 19p13.2). *JAK2*^{V617F} is present in almost all patients with PV, and in about 50–60% of those with ET or PMF; *CALR* is typically absent in PV, and present in 20–25% ET and PMF. *MPL* mutation also tends to be absent in PV and present in 3–4% of ET and 6–7% of PMF; about 15% of all patients with ET and PMF are considered negative for all the driver mutations and labelled 'triple negative' MPN. In addition to these mutations, several other somatic mutations have now been characterized, such as the epigenetic genes (*ASXL1, TET2, EZH2, IDH1, IDH2, DNMT3A*), RNA splicing genes (*SRSF2, U2AF1, U2AF2, SF3B1*) or transcription regulatory genes (*TP53, IKZF1, NF-E2, CUX1*). Though the precise contribution of each mutation remains an enigma, preliminary data suggests their prognostic and predictive value, and if validated robustly, should help personalize assessment of the risk of survival, from risk of thrombosis and from risk of transformation (Chapters 8–10).

Treatment goals of MPN

The drug ruxolitinib, a type I JAK1/2 inhibitor, was rationally designed to inhibit the constitutive JAK2 signalling that is generally believed to lead to the development of MPN. Following the qualified success in some patients with MF, who achieve control of disease-related symptoms and splenomegaly, several other type I JAK2 inhibitors and other candidate agents which target pathways activated by the dysfunctional JAK2 signalling, such as STAT, PI3K/AKT, and MEK/ERK, and the associated NF-κB inflammatory pathways, are now being tested in clinical trials. Each of these could prove valuable, even after resistance to ruxolitinib as a single agent has developed. Consequently, the MPN research community is facing the issue of testing a high number of agents with trials whose outcomes should measure clinically relevant benefits for the patients. This is a daunting task with multiple variables, both disease and treatment related, and adds much to the complexity of designing clinical trials for patients with MPN.

The design of clinical trials in MPN has evolved during the time to shape the growing understanding of disease biology, clinical and biological predictors of response, and benefit of therapies. In this process, the outcomes of the trials have been tailored to disease subtypes and goal of treatments. In PV and ET patients, the goal of therapy is to avoid first occurrence and/

or recurrence of thrombotic and bleeding complications. This should be obtained with drugs that do not increase the risk of acute leukaemia and post-PV/ET MF. In MF patients at a stage of early disease, like those with a prefibrotic bone marrow picture and with low risk of progression, the key is to avoid overtreatment. In MF at a stage of overt disease and with high risk of disease progression, the goal of therapy is prolongation of survival and, if possible, cure. In these patients, systematic therapies are targeted to managing anaemia, splenomegaly, and improving quality of life. Most, if not all, of these efforts relied on the historical Lille risk score, first introduced in 1996, the International Prognostic Scoring System (IPSS), dynamic-IPSS (DIPSS) or the DIPSS plus (DIPSS plus cytogenetic information) prognostic system for the risk stratification of MF patients eligible for clinical trials. Parenthetically, none of these risk scores were developed for patients with MF; rather, the risk scores were developed and tested exclusively in patients with PMF, and thereafter simply extrapolated into the treatment-decision-making process for all MF patients, including those with post-ET MF or post-PV MF. These risk stratification methods have also been tested in intermediate and high-risk MF patients being considered for allo-SCT, currently the only therapy which can accord long-term remission, and possible cure. Though comparative studies have suggested the usefulness of the various scoring systems, most experts use these in combination with a transplant-specific risk score (Chapter 16). Clearly such efforts are important, given the older age of MF patients and the increased risk of comorbid conditions, which contribute to the excessive historical non-relapse transplant mortality.

At present, the very considerable advances in the understanding of the genetic and epigenetic landscape of MPN, is only just being tested with considerable enthusiasm to personalize the risk stratification process, in particular for patients with MF. As an illustration, the ReTHINK study was designed to investigate the potential benefits of ruxolitinib in patients with early non-symptomatic MF who harboured at least one high molecular risk (HMR) mutation and for whom ruxolitinib is currently not used (ClinicalTrials.gov Identifier: NCT02598297). Primary objective was to evaluate the clinical benefit of ruxolitinib in delaying progression of MF from early disease to more advanced disease stages. The trial was, however, discontinued for difficulties in the enrolment of patients. The role of genomic characteristics in the progression and transformation of MF to acute leukaemia, irrespective of being clonal or subclonal, has now been reported in several studies. Indeed, recent work from Green and Campbell laboratories (Cambridge, UK) demonstrate the superior clinical performance of a high-risk mutational score, compared with the conventional IPSS or DIPSS risk scores. The group is now validating an online genomic application that will enable clinical predictions based on clinical, laboratory, and genomic features of newly diagnosed patients with MPN which may be useful in treatment and clinical trial discussions (https://cancer.sanger.ac.uk/mpn-multistage).

Clinical trials in MPN measuring overall survival (OS)

OS is an unambiguous outcome measure and a precise endpoint that measures patients alive after a fixed duration of time. In an indolent disease such as ET or PV, with a good prognosis and a median OS of more than 15 years, and a tendency to late transformations, the assessment of a therapeutic benefit in terms of OS is probably not realistic, and short-term, more clinically meaningful measures of benefit might represent agreeable surrogate endpoints. have been recommended. In contrast, OS is probably a reasonable and realistic primary clinical outcome endpoint for patients with MF, who have a heterogeneous disease with an expected median survival of 5 years (range: 2.2–11.2 years). Indeed, the ELN/IWG-MRT working group recommended that for phase III trials in MF, the primary endpoint should be a time-to-event (TTE) endpoint, such as OS or PFS. That said, no clinical trial in MF had OS as primary endpoint so far. OS was the secondary endpoint of a prospective phase IIB, randomized, double-blind, multicentre, placebo-controlled trial enrolling patients with advanced MF with anaemia published in 2006. Fifty-two (52) patients with MF from 19 French hospitals were randomized to receive either thalidomide or placebo. The number of patients required in each arm was calculated according to the first outcome criterion (response on anaemia): thus, the trial was not powered to detect differences in OS. At the time of therapy assessment (day 180), 14 patients were dead (8 in the thalidomide group and 6 in the placebo group), and the median OS was not significantly different between the two groups.

OS was also a secondary endpoint in the two seminal trials which tested the drug, ruxolitinib, a JAK1 and type I JAK2 inhibitor, with a short half-life, in patients with intermediate and high-grade MF. The two randomized phase III trials, *COMFORT* I and II, had some study design and endpoint differences, which ultimately impact the licensing and clinical use of the drug. The study results were published in 2012, leading to the drug being licensed by the US Food and Drug Administration (FDA) for patients with intermediate-2 and high-grade MF, and the European Medicines Agency (EMA) for patients with significant constitutional symptoms and splenomegaly. *COMFORT* I was a largely US-based study in which over 300 patients with intermediate-2 or high-risk MF with splenomegaly, who were considered to require treatment for disease-related symptoms, but were not candidates for conventional therapies, were randomized (1:1) to either receive ruxolitinib or a placebo. *COMFORT* II was an open-label, international study in over 200 MF patients, with similar clinical features were randomized (2:1) to receive either ruxolitinib or best available therapy (BAT). The number of events (death) at different follow-up times in patients treated with ruxolitinib, placebo, or BAT in *COMFORT* I and *COMFORT* II trial is depicted in Table 18.1. By using Grading of Evidence, Assessment, Development and Evaluation (GRADE) methodology, the confidence in estimates of effect on OS was rated by analysing these results for precision. Pooling hazard ratios (HRs) and confidence intervals for mortality, a statistically significant benefit associated with ruxolitinib treatment at late follow-up was documented. However, by applying the criterion of 'optimal information size' (OIS), which suggests

Table 18.1 Number of events (death) at different follow-up times in patients treated with ruxolitinib or placebo/BAT in COMFORT I and COMFORT II trials

	Ruxolitinib		Placebo/BAT			
	N. events	Total treated	N. events	Total treated	HR	P
At data cut off						
COMFORT I	10 (6.5%)	155	14 (9.1%)	154	0.67 (0.30–1.50)	NS
COMFORT II	6 (4%)	146	4 (5%)	73	0.70 (0.20–2.39)	NS
Median follow-up: 55 weeks (COMFORT I); 61.1 weeks (COMFORT II)						
COMFORT I	13 (8.4%)	155	24 (15.6%)	154	0.50 (0.25–0.98)	0.04
COMFORT II	11 (8%)	146	4 (5%)	73	1.01 (0.32–3.24)	NS
Median follow-up: 2 years (COMFORT I), 3 years (COMFORT II)						
COMFORT I	27 (17.4%)	155	41 (26.6%)	154	0.58 (0.36–0.95)	0.03
COMFORT II	29 (19.9%)	146	22 (30.1%)	73	0.48 (0.28–0.85)	0.009

Reproduced with permission from Barosi G, et al. (2015). Critical appraisal of the role of ruxolitinib in myeloproliferative neoplasm-associated myelofibrosis. *Onco Targets Ther*. 18(8):1091–102. DOI: 10.2147/OTT.S31916.

precision is only achievable when numbers of subjects in a systematic review is greater than number of subjects estimated by a conventionally calculated sample size for one, appropriately powered trial, OIS resulted to be of 471 persons per arm or 942 total. This was almost twice as large as the 528 subjects in the combined *COMFORT* I and *COMFORT* II trials. The longer-term data confirm the qualified success of ruxolitinib, and when the rank-preserving structural failure time (RPSFT) model was used in order to correct the OS estimates for crossover, there appears to be a modest survival benefit for ruxolitinib over placebo and BAT, in particular for patients in whom some histological features of improvement in the bone marrow fibrosis had been observed. However, the accuracy of the RPSFT model was challenged because there is no tangible reality behind the statistical model against which to confront the estimated results.

In summary, both the French thalidomide study and the *COMFORT* studies, highlighted that the detection of differences in OS in randomized trials with MF is a complex task, with confounding results related to sample size. Moreover, critical appraisals of evidence of *COMFORT* trials revealed that a number of additional issues make OS a cumbersome method of measuring the therapy benefit in MF. Since OS comprises both PFS and survival after progression, potential interventions available at disease progression, such as crossover into a different arm of the trial, treatment with an alternative drug, continuation with the same drug, or no further treatment, make it difficult to assess the effect of the initial intervention on OS. Moreover, uncontrolled follow-ups are exposed to several sources of bias that make them close to observational studies with regard to the quality of the evidence on the magnitude of treatment effect. It is of interest to note that the subsequent phase 3 randomized trials testing the next generation type I JAK2 inhibitors, do not include OS as a designated primary or secondary endpoint, as a recognition that in MF, in spite of its objective feature and great clinical relevance, OS is not necessarily an unequivocal measure of therapeutic benefit. The ELN/IWG-MRT working group has stressed the importance that future randomized trials with OS as the primary endpoint should contrast the risk a high number of potential biases.

Clinical trials in MPN measuring progression-free survival (PFS)

PFS, defined as time from randomization to disease progression or death, is frequently used in cancer to identify benefit earlier and to implicitly assess OS. Its advantage with respect to OS is that it potentially allows a direct assessment of the effect of the intervention on disease control.

PFS has been used as an additional secondary endpoint in *COMFORT* II, but not *COMFORT* I, trial. It is of interest to note that at the week 48 milestone in the COMFORT II trial, about a third of the ruxolitinib-treated cohort had progression events, compared with 26% in the group receiving BAT (hazard ratio for progression with ruxolitinib, 0.81; 95% CI, 0.47 to 1) and when the OS analysis was performed at the study milestone, 6 events (4%) were noted in the ruxolitinib-treated cohort, as compared with

4 events (5%) in the patients receiving BAT (HR, 0.70; 95% CI, 0.20–2.249). This observation suggests that in the context of the *COMFORT* II study, PFS has greater impact with respect to OS; however, the reflection of benefit of PFS on OS in this category of patients has still to be demonstrated.

An important issue of PFS as an endpoint of trials in MF is the definition of disease progression. In the *COMFORT* II trial, compared with *COMFORT* I, disease progression was defined as having any of the following occurrences: an increase in spleen volume of ≥25% from the on-study nadir (including baseline), splenic irradiation, or splenectomy, leukaemic transformation defined by an increase in peripheral blood blast percentage to ≥20% that was sustained for ≥8 weeks or bone marrow blast count ≥20%, and death. This definition was quite similar to the IWG-MRT definition of disease progression. However, when this definition is used as a surrogate endpoint for death, a criterion could be that it would include two prognostically different events. As a matter of fact, progression in splenomegaly belongs to the natural history of the disease and its detrimental prognostic value is poorly documented. At variance, blast transformation occurs in 10–20% of the patients with MF and its negative prognostic evidence is strongly documented.

In conclusion, the inherent clinical benefit of increasing PFS in MF has not yet fully exploited by clinical trials. A more focused definition of progression specifically targeted to biologically significant outcome measures seems to be necessary for this goal.

Clinical trials in MPN measuring objective response rate (ORR)

In most cancers, the ORR includes the proportion of patients who have a partial (PR) and complete response (CR). In patients with MPN, in particular MF, the relevance of such response categories is not clear. In general, it is considered that these categories might not to be sufficient to capture the whole range of responses, and the notion of including clinical improvement (CI) was suggested by the ELN/IWG-MRT. CI helps to define the response on a single aspect of the disease, such as splenomegaly, anaemia, or disease-related symptoms. Several phase II trials documented that molecularly targeted agents resulted in significant ORR in MPN. For example, 16 of 25 anaemic patients (64%) with MF achieved a CR with Peg-interferon alpha (IFNα)-2a; all 37 evaluable patients with PV had haematologic response, including 94.6% CRs with IFNα. It has been proposed by the ELN/IWG-MRT working group that ORR is an excellent and reliable endpoint for phase II efficacy trials in MPN, but not useful in phase III comparative trials. The recommendation reflects the ongoing debate on the precise relevance of ORR and its merit, and impact, on treatment, compared to being a meaningful surrogate endpoint for OS and disease control. This is particularly relevant in MPN were the response criteria are heterogeneous, and reflect improvement in different dimensions and characteristics of the disease.

As an illustration, response in splenomegaly was the primary endpoint in the two *COMFORT* randomized trials. In *COMFORT* I, the proportion of

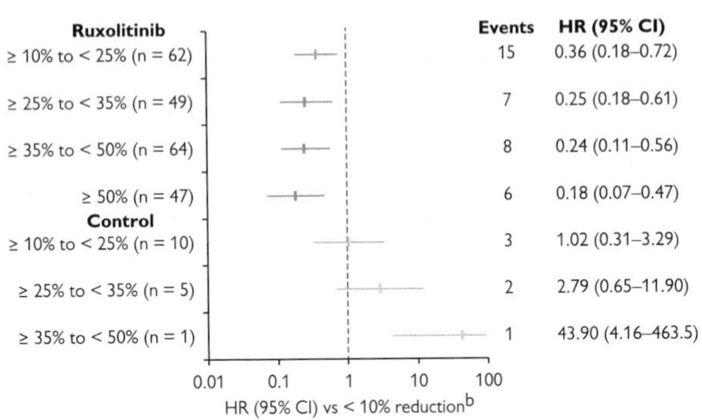

[a]Includes patients known to be alive at week 24.

[b]Category includes patients with a < 10% reduction from baseline in spleen volume at week 24 or no assessment (ruxolitinib, n = 64; control, n = 189); among these patients, there were 26 deaths (events) in the pooled ruxolitinib group and 63 deaths in the control group.

Figure 18.1 Analysis of pooled results (Terreri et al. 2013; Abgrall et al. 2006; and Barosi et al. 2012) of COMFORT I and COMFORT II trials. Forest plot of odds ratios with its 95% CI for the incidence of death among patients taking ruxolitinib versus control. HR for survival were correlated with spleen response.

Reproduced with permission from Vannucchi A, et al. (2015). A pooled overall survival analysis of the COMFORT studies: 2 randomized phase 3 trials of ruxolitinib for the treatment of myelofibrosis. *Haematologica*. 100(9):1139–45. DOI: 10.3324/haematol.2014.119545. Copyright © 2015 Ferrata Storti Foundation.

patients who met the primary endpoint of a reduction of 35% or more in spleen volume, as measured by MRI or computed tomography (CT) scans, at week 24, was 41.9% in the ruxolitinib group as compared with 0.7% in the placebo group (odds ratio, 134.4). In contrast, this observation was considered a secondary endpoint in the *COMFORT* II trial. In the *COMFORT* II trial, the primary endpoint was a reduction of 35% or more in spleen volume at 48 weeks after randomization, which was confirmed in 28% of the ruxolitinib-treated cohort, compared with only 1 of 72 patients receiving BAT. The longer-term follow-up, at about 3 years, confirmed the durability of these responses and also observed that about one-half of the study cohort, who remained on ruxolitinib, and had post-baseline spleen assessments, achieved a spleen response according to the protocol. Spleen symptom reduction with ruxolitinib was associated with a modest improvement of survival as just discussed (Figure 18.1). These results would drive to consider spleen and symptoms response as representative of a significant clinical benefit. Indeed, the randomized trials with next generation JAK2 inhibitors have continued to use the spleen response as the primary endpoint. However, it is important to recognize that despite these useful ORRs, the discontinuation rate of the drug appears high, with a median duration of therapy being 3 years, and some patients develop resistance. Furthermore, there have been some concerns highlighted by a recent Austrian-French collaborative study assessing over 600 patients with MPN who were noted to have a 16-fold increase in the risk of developing an aggressive extranodal B-cell lymphoma while receiving a type I JAK2 inhibitor, and requires further study. The patients at risk appear to have a pre-existing B-cell clone and it has been hypothesized that the secondary malignancy in these patients could be related to the drug's immune suppression. The drug also results in cytopenias and increased risk of opportunistic infections.

The pooled analysis of the results from *COMFORT* trials observed 24% deaths in the ruxolitinib cohort, compared with 33% in the control group. These results, however, need to be reconciled with those of *COMFORT* II trial in which PFS was not significantly different in patients receiving ruxolitinib or BAT in spite of the fact that they had quite different responses on the spleen size conducted at the same time. In conclusion, the available evidence is not enough to firmly validate the surrogacy principle of ORR in MF with respect to TTE endpoints, such as PFS or OS.

Ruxolitinib has now been tested against conventional therapy (hydroxyurea/hydroxycarbamide) in patients with PV, who either had an inadequate response to, or were not able to tolerate hydroxyurea associated side effects, in the randomized *RESPONSE* trial. This trial used ORR of at least 35% reduction in spleen volume at week 32, as determined by MRI/CT scans, and haematocrit control through week 32 as the composite primary endpoints. At the 32-week milestone, 21% of the ruxolitinib-treated cohort, compared to 1% of conventional therapy were noted to have met the primary endpoint ($p < 0.001$).

These randomized phase III studies provide some rationale as to the rationale for the utility of ORR as a reliable and clinically useful primary endpoint in trials with MPN. This endpoint is also recognized as a keynote surrogate endpoint in such trials by the regulatory bodies and often used for accelerated approval of drugs. In fact, ruxolitinib was licensed by both the FDA and EMA for use in selected patients with MF, based on the ORR from the two *COMFORT* studies, and for use in patients with PV based on the ORR from the *RESPONSE* study. It is of some interest that the drug's major effect is the suppression of the inflammatory cytokine production, a principal feature resulting in MPN-related symptoms, plus myelosuppression. And it has been recognized that the drug probably does not exert significant disease-modifying effects, with a minor effect on bone marrow fibrosis and *JAK2*^{V617F} allelic burden, properties which would impact OS.

In patients with ET, where the principal goal of therapy is to avoid the occurrence of thrombotic events, a correlation between attainment of haematological response, as demonstrated by the normalization of platelet count and leucocytes, and disease-related symptoms. Two interesting historical retrospective studies, which impact modern clinical trials viewpoints for patients with ET are those conducted by Hernandez-Bolunda et al. and Carobbio et al. The former study assessed the utility of haematological responses and observed that in a cohort of 166 ET patients who were treated with hydroxyurea for a median of 4.5 years, in the vast majority who achieved complete remissions, who comprised 134 of the 166 study cohort, there was no significant benefit from a lower incidence of thrombosis or an improved survival, and therefore no effect on the clinical outcomes of the patients. The Carobbio study examined 416 patients with ET treated with hydroxyurea for at least 12 months. Impressive haematological responses were again achieved in the majority of the study cohort, and following a longer-term follow-up of just under 4 years, there was no significant impact on the risk of thrombosis nor the natural history.

To overcome the discrepancies between attainment of ORR and clinical benefit in patients with ET, new response criteria were issued in 2013. They were based on the concept that response to therapies in ET patients should also capture the long-term effects on clinically relevant outcomes. The definition of response required normalization of symptoms and signs of the disease, remission of peripheral blood counts, absence of vascular events without signs of progression of disease, and bone marrow histological abnormalities. A patient-reported quality-of-life instrument was used for the definition of normalization of symptoms through an ad hoc specific questionnaire (Myeloproliferative Neoplasm-Symptoms Assessment Form Total Symptom Score [MPN-SAF TSS]). However, after the revision of response criteria, no trial in ET has been designed adopting the new criteria as endpoint.

Clinical trials in MPN measuring time-to-vascular-event (TTE)

Direct measures of benefit on the vascular outcomes have been recommended by the ELN/IWG-MRT working group and others, and have been used in the clinical research of MPN. Here in we discuss some of the keynote trials in MPN, primarily ET and PV, assessing TTE.

Cortelazzo et al. were the first to demonstrate the use of hydroxyurea in preventing high-risk ET patients from thrombotic events. In 1996, they assessed TTE in a randomized study enrolling 114 ET patients who were assigned to receive hydroxyurea or some other therapy. After a follow-up of 27 months, 3.6% of the hydroxyurea cohort experienced thrombotic events, compared with 24% of the control arm ($p = 0.003$).

Thereafter, in 2004, Landolfi et al. assessed the potential antithrombotic role of low-dose aspirin in about 500 patients with PV, in-a double-blind, placebo-controlled, randomized *ECLAP* study. Following a mean duration of follow-up was about three years, treatment with low-dose aspirin, as compared with placebo, was found to reduce the risk of the combined primary endpoint of thrombotic cardiovascular and stroke-related deaths. This study provided evidence that low-dose aspirin can safely prevent thrombotic complications in patients with PV who have no contraindications to such treatment and resulted in a significant treatment paradigm shift in PV. Thereafter, a year later, Harrison et al conducted a randomized study assessing over 800 patients with ET who were at high risk for vascular events to receive low-dose aspirin plus either anagrelide or hydroxyurea (*PT-1* trial). The composite primary endpoint was the actuarial risk of arterial thrombosis, venous thrombosis, serious haemorrhage, or death from thrombotic or haemorrhagic causes. Following a median follow-up of 39 months, the anagrelide cohort were noted to be significantly more likely to be associated with an arterial thrombotic event (p = 0.004), serious haemorrhage (p = 0.008), or transformation to MF (p = 0.001), but a decreased rate of venous thromboembolism (p = 0.006), compared with those receiving hydroxyurea group.

The efficacy and tolerability of anagrelide has also been compared with hydroxyurea in a prospective randomized non-inferiority phase III *ANAHYDRET* study. The study assessed about 260 high-risk ET patients and concluded that there were no major differences between the two study cohorts with regards to arterial or venous thrombosis or haemorrhage, and anagrelide was not inferior compared with hydroxyurea in the prevention of thrombotic complications in patients with ET. Then in 2014 Marchioli et al. investigated over 360 patients with PV in the pivotal *CYTO-PV* trial which assessed the importance of achieving and maintaining a target haematocrit of <45% versus 45–50%. The primary composite endpoint was the time until death from cardiovascular causes or major thrombotic events. Following a median follow-up of 31 months, the primary endpoint was observed in 2.7% of the low-haematocrit cohort and 9.8% of the higher-haematocrit group (hazard ratio in the high-haematocrit group, 3.91). A common denominator in these pivotal though simple trials was the notion of structuring a robust composite endpoint to address the keynote questions in patients with ET and PV.

Clinical trials in MPN measuring patient-reported outcomes (PROs)

It is generally recognized that PRO measures constitute important clinical decision-making tools provided they address more than just disease-related symptoms. It is therefore important that well-validated methods are employed to assess HRQoL issues and efforts should be enforced to ensure the best patient care and address the various questions appropriately. The questions now encompass the effect of the illness on an individual's physical, psychological, social, and somatic functioning and general well-being. Symptom control refers to alleviation of one or more symptoms and is complementary to HRQoL. PROs have garnered a greater influence as established, clinically relevant endpoints in a variety of solid cancers. The FDA, and now other regulatory agencies increasingly recognize PROs as a direct measure of clinical benefit to patients and as independent endpoints constitute important consideration in drug approval. The importance of PROs is critical in defining clinical benefit from the candidate drug and also the interpretation of any survival gains, OS, or PFS. PROs are particularly useful in incurable diseases where palliation of symptom-burden is critical. As an illustration, both of the *COMFORT* trials in MF included PROs as a secondary endpoint, though the methodologies employed were different; the *RESPONSE* trial for PV also incorporated PROs measurements to be performed at the 32-week primary endpoint. In *COMFORT* I trial, the modified Myelofibrosis Symptom Assessment Form (MF-SAF) was used. Patients were required to have achieved a reduction in the total symptom score of 50% or more from baseline to week 24. The study cohort achieving this endpoint was significantly higher in the ruxolitinib group, compared with the placebo group (45.9% vs. 5.3%; odds ratio, 15.3). In *COMFORT* II, symptoms and quality of life were assessed using the European Organization for Research and Treatment of Cancer (EORTC) quality-of-life questionnaire core model (QLQ-C30) and the Functional Assessment of Cancer Therapy–Lymphoma (FACT-Lym) scale. Results documented that based on the EORTC-QLQ-C30, treatment-induced differences in physical and role functioning, fatigue, and appetite loss significantly favoured ruxolitinib versus BAT from week 8 ($p < 0.05$) up to week 48 ($p < 0.05$).

In the *RESPONSE* study, PROs measures used the Myeloproliferative Neoplasm Symptom Assessment Form (MPN-SAF) patient diary to assess 14 PV-related symptoms, the European Organisation for Research and Treatment of Cancer Quality of Life Questionnaire (EORTC-QLQ-C30), the Pruritus Symptom Impact Scale, and the Patient Global Impression of Change; furthermore, scores for individual symptoms and symptom clusters using the MPN-SAF patient diary were obtained for all patients. At the primary endpoint of the study, almost one-half of all ruxolitinib-treated PV patients, compared to 5% in the control arm, reported at least a 50% reduction in the 14-item MPN-SAF total symptom score. Additionally, most of the ruxolitinib-treated cohort experienced greater reductions in all symptom clusters and a decrease in nearly all individual symptoms, compared with the control arm, who experienced an increase in many symptoms. Improvements were observed in the EORTC-QLQ-C30 global health scores, the Pruritis Symptom Impact Scale, and the Patient Global Impression of Change, whereas no major improvements were noted in the controls.

A key feature of the PROs in all of the aforementioned trials was the interactions with stakeholders, including regulatory agencies, to ensure accountability and responsible governance, and ultimately accorded full approval of the drug for the qualified indications. To be useful in MPN clinical trials, PROs must have acceptable reliability and validity. Responsiveness, the major dimension of validity, is determined by evaluating the relationship between changes in clinical- and patient-based endpoints and changes in the PRO scores over time. Arguably, improvement in HRQoL, delay in time to symptom progression and of course symptom improvement collectively provides a powerful composite to serve as a major endpoint in incurable diseases, such as MPN. A recent appraisal of 535 MPN trials observed an increasing incorporation of PROs as secondary endpoints, rather than primary endpoints. Although much has been achieved with the regards to the appreciation and utility of PROs in MPN trials, many weaknesses remain—to mention a few, analysis and interpretation of the effect of treatment of symptom-burden, and collecting and analysing information after the candidate trial and during subsequent treatment.

Conclusion and future directions

In MPN, heterogeneity of disease phenotype, differences in natural history and outcomes need a disease targeted, individualized design of clinical trials and, therefore endpoints. Recently, a working group, comprised of members from ELN and IWG-MRT, published consensus-based recommendations regarding trial design, patient selection, and definition of relevant endpoints for MPN with the objective to facilitate communication between academic investigators, regulatory agencies, and drug companies. Herein, we have analysed how published phase III randomized trials in MPN met the recommendations issued by the working group.

The detailed review of the use of different endpoints in the evaluation of traditional (e.g. aspirin and phlebotomy in PV) as well as innovative (e.g. ruxolitinib in MF and PV) interventions, clearly highlighted the need for well predefined, but flexible approaches in the selection of primary and secondary endpoints. While the adequacy of the sample size for relatively rare disease remains the principal challenge, the rules to be followed in MPN closely overlap with the wisdom which has been gained over the years also in other areas, such as oncology.

Although the demonstration of an OS or PFS benefit is the preferred objective for phase III trials in MPN, a number of randomized clinical trials in these disorders have used surrogate primary endpoints, like ORR, and were grounded on evidence of efficacy by taking PROs as secondary endpoints. A major reason for the use of surrogate endpoints in trials with MPN is the fact that regulatory bodies, such as the FDA and the EMA, recognize such endpoints as useful tools in specific disease settings. The major example was spleen response and improvement in PRO in order to approve ruxolitinib use in MF. In MPN, however, this policy contrasts with the objective of trials with new drugs recommended by clinicians who claimed none of the candidate surrogate endpoints, molecular response, pathological response, PROs, or ORR was deemed to have adequate validation to be used in phase III trials for new drugs development

The results of ORR and PROs as secondary endpoints of trials in MPN may aid clinical decision-making and influence healthcare policy. However, they need to be methodologically and clinically validated. Detailed instructions on the PRO rationale, methods for data collection methods, training, and management are essential to produce consistent data and avoiding biases. Evidence on the correlation between ORR and clinical benefits for patients presented in this chapter, drives to conclude that the rationale for using ORR is present in PV, but is lacking in ET and MF. Moreover, no assessment of the PRO measures utilized in clinical trials in terms of their psychometric qualities and robustness has been performed.

In conclusion, the design of trials for new agents continues to be a challenge in clinical research of MPN. An ideal objective should be that hard clinical endpoints (OS, PFS and TTE) should be consistent and combined with validated PROs, that are comprehensive expression of the safety and acceptability of new treatments. Surrogate endpoints should be consistently associated with hard outcomes in order to produce clinically applicable results. Explicit reasons of the criteria adopted to comply with the aforementioned rules could favour the comparability of results. Not only will an optimal choice of endpoints help to ensure accountability, but also it will help prioritize the best use of resources.

Further reading

Abgrall JF, Guibaud I, Bastie JN, et al. Thalidomide versus placebo in myeloid metaplasia with myelofibrosis: a prospective, randomized, double-blind, multicenter study. *Haematologica.* 2006;91:1027–32.

Baerlocher, GM, Oppliger Leibundgut E, et al. Imetelstat rapidly induces and maintains substantial hematologic and molecular responses in patients with essential thrombocythemia (ET) who are refractory or intolerant to prior therapy: preliminary phase II results. *Blood.* 2012;120: Abstract 179.

Barbui T, Barosi G, Birgegard G, et al. Philadelphia-negative classical myeloproliferative neoplasms: critical concepts and management recommendations from European Leukemia Net. *J Clin Oncol.* 2011;29:761–70.

Barbui T, Thiele J, Passamonti F, et al. Survival and disease progression in essential thrombocythemia are significantly influenced by accurate morphologic diagnosis: an international study. *J Clin Oncol.* 2011;29:3179–84.

Barosi G, Birgegard G, Finazzi G, et al. Response criteria for essential thrombocythemia and polycythemia vera: result of a European Leukemia Net consensus conference. *Blood.* 2009;113:4829–33.

Barosi G, Mesa R, Finazzi G, et al. Revised response criteria for polycythemia vera and essential thrombocythemia: an ELN and IWG-MRT consensus project. *Blood.* 2013;121:4778–81.

Barosi G, Rosti V, Gale RP. Critical appraisal of the role of ruxolitinib in myeloproliferative neoplasm-associated myelofibrosis. *Onco Targets Ther.* 2015;8:1091–102.

Barosi G, Rosti V, Massa M, et al. Spleen neoangiogenesis in patients with myelofibrosis with myeloid metaplasia. *Br J Haemato.* 2004;124:618–25.

Barosi G, Tefferi A, Barbui T. Do current response criteria in classical Ph-negative myeloproliferative neoplasms capture benefit for patients? *Leukemia.* 2012;26:1148–9.

Barosi G, Tefferi A, Besses C, et al. Clinical end points for drug treatment trials in BCR-ABL1-negative classic myeloproliferative neoplasms: consensus statements from European LeukemiaNET (ELN) and International Working Group—Myeloproliferative Neoplasms Research and Treatment (IWG-MRT). *Leukemia.* 2015;29:20–6.

Baxter EJ, Scott LM, Campbell PJ, et al. Acquired mutation of the tyrosine kinase JAK2 in human myeloproliferative disorders. *Lancet.* 2005;365:1054–61.

Bogani C, Bartalucci N, Martinelli S, et al. mTOR inhibitors alone and in combination with JAK2 inhibitors effectively inhibit cells of myeloproliferative neoplasms. *PLoS One.* 2013;8:e54826.

Carobbio A, Finazzi G, Antonioli E, et al. Hydroxyurea in essential thrombocythemia: rate and clinical relevance of responses by European LeukemiaNet criteria. *Blood.* 2010;116:1051–5.

Cervantes F, Dupriez B, Pereira A, et al. New prognostic scoring system for primary myelofibrosis based on a study of the International Working Group for Myelofibrosis Research and Treatment. *Blood.* 2009;113:2895–901.

Cervantes F, Pereira A. Does ruxolitinib prolong the survival of patients with myelofibrosis? *Blood.* 2017;129:832–7.

Cervantes F, Vannucchi AM, Kiladjian JJ, et al. COMFORT-II investigators. Three-year efficacy, safety, and survival findings from COMFORT-II, a phase 3 study comparing ruxolitinib with best available therapy for myelofibrosis. *Blood.* 2013;122:4047–53.

Cortelazzo S, Finazzi G, Ruggeri M, et al. Hydroxyurea for patients with essential thrombocythemia and a high risk of thrombosis. *N Engl J Med.* 1995;332:1132–6.

Deisseroth A, Kaminskas E, Grillo J, et al. U.S. Food and Drug Administration approval: ruxolitinib for the treatment of patients with intermediate and high-risk myelofibrosis. *Clin Cancer Res.* 2012;18:3212–17.

Fiskus W, Verstovsek S, Manshouri T, et al. Dual PI3K/AKT/mTOR inhibitor BEZ235 synergistically enhances the activity of JAK2 inhibitor against cultured and primary human myeloproliferative neoplasm cells. *Mol Cancer Ther.* 2013;12:577–88.

Gangat N, Caramazza D, Vaidya R, et al. DIPSS plus: a refined Dynamic International Prognostic Scoring System for primary myelofibrosis that incorporates prognostic information from karyotype, platelet count, and transfusion status. *J Clin Oncol*. 2011;29:392–7.

Gisslinger H, Gotic M, Holowiecki J, et al. Anagrelide compared with hydroxyurea in WHO-classified essential thrombocythemia: the ANAHYDRET Study, a randomized controlled trial. *Blood*. 2013;121:1720–8.

Guglielmelli P, Barosi G, Rambaldi A, et al. Safety and efficacy of everolimus, a mTOR inhibitor, as single agent in a phase 1/2 study in patients with myelofibrosis. *Blood*. 2011;118:2069–76.

Guglielmelli P, Lasho TL, Rotunno G, et al. MIPSS70: mutation-enhanced international prognostic score system for transplantation-age patients with primary myelofibrosis. *J Clin Oncol*. 2018;36:310–18.

Guyatt GH, Oxman AD, Kunz R, et al. GRADE guidelines 6. Rating the quality of evidence--imprecision. *J Clin Epidemiol*. 2011;64:1283–93.

Harrison C, Kiladjian JJ, Al-Ali HK, et al. JAK inhibition with ruxolitinib versus best available therapy for myelofibrosis. *N Engl J Med*. 2012;366:787–98.

Harrison CN, Campbell PJ, Buck G, et al. Hydroxyurea compared with anagrelide in high-risk essential thrombocythemia. *N Engl J Med*. 2005;353:33–45.

Harrison CN, Vannucchi AM, Kiladjian JJ, et al. Long-term findings from COMFORT-II, a phase 3 study of ruxolitinib vs best available therapy for myelofibrosis. *Leukemia*. 2016;30:1701–7.

Harrison CN, Vannucchi AM, Platzbecker U, et al. Momelotinib versus best available therapy in patients with myelofibrosis previously treated with ruxolitinib (SIMPLIFY 2): a randomised, open-label, phase 3 trial. *Lancet Haematol*. 2018;5:e73–e81.

Hernández-Boluda JC, Pereira A, Cervantes F, et al. Clinical evaluation of the European LeukemiaNet response criteria in patients with essential thrombocythemia treated with anagrelide. *Ann Hematol*. 2013;92:771–5.

Ianotto JC, Boyer-Perrard F, Gyan E, et al. Efficacy and safety of pegylated-interferon α-2a in myelofibrosis: a study by the FIM and GEM French cooperative groups. *Br J Haematol*. 2013;162:783–91.

ICH Harmonised Tripartite Guideline. Statistical principles for clinical trials. International Conference on Harmonisation E9 Expert Working Group. *Stat Med*. 1999;18:1905–42.

James C, Ugo V, Le Couédic JP, et al. A unique clonal JAK2 mutation leading to constitutive signalling causes polycythaemia vera. *Nature*. 2005;434:1144–8.

Joly F, Vardy J, Pintilie M, Tannock IF. Quality of life and/or symptom control in randomized clinical trials for patients with advanced cancer. *Ann Oncol*. 2007;18:1935–42.

Kiladjian JJ, Cassinat B, Chevret S, et al. Pegylated interferon-alfa-2a induces complete hematologic and molecular responses with low toxicity in polycythemia vera. *Blood*. 2008;112:3065–72.

Klampfl T, Gisslinger H, Harutyunyan AS, et al. Somatic mutations of calreticulin in myeloproliferative neoplasms. *N Engl J Med*. 2013;369:2379–90.

Kralovics R, Passamonti F, Buser AS, et al. A gain-of-function mutation of JAK2 in myeloproliferative disorders. *N Engl J Med*. 2005;352:1779–90.

Kundranda MN, Tibes R, Mesa RA. Transformation of a chronic myeloproliferative neoplasm to acute myelogenous leukemia: does anything work? *Curr Hematol Malig Rep*. 2012;7:78–86.

Kyte D, Duffy H, Fletcher B, et al. Systematic evaluation of the patient-reported outcome (PRO) content of clinical trial protocols. *PLoS One*. 2014;9:e110229.

Landolfi R, Marchioli R, Kutti J, et al. Efficacy and safety of low-dose aspirin in polycythemia vera. *N Engl J Med*. 2004;350:114–24.

Levine RL, Wadleigh M, Cools J, et al. Activating mutation in the tyrosine kinase JAK2 in polycythemia vera, essential thrombocythemia, and myeloid metaplasia with myelofibrosis. *Cancer Cell*. 2005;7:387–97.

Marchioli R, Finazzi G, Specchia G, et al. Cardiovascular events and intensity of treatment in polycythemia vera. *N Engl J Med*. 2013;368:22–33.

Mascarenhas J, Hoffman R, Talpaz M, et al. Pacritinib vs best available therapy, including ruxolitinib, in patients with myelofibrosis: a randomized clinical trial. *JAMA Oncol*. 2013;4:652–9.

Mesa RA, Kiladjian JJ, Catalano JV, et al. SIMPLIFY-1: a phase III randomized trial of momelotinib versus ruxolitinib in Janus kinase inhibitor-naïve patients with myelofibrosis. *J Clin Oncol*. 2017;35:3844–50.

Mesa RA, Vannucchi AM, Mead A, et al. Pacritinib versus best available therapy for the treatment of myelofibrosis irrespective of baseline cytopenias (PERSIST-1): an international, randomised, phase 3 trial. *Lancet Haematol*. 2017;4:e225–36.

Mullally A, Lane SW, Ball B, et al. Physiological Jak2V617F expression causes a lethal myeloproliferative neoplasm with differential effects on hematopoietic stem and progenitor cells. *Cancer Cell.* 2010;17:584–96.

Nangalia J, Massie CE, Baxter EJ, et al. Somatic CALR mutations in myeloproliferative neoplasms with nonmutated JAK2. *N Engl J Med.* 2013;369:2391–405.

Pang M, Zhuang S. Histone deacetylase: a potential therapeutic target for fibrotic disorders. *J Pharmacol Exp Ther.* 2010;335:266–72.

Pardanani A, Harrison C, Cortes JE, et al. Safety and efficacy of Fedratinib in patients with primary or secondary myelofibrosis: a randomized clinical trial. *JAMA Oncol.* 2015;1:643–51.

Passamonti F, Cervantes F, Vannucchi AM, et al. A dynamic prognostic model to predict survival in primary myelofibrosis: a study by the IWG-MRT (International Working Group for Myeloproliferative Neoplasms Research and Treatment). *Blood.* 2010;115:1703–8.

Pazdur R. Endpoints for assessing drug activity in clinical trials. *Oncologist.* 2008;13 Suppl 2:19–21.

Pearson TC, Wetherley-Mein G. Vascular occlusive episodes and venous haematocrit in primary proliferative polycythaemia. *Lancet.* 1978;2:1219–22.

Quintás-Cardama A, Kantarjian H, Estrov Z, et al. Therapy with the histone deacetylase inhibitor pracinostat for patients with myelofibrosis. *Leuk Res.* 2012;36:1124–7.

Quintás-Cardama A, Verstovsek S. Molecular pathways: Jak/STAT pathway: mutations, inhibitors, and resistance. *Clin Cancer Res.* 2013;19:1933–40.

Rambaldi A, Dellacasa CM, Finazzi G, et al. A pilot study of the histone-deacetylase inhibitor givinostat in patients with JAK2V617F positive chronic myeloproliferative neoplasms. *Br J Haematol.* 2010;150:446–55.

Rampal R, Al-Shahrour F, Abdel-Wahab O, et al. Integrated genomic analysis illustrates the central role of JAK-STAT pathway activation in myeloproliferative neoplasm pathogenesis. *Blood.* 2014;123:e123–33.

Revicki D, Hays RD, Cella D, Sloan J. Recommended methods for determining responsiveness and minimally important differences for patient-reported outcomes. *J Clin Epidemiol.* 2008;61:102–9.

Revicki DA, Osoba D, Fairclough D, et al. Recommendations on health-related quality of life research to support labeling and promotional claims in the United States. *Qual Life Res.* 2000;9:887–900.

Samuelsson J, Hasselbalch H, Bruserud O, et al. A phase II trial of pegylated interferon alpha-2b therapy for polycythemia vera and essential thrombocythemia: feasibility, clinical and biologic effects, and impact on quality of life. *Cancer.* 2006;106:2397–405.

Swerdlow SH, Campo E, Harris NL, et al. (eds.). WHO Classification of Tumours of Haemopoietic and Lymphoid Tissues. Lyon, France: IARC, 2008.

Tabarroki A, Tiu RV. Immunomodulatory agents in myelofibrosis. *Expert Opin Investig Drugs.* 2012;21:1141–54.

Tefferi A, Cervantes F, Mesa R, et al. Revised response criteria for myelofibrosis: International Working Group—Myeloproliferative Neoplasms Research and Treatment (IWG-MRT) and European LeukemiaNet (ELN) consensus report. *Blood.* 2013;122:1395–8.

Tefferi A, Guglielmelli P, Lasho TL, et al. MIPSS70+ version 2.0: mutation and karyotype-enhanced international prognostic scoring system for primary myelofibrosis. *J Clin Oncol.* 2018;36:1769–70.

Tefferi A, Rumi E, Finazzi G, et al. Survival and prognosis among 1545 patients with contemporary polycythemia vera: an international study. *Leukemia.* 2013;27:1874–81.

Tefferi A. Primary myelofibrosis: 2013 update on diagnosis, risk-stratification, and management. *Am J Hematol.* 2013;88:141–50.

Thepot S, Itzykson R, Seegers V, et al. Treatment of progression of Philadelphia-negative myeloproliferative neoplasms to myelodysplastic syndrome or acute myeloid leukemia by azacitidine: a report on 54 cases on the behalf of the Groupe Francophone des Myelodysplasies (GFM). *Blood.* 2010;116:3735–42.

Thomas DJ, Marshall J, Russell RW, et al. Effect of haematocrit on cerebral blood-flow in man. *Lancet.* 1977;2:941–43.

Vainchenker W, Delhommeau F, Constantinescu SN, et al. New mutations and pathogenesis of myeloproliferative neoplasms. *Blood.* 2011;18:1723–35.

Vannucchi A, Kantarjian H, Kiladjian JJ, et al. A pooled overall survival analysis of the COMFORT studies: 2 randomized phase 3 trials of ruxolitinib for the treatment of myelofibrosis. *Blood.* 2013;122(21):2820.

Vannucchi AM, Kantarjian HM, Kiladjian JJ, et al. A pooled analysis of overall survival in COMFORT-I and COMFORT-II, 2 randomized phase 3 trials of ruxolitinib for the treatment of myelofibrosis. *Haematologica.* 2015;100:1139–45.

Vannucchi AM, Kiladjian JJ, Griesshammer M, et al. Ruxolitinib versus standard therapy for the treatment of polycythemia vera. *N Engl J Med*. 2015;372:426–35.
Verstovsek S, Mesa RA, Gotlib J, et al. A double-blind, placebo-controlled trial of ruxolitinib for myelofibrosis. *N Engl J Med*. 2012;366:799–807.
Verstovsek S, Mesa RA, Gotlib J, et al. Efficacy, safety and survival with ruxolitinib in patients with myelofibrosis: results of a median 2-year follow-up of COMFORT-I. *Haematologica*. 2013;98:1865–71.
Verstovsek S, Mesa RA, Gotlib J, et al. Efficacy, safety, and survival with ruxolitinib in patients with myelofibrosis: results of a median 3-year follow-up of COMFORT-I. *Haematologica*. 2015;100:479–88.
Visser O, Trama A, Maynadié M, et al. RARECARE Working Group. Incidence, survival and prevalence of myeloid malignancies in Europe. *Eur J Cancer*. 2012;48:3257–66.
Wang X, Prakash S, Lu M, et al. Spleens of myelofibrosis patients contain malignant hematopoietic stem cells. *J Clin Invest*. 2012;122:3888–99.
Wang X, Ye F, Tripodi J, et al. JAK2 inhibitors do not affect stem cells present in the spleens of patients with myelofibrosis. *Blood*. 2014;124:2987–95.
Wilson MK, Karakasis K, Oza AM. Outcomes and endpoints in trials of cancer treatment: the past, present, and future. *Lancet Oncol*. 2015;16:e32–42.

Index

Note: Tables, figures and boxes are indicated by *t*, *f* and *b* following the page number

Numbers

5q-syndrome 158
8p11 leukaemia-lymphoma syndrome, pathogenesis 33*f*
24-hour urine studies, systemic mastocytosis 177–8

A

abdominal vein thrombosis 117*b*
ABL1-BCR fusion gene 96, 7
ABL1 mutations 194
ABL gene, break points 99*f*, 237*f*
accelerated phase of CML, WHO diagnostic criteria 95*b*
acute lymphoblastic leukaemia (ALL)
  P190 protein 69–70
  Ph-positive 98–100
acute myeloid leukaemia (AML) *see* leukaemic transformation
additional cytogenetic abnormalities (ACAs)
  chronic myeloid leukaemia 96–7, 98–100
    prognostic significance 68–9, 73–4
  systemic mastocytosis 175
adenosine deaminase, role in leukaemic transformation 225
adverse effects of treatment
  anagrelide 161
  avapritinib 186
  cladribine 183
  danazol 144*b*
  erythropoiesis-stimulating agents 144*b*
  hydroxyurea (hydroxycarbamide) 119, 120, 121*t*, 143–4
  interferons 182
  lenalidomide 144*b*
  masitinib 184
  midostaurin 185
  ruxolitinib 142–3, 144*b*
  thalidomide 144*b*
  tyrosine kinase inhibitors 107, 108*t*
AFFIRM score 277–8
age, prognostic significance in CML 64–7, 71–2
aggressive systemic mastocytosis (ASM) 170*b*, 172
  serum tryptase level 174–5
  treatment algorithm 181*f*
alkylating agents, risk of leukaemic transformation 155
allele-specific PCR 243
allogeneic stem cell transplantation (all-SCT) 94, 250
  in atypical chronic myeloid leukaemia 201
  in BCR-ABL1-negative MPN 255–63
  in BCR-ABL1-positive MPN 250–5
    indications for CML in CP 250–2
  in chronic myeloid leukaemia 109–10, 251*f*
    conditioning regimens 253–4
    donor types 254
    indications in CP 250–2
    post-procedure monitoring 254–5
    prognostic factors for outcomes 252–3
    recent results 252
    stem cell sources 254
    summary 255
    survival 253*f*
  in juvenile myelomonocytic leukaemia 200
  in leukaemic transformation 230*t*, 231
  in MPN-eo 215*t*, 216
  in myelofibrosis 139–49, 255–63
    after leukaemic transformation 262–3
    bone marrow fibrosis regression 257–60, 260*t*
    clinical trials 258*t*
    development in Europe 260*f*
    donor source 261
    molecular markers and residual disease 257
    relapse management 263
    results 256–7
    role of disease risk scores 261, 262*f*
    splenectomy and spleen size reduction 262
  in systemic mastocytosis 186–7
anaemia 131
  management 140–1, 144*b*
anagrelide
  adverse effects 161
  in essential thrombocytosis 160–1, 297
    combination with low-dose aspirin 159–60
  mechanism of action 161
ANAHYDRET study 160–1, 297
anaphylaxis management 180
anaphylaxis risk, systemic mastocytosis 179–80
androgen therapy, in anaemia 140, 144*b*
anti-CD30 therapy 188
anticoagulation 162
antihistamines 180
antiplatelet therapy 162*f*
  high-risk patients 162
  low-risk patients 163
  see also aspirin
arterial thrombosis 154–5
asciminib 108–9
aspirin
  in erythromelalgia 155
  in essential thrombocytosis 162*f*
    high-risk patients 159–60, 162
    low-risk patients 163
    during pregnancy 165
  in polycythaemia vera 115, 118, 122–3
    ECLAP study 296–7
    low thrombotic risk patients 119

ASXL1 mutations 26, 27, 28, 29*t*, 37, 88*t*
frequency in PMF 90*t*
and leukaemic transformation 225–7, 227*t*
myelodysplastic/myeloproliferative overlap neoplasms 194, 195*t*
CMML 195–7
MDS/MPN-RS-T 201
prognostic significance 89–90, 116, 137
in systemic mastocytosis 175, 179, 187
atypical chronic myeloid leukaemia (aCML) 203
clinical features 194–5, 200
CSF3R mutations 244–5
cytogenetics 27
diagnosis 200
genetics 194, 200
somatic mutations 29*t*
pathogenesis 33*f*, 35
treatment 201
WHO diagnostic criteria 193*t*
Auer rods 197
avapritinib 186
azacytidine
in chronic myelomonocytic leukaemia 197–8
in leukaemic transformation 230, 230*t*

B

B2A2 transcript 69–70
B3A2 transcript 69–70
BCR-ABL1 fusion gene 20*f*, 20–1, 94, 96–7, 98*f*, 235
detection of 96, 97*f*
isoforms 236–7, 237*f*
and leukaemic transformation 225
molecular biology 21*f*, 98–100, 99*f*
monitoring
clinical applications 238
DNA PCR 245
FISH 236
post-transplantation 254–5
reverse transcription PCR 236–8
Sanger sequencing 241
transcript type and transcript level 69–70
treatment response assessment 239*t*, 240–1
see *also* Philadelphia chromosome
BCR-ABL1 fusion protein 34–5
tyrosine kinase activity 34–5
BCR-ABL1-negative MPN 2
allogenic stem cell transplantation 255–63
BCR gene, break points 99*f*, 237*f*
BELA study 105
Bennett, John 4, 5*f*
beta-catenin pathway 225, 226*f*
Beutler, Ernest 7–8
B-findings, systemic mastocytosis 170*b*
BFORE study 105
BIM polymorphism 71
bisphosphonates 180
Bizzozero, Giulio 4
blast crisis (BC) 223
chronic myeloid leukaemia 95
molecular biology 98–100
definition 223–4
somatic mutations 29*t*
see *also* leukaemic transformation
Block, M.H. 9
BLU-285 188
bone marrow mastocytosis 169–71
bone marrow morphology 46–7, 48*f*
chronic myeloid leukaemia 96
chronic myelomonocytic leukaemia 197
essential thrombocytosis 53*t*, 56–8
differentiation from pre-PMF 52
mast cell leukaemia 172–3
MPN-eo 211, 214*t*
myelofibrosis 53*t*, 55–6, 132, 135*t*
prefibrotic 47*b*, 55*f*, 156–8
polycythaemia vera 53*t*, 58–60, 117*b*
standardization 50–1
systemic mastocytosis 170*b*
WHO diagnostic criteria 53*t*
bone marrow transplantation
historical background 11
see *also* allogeneic stem cell transplantation
bosutinib 12, 105
adverse effects 107, 108*t*
clinical trials 105
discontinuing therapy 110
molecular structure 102*f*
see *also* tyrosine kinase inhibitors
Boveri, Theodore 7
brentuximab vedotin 188
buparlisib 147*t*
Burkhardt, R. 9
busulfan
in essential thrombocytosis 162
introduction of 3*f*, 9–10
and leukaemic transformation risk 224
in myelofibrosis 143–4, 144*b*
prior to allo-SCT 253–4, 256–7, 258*t*

C

calcium supplementation 180
CALR (calreticulin) mutations 23, 29*t*, 36, 80, 89–90, 288
essential thrombocytosis 152–3, 155
risk of myelofibrotic transformation 155
frequency 24*f*
monitoring 244
murine models 38
myelodysplastic/myeloproliferative overlap neoplasms 194, 195*t*
MDS/MPN-RS-T 201
myelofibrosis 128
post-transplantation 257
prognostic significance 83, 85–6, 87*f*, 137
subclonal mutations 88*t*
thrombosis risk 155
cardiac involvement, MPN-eo 211
CBL mutations 22–3, 27, 28, 29*t*, 88*t*
myelodysplastic/myeloproliferative overlap neoplasms 195*t*
juvenile myelomonocytic leukaemia 199
systemic mastocytosis 175
CCA/Ph⁺
clonal evolution 22
prognostic significance 68–9
CD25 expression
mast cell activation syndrome 173

systemic mastocytosis 169, 170*t*
CD30 expression, systemic mastocytosis 174
CD34 expression, systemic mastocytosis 174
CDKN2A mutations 98–100
cerebral vein thrombosis 117*b*
C-findings, systemic mastocytosis 170*b*
children
chronic myeloid leukaemia 94
dasatinib 105
epidemiology 95
cutaneous mastocytosis 169, 178–9
essential thrombocytosis 166
juvenile myelomonocytic leukaemia 199–200
chromosome abnormalities
myelodysplastic/myeloproliferative overlap neoplasms 194
CMML 195–7
juvenile myelomonocytic leukaemia 199
MPN-U 202
role in leukaemic transformation 225–7, 228
trisomy 8 27, 28
see also Philadelphia chromosome
chromosome banding analysis (CBA) 68
chronic eosinophilic leukaemia (CEL) 209
pathogenesis 33*f*
somatic mutations 29*t*
WHO classification 2016 206*t*, 207, 208*f*
chronic eosinophilic syndrome (CES) 269*t*
chronic mast cell leukaemia 172–3
chronic myeloid leukaemia (CML) 94
accelerated phase, WHO diagnostic criteria 95*b*
adverse effects of treatment 107, 108*t*
aetiology 95
allogeneic stem cell transplantation 250–5, 251*f*
conditioning regimens 253–4
donor types 254
indications in CP 250–2
post-procedure monitoring 254–5
prognostic factors for outcomes 252–3
recent results 252
stem cell sources 254
summary 255
survival 253*f*
atypical *see* atypical chronic myeloid leukaemia
clinical features and diagnosis 96*f*, 96, 97*f*
clonal evolution 17–18
cytogenetics 96–7
disease persistence, causes 70
epidemiology 95
future prospects 111
genomic landscape
BCR-ABL translocation 20–2, 21*f*
CSF3R mutations 244–5
clonal cytogenetic evolution 22
mutation types 19–20
historical background 3*f*, 4, 7–8, 9–10, 11, 12
leukaemic transformation 109–10, 223
genetics and biology 225–8, 226*f*, 227*t*, 228*f*
incidence 223–4
risk factors 224, 224*t*
role of activated β-catenin 226*f*
treatment 230–1
management 101–2, 109–10
discontinuing TKI therapy 110
first-generation TKI 102–5
in imatinib failure 111*f*
investigational approaches 108–9, 109*f*
monitoring TKI therapy 101*b*
second-generation TKIs 105
third-generation TKIs 106
see also allogeneic stem cell transplantation
molecular biology 98–100
monitoring
BCR-ABL1 fusion gene 236–8
Philadelphia chromosome 235
treatment response assessment 238–41, 239*t*
natural history 95
pathogenesis 33*f*, 34–5
cooperating mutations 37
prognostic factors 70, 73–5, 74*b*, 100
age 64–7, 71–2
comorbidities 71–2
cytogenetics 68–9
gene expression profile screening 70
pharmacological 71
on second-line treatment 72
transcript type and transcript level 69–70
prognostic scores 64–8
baseline prognostic factors 65*t*
response and outcome by risk 66*t*
survival over time 94*f*
thrombocytosis 158
chronic myelomonocytic leukaemia (CMML) 203
classification 197
clinical features 194–5, 197
diagnosis 197
WHO diagnostic criteria 193*t*
epidemiology 192–4
genomic landscape 28, 194, 195–7, 195*t*
somatic mutations 29*t*
leukemic transformation 225
pathogenesis 33*f*
prognostic factors 197–8
risk stratification 197
treatment 197–8
chronic neutrophilic leukaemia (CNL)
cytogenetics 27
genomic landscape, somatic mutations 29*t*
leukaemic transformation 228
P230 protein 69–70
pathogenesis 33*f*, 35
Ph-positive 98–100
cladribine 183
in MPN-eo 215*t*
'classic' MPN 2, 46, 114, 152
genomic landscape 22–3
classification *see* World Health Organization classification (2016)

clinical features
  atypical chronic myeloid leukaemia 194–5, 200
  chronic myeloid leukaemia 96*f*, 96, 97*f*
  chronic myelomonocytic leukaemia 194–5, 197
  essential thrombocytosis 153–5
  juvenile myelomonocytic leukaemia 194–5
  leukaemic transformation 228–9
  MPN-eo 210–12
  myelodysplastic/ myeloproliferative overlap neoplasms 194–5
  myelofibrosis 55–6, 130–1
  polycythaemia vera
    symptom-burden 114–15
    thrombosis 115
  systemic mastocytosis 168
clinical trials, endpoints 287–8, 299–300
  overall response rate 293–6
  overall survival 290–2, 291*t*
  patient-reported outcomes 297–8
  progression-free survival 292–3
  time-to-vascular-event 296–7
clonal diversity 17–18, 18*f*
clonal endothelial progenitor cells (cEPC) 129
clonal evolution 17–18, 18*f*
  in CML 22
clonal haematopoiesis 17
clonal succession 17–18, 18*f*
cohesin complex mutations 27, 29*t*
COMFORT studies
  COMFORT I 141–2, 242–3, 280, 282*t*
    overall survival as an endpoint 290–2, 291*t*
  COMFORT II 79, 141–2, 242–3
    overall survival as an endpoint 290–2, 291*t*
    progression-free survival as an endpoint 292–3
    overall response rate 293–5, 294*f*
    use of PROs 297–8
comorbidities, prognostic significance 71–2
complete haematologic response 238
complete molecular remission (CMR) 240
Conan Doyle, Arthur 4, 5*f*
conditioning regimens, allo-SCT
  in CML 253
  in myelofibrosis 256–7, 258*t*
congenital erythrocytosis 24–5
Conley, C.L. 8–9
constitutional symptoms, myelofibrosis 130
CONTINUATION-PV trial 120
cooperating mutations 37
cord blood transplants
  CML 254
  myelofibrosis 261
cromolyn sodium 180
CSF3R mutations 27, 29*t*, 35
  monitoring 244–5
  myelodysplastic/ myeloproliferative overlap neoplasms 195*t*
    aCML 200
cutaneous mastocytosis (CM) 169, 178–9, 268
  symptoms 269*t*
  treatment 181
CXCl12 129
cyclophosphamide (CTX)
  GvHD prophylaxis 254
  prior to allo-SCT 253
cytarabine 9–10
cytogenetic abnormalities 68–9
cytogenetic analysis 235–6
  MPN-eo 212–13, 214*t*
cytogenetic response assessment 238–40, 239*t*
cytokine pathway mutations 22–3
  JAK/STAT signalling 22–3
cytokines
  correlation with disease burden 271
  prognostic significance in myelofibrosis 139
  role in myelofibrosis 128*f*, 129–30
CYTO-PV (Cytoreductive Therapy in PV) study 115, 118–19, 297

D

Dameshek, William 2, 7, 10, 16–17
danazol
  anaemia management 140, 144*b*
  and risk of leukaemic transformation 224
dasatinib 12, 105
  adverse effects 107, 108*t*
  in atypical chronic myeloid leukaemia 201
  clinical trials 105, 106*t*
  discontinuing therapy 110
  dose 74
  in leukaemic transformation 230–1
  molecular structure 102*f*
  pharmacokinetics 71
  in systemic mastocytosis 183–4
  see also tyrosine kinase inhibitors
DASISION study 105
DCC-2618 186
decitabine
  in chronic myelomonocytic leukaemia 197–8
  in leukaemic transformation 230, 230*t*
del (7q) 28
del (9q-) 68–9
del (20q) 27
denosumab 180
developing countries, diagnosis and monitoring issues 246–7
diagnosis 157*f*
  chronic myeloid leukaemia 96
  in developing countries 246–7
  essential thrombocytosis 53*t*, 56–8, 153–6, 157*b*
  initial stages of MPN 51
  MPN-eo 214*t*
    clinical features 210–12
    cytogenetics and molecular analyses 212–13
    T-cell clonality analyses 213
  myelodysplastic/ myeloproliferative overlap neoplasms
    aCML 200
    CMML 197
    JMML 200
  myelofibrosis 53*t*, 55–6, 133

polycythaemia vera 53*t*, 58–60, 116
WHO diagnostic criteria 117*b*
systemic mastocytosis 169, 174–8
WHO diagnostic criteria 53*t*
digital PCR 245–6
Di Guglielmo, Giovanni 6
disease burden 268
assessment 276–9
PROs as trial endpoints 281–3
PRO validation for FDA/EMA submission 280–1
assessment tools 272–6
prognostic tools 272
symptom assessment tools 273*t*, 276
impact on quality of life 271
myelofibrosis 268
relationship to risk scores 270–1
spectrum of 270–1
systemic mastocytosis 268–70, 272
disease persistence, causes 70
DNA PCR 245
DNMT3A mutations 25–6, 28, 29*t*, 37, 88*t*
and leukaemic transformation 227*t*
myelodysplastic/myeloproliferative overlap neoplasms 195*t*
systemic mastocytosis 175
Donne, Alfred 4
donor lymphocyte infusions (DLIs) 254–5, 256–7, 263
Druker, Brian 9–10
dual-energy X-ray absorptiometry (DEXA) scans 177–8
dynamic International Prognostic Scoring System (DIPSS) 137, 138*t*, 224, 261, 276

E

e13a2 (b2a2) isoform, *BCR-ABL1* 236–7
e14a2 (b3a2) isoform, *BCR-ABL1* 236–7
ECLAP (European Collaboration on Low-dose Aspirin in Polycythaemia Vera) study 115, 116, 118, 119–20, 296–7
EED mutations 88*t*
myelodysplastic/myeloproliferative overlap neoplasms 194
Ehrlich, Paul 2, 4
ELTS (EUTOS Long Term Survival Score) 64, 67–8
elzonris 198
endogenous erythroid colonies (EECs), historical background 9
endonuclease digestion 243
ENESTnd study 105
eosinophilia 205
clonal, as a consequence of point mutations 209
eosinophilia-associated MPN (MPN-eo) 205
chronic eosinophilic leukaemia-NOS 209
clinical features 210–12
bone marrow morphology 211
organ involvement 211–12
peripheral blood 210
cytogenetics and molecular analyses 212–13
T-cell clonality analyses 213
diagnostic procedures 214*t*
treatment 214–18, 215*t*
FIP1L1-PDGFRA positive MLN-eo in chronic phase 214–17
other *PDGFR* fusion genes in chronic phase 217
other TK fusion genes 218
PDGFR fusion genes in blast phase 217, 218*f*
tyrosine kinase fusion genes 207, 208*f*
WHO classification 2016 206*t*
eosinophils, normal range 205
EPIC study 106, 107, 111*f*
epidemiology
chronic myeloid leukaemia 95
essential thrombocytosis 153
myelodysplastic/myeloproliferative overlap neoplasms 192–4
polycythaemia vera 114
primary myelofibrosis 127
epidermal growth factor (EGF), role in fibrosis 128*f*, 129–30
epigenetic modifiers, mutations 25–6
EpoR mutations 24–5
Epstein, Emil 7, 9
erythromelalgia 155
erythropoiesis-stimulating agents (ESA) 141, 144*b*
erythropoietin (EPO), serum levels 58–9
in essential thrombocytosis 154
essential thrombocytosis (ET) 152, 166, 287
bone marrow morphology 48*f*, 56–8
in children 166
classification, importance of 57
clinical features 153–6, 269*t*
haemorrhagic complications 155
thrombotic complications 154–5
thrombotic risk factors 154
vasomotor symptoms 155
clinical trials
measuring overall response rate 295–6
measuring time-to-vascular-event 296, 297
diagnosis 153–6
WHO diagnostic criteria 53*t*, 81*t*, 157*b*
differential diagnosis 52, 156–8
disease burden 270–1
disease transformation
acute myeloid leukaemia 156, 223
myelofibrosis 155
polycythaemia vera 156
epidemiology 153
genomic landscape 22–3
JAK2 mutations 59
MPL mutations 244
mutation frequencies 24*f*, 83*f*
somatic mutations 29*t*

essential thrombocytosis (ET) *(Contd.)*
historical background 9
management 159–62, 277
anagrelide 159–61
antiplatelet therapy 162*f*, 162
busulfan 162
cardiovascular risk factors assessment 163
goals of therapy 159
high-risk patients 159–62
hydroxyurea (hydroxycarbamide) 159–60, 161
interferon 161
intermediate-risk patients 163
low-dose aspirin 159–60, 162
low-risk patients 163
practical tips 164*b*
during pregnancy 165
risk-adapted approach 159–64
surgery 165
symptom burden assessment 163
treatment efficacy evaluation 163–4
treatment resistance/intolerance 164*b*, 164
treatment targets 164
myelofibrotic progression
diagnosis 133, 134*t*
epidemiology 127
WHO diagnostic criteria 57*t*
pathogenesis 33*f*
JAK2 mutations 35–6, 38*f*
MPL mutations 37
pathophysiology and molecular biology 152–3
prognostic tools 272
response criteria 296
risk stratification 85–6, 159–64, 160*t*
IPSET score 86*t*
ETNK1 mutations
myelodysplastic/myeloproliferative overlap neoplasms, aCML 200
in systemic mastocytosis 175
ETV6-ABL1 fusion gene 207, 208*f*, 218
ETV6-ACSL6 fusion gene 209
ETV6-FLT3 fusion gene 218
ETV6 mutations
myelodysplastic/myeloproliferative overlap neoplasms 195*t*
systemic mastocytosis 175
European Competency Network on Mastocytosis (ECNM) registry 187–8
European Group for Blood and Bone Marrow Transplantation (EBMT) risk score 252
European LeukemiaNet (ELN) 64–8, 100
TKI treatment response guidelines 101*t*
EURO score 64–8, 100*t*
baseline prognostic factors 65*t*
response and outcome by risk 66*t*
Euro-SKI study 110
EUTOS (European Treatment and Outcome Study) score 64–8, 100*t*
baseline prognostic factors 65*t*
response and outcome by risk 66*t*
EUTOS Long Term Survival (ELTS) score 64, 67–8
EV1 overexpression 98–100
extramedullary haematopoiesis 130–1
EZH2 mutations 26, 27, 37, 88*t*
and leukaemic transformation 227*t*
myelodysplastic/myeloproliferative overlap neoplasms 194, 195*t*
primary myelofibrosis 90*t*
prognostic significance 89–90, 137
systemic mastocytosis 175

F

familial predisposition 24
germ-line mutations 24–5
mRNA splicing gene mutations 26
mutations in epigenetic modifiers and transcription factors 25–6
mutations in genes regulating genome stability 27
fatigue 271
myelofibrosis 130
FGFR1 fusion genes 35
MPN-eo 218
myelodysplastic/myeloproliferative overlap neoplasms 194
Fialkow, Phillip 7–8
fibroblast growth factor (FGF), role in fibrosis 128*f*, 129–30
FIP1L1-PDGFRA fusion gene 207, 208*f*
screening for 212
FIP1L1-PDGFRA positive MLN-eo in chronic phase, treatment 214–17
first-generation TKI 102–5
FLT3 inhibitors 230
FLT3 mutations 28, 29*t*
fludarabine, prior to allo-SCT 256–7, 258*t*
fluorescence *in situ* hybridization (FISH) 236
fluoxymesterone, anaemia management 140
Fowler, Thomas 4

G

Galton, David 9–10
gastrointestinal tract biopsies 177–8
gemtuzumab ozogamicin 188
gender differences
in disease burden 271
MPN-eo 210
gene expression profile (GEP) screening 70
genomic landscape 16–17, 288
chronic myeloid leukaemia 27
chronic myelomonocytic leukaemia 20–2, 28, 96–7
classical MPN 22–3
clonal evolution, diversity, and succession 17–18, 18*f*
clonal haematopoiesis 17
essential thrombocytosis 152–3
familial predisposition 24
germ-line mutations 24–5
mRNA splicing gene mutations 26
mutations in epigenetic modifiers

and transcription factors 25–6
mutations in genes regulating genome stability 27
and leukaemic transformation 225–8
myelodysplastic/ myeloproliferative overlap neoplasms 194, 195*t*
CMML 195–7
primary myelofibrosis 128–9
somatic mutations 29*t*
systemic mastocytosis 28
types of mutations 19–20
germ-line mutations 24–5
GIMEMA (Gruppo Italiano Malattie Ematologiche dell' Adulto) data set 64–7
givinostat 121–2
GM-CSF sensitivity
chronic myelomonocytic leukaemia 197
juvenile myelomonocytic leukaemia 199
Goedel, Alfred 7, 9
Goldman, John 11
graft-versus-host disease (GvHD), CTX prophylaxis 254
Gunz, F.W. 9

H

haematocrit targets, polycythaemia vera 118–19
during pregnancy 123*b*
haematopoiesis
clonal 17
JAK/STAT signalling 22–3
haematopoietic cell transplantation comorbidity index (HSCT-CI) 252
haematopoietic niche 129
haematopoietic stem cells (HSCs), effect of *JAK2*^{V617F} 41–2
haematopoietic stem cell transplantation (HSCT) 94
in chronic myeloid leukaemia 109–10
in myelofibrosis 146–8
ruxolitinib therapy 146–8
in systemic mastocytosis 186–7
see also allogeneic stem cell transplantation
haemoglobin thresholds, polycythaemia vera 46, 58–9, 116, 117*b*
haemorrhage risk
essential thrombocytosis 155
pre-PMF 52
Harrison, C.V. 7
headache 155
heparin activity, systemic mastocytosis 177–8
hepatomegaly
imaging studies 177–8
myelofibrosis 130
systemic mastocytosis 170*b*
hereditary alpha-tryptasemia 173
hereditary thrombocytosis 24–5
Heuck, Gustav 4
Hewson, William 2
histone deacetylase (HDAC) inhibitors 121–2
historical background 2
CML, milestones in study and treatment 3*f*
seventeenth and eighteenth centuries 2
nineteenth century 4–6
twentieth century 6–11
twenty-first century 11–12
Hooke, Robert 2
HOXA9, HOXA10, and leukaemic transformation 225
human leukocyte antigen (HLA) testing
indications 250–2
systemic mastocytosis 177–8
Hungerford, David 7, 20–1
hydroxyurea (hydroxycarbamide)
adverse effects 120, 121*t*, 143–4
busulfan 144*b*
in chronic myelomonocytic leukaemia 197–8
criteria of clinical resistance and intolerance 121*t*
in essential thrombocytosis 159, 161
clinical trials 295–6
combination with low-dose aspirin 159–60
resistance/intolerance 164*b*, 164
introduction of 9–10
melphalan 144*b*
in MPN-eo 215*t*
in myelofibrosis 143–4, 144*b*
in polycythaemia vera 118, 119–20, 122–3
and risk of leukaemic transformation 224
WHO diagnostic criteria 156
hypereosinophilia 205, 211
hypereosinophilia of unknown significance (HE_{US}) 205
TK fusion genes 207
hypereosinophilic syndrome (HES) 205
pathogenesis 35
hyperkalaemia, essential thrombocytosis 154

I

IDH1/2 mutations 26, 27, 28, 29*t*, 37, 88*t*
and leukaemic transformation 225–7, 227*t*
myelodysplastic/ myeloproliferative overlap neoplasms 194, 195*t*
primary myelofibrosis 90*t*
prognostic significance 89–90, 116
idiopathic myelofibrosis (IMF) *see* primary myelofibrosis
IKZF1 inactivation 26, 29*t*, 88*t*
imaging studies, systemic mastocytosis 177–8
imatinib 12, 35, 238
ACA, prediction of treatment response 68–9
adverse effects 107, 108*t*
discontinuing therapy 110, 217
dose 74
high dose 102–5
introduction of 9–10, 102–5
in leukaemic transformation 230–1
in MDS/ MPN-RS-T 201–2
mechanism of action 103*f*
molecular structure 102*f*
in MPN-eo
blast phase disease 217, 218*f*
chronic phase disease 214–17, 215*t*
ETV6-ABL1 and *ETV6-FLT3* positive disease 218
secondary resistance, 216*f*
pharmacogenetics 71

imatinib (*Contd.*)
pharmacokinetics 71
plasma level measurement 71
post-transplantation 254–5
resistance to 102–5, 216*f*
subsequent allo-SCT 252
in systemic mastocytosis 184
treatment response 67*t*
imatinib failure, treatment algorithm 111*f*
imetelstat 147*t*
immunoglobulin E (IgE) levels 210
INCB039110 147*t*
indolent phase 223
indolent systemic mastocytosis (ISM) 169–71, 170*b*
prognosis 179
serum tryptase level 174–5
treatment algorithm 181*f*
inflammatory cytokines 38
initial stage MPN
diagnosis 51
polycythaemia vera, bone marrow morphology 59–60
see *also* prefibrotic PMF
interferons
in atypical chronic myeloid leukaemia 201
in chronic myeloid leukaemia 108–9
in essential thrombocytosis 161
introduction of 9–10
in MPN-eo 215*t*
in polycythaemia vera 120, 122–3, 242
in systemic mastocytosis 180, 182
use during pregnancy 165
interleukin levels, prognostic significance in myelofibrosis 139
International Prognostic Scoring System (IPSS) 137, 138*t*, 261, 276
International Prognostic Scoring System for Essential Thrombocythemia (IPSET) score 86*t*, 159, 272
IPSET-thrombosis 154
International Working Group for Myeloproliferative Neoplasm Research and Treatment (WG-MRT) criteria 276
IRIS study 105, 107
IRIS trial 238–40
iron chelation 141
isochromosome 17p 22

J

JAK2 35–6
JAK2 fusion genes, MPN-eo 218
JAK2 inhibitors 118
in atypical chronic myeloid leukaemia 201
historical background 11, 12
in MDS/MPN-RS-T 201–2
in MPN-eo 215*t*, 218
in myelofibrosis 141–3
prior to allo-SCT 262
see *also* ruxolitinib
JAK2 mutations 28, 29*t*, 35–6, 36*f*, 59, 80, 241–2
exon 12 22–3
familial predisposition 24
frequency 24*f*
JAK2^{V617F} 22–3, 27, 36, 37, 288
allele burden 242–3
concomitant loss of *TET2* 42–3
effect on HSCs 41–2
essential thrombo cytosis 152–3
heterozygous or homozygous status 84, 242
influence of STATs 40
laboratory assays 243
murine models 38–9, 40, 41–3
phenotype determination 37–8, 38*f*
reduction of allele burden 84–5
serum level monitoring 84–5
thrombosis risk 85–6, 154
and leukaemic transformation 227–8, 228*f*
monitoring 241–3, 244
MPN-eo 212
myelodysplastic/myeloproliferative overlap neoplasms 194, 195*t*
MDS/MPN-RS-T 201
MPN-U 202
myelofibrosis 128
post-transplantation 257
polycythaemia vera 116
allelic burden, prognostic significance 116
prognostic significance 80, 84–5, 87*f*, 137
subclonal mutations 88*t*
systemic mastocytosis 175
and *TET2* mutation 25–6
JAK3 mutations, myelodysplastic/myeloproliferative overlap neoplasms 195*t*
juvenile myelomonocytic leukaemia 199
JAK/STAT pathway activation, primary myelofibrosis 128–9
JAK/STAT signalling 22–3
effect of *CALR* mutations 23
Janus kinase (JAK) family 241–2
JARID mutation 88*t*
juvenile myelomonocytic leukaemia (JMML) 203
clinical features 194–5
diagnosis 200
WHO diagnostic criteria 193*t*
epidemiology 192–4
genetics 194, 199
treatment 200

K

ketotifen, in systemic mastocytosis 180
KIT D816 inhibitors 186, 188
KIT gene structure and mutations 176–7*f*
KIT mutation analysis 175–7
KIT mutations 28, 29*t*, 35, 171, 175
mast cell activation syndrome 173
MPN-eo 212
prognostic significance 179
SM with associated haematological neoplasms 172
well-differentiated SM 173
K/N RAS mutations

myelodysplastic/ myeloproliferative overlap neoplasms 195*t*
in systemic mastocytosis 175
KRAS mutations 27, 28, 29*t*
juvenile myelomonocytic leukaemia 199

L

LAST study 110
Lawrence, J.H. 10
Leeuwenhoek, Anton van 2
lenalidomide
in anaemia 141, 144*b*
in MDS/ MPN-RS-T 201–2
leukaemic transformation 223, 268
clinical features 228–9
in essential thrombocytosis 156
genetics and biology 225–8, 226*f*, 227*t*, 228*f*
incidence 223–4, 225
key points 229*b*
murine models 228
in myelofibrosis 132–3
allogeneic stem cell transplantation 262–3
in polycythaemia vera 116
risk factors 119–20
prognosis 229–30
risk factors 119–20, 224, 224*t*
risk stratification 87–90, 88*f*, 90*f*
treatment 230–1, 230*t*
leukotriene receptor antagonists 180
Lieutaud, Joseph 2
LNK mutations 22–3, 29*t*, 36*f*
and leukaemic transformation 227*t*
loss of heterozygosity (LOH) 19*f*
low-molecular-weight heparin (LMWH)
ET management during pregnancy 165
PV management during pregnancy 123*b*
lymph node involvement 212
Lyon, Mary 7–8

M

MAJIC-ET trial 164
major molecular response (MMR) 240
masitinib 184
mast cell activation, systemic mastocytosis 179–80
mast cell activation syndrome (MCAS) 173
diagnostic decision-making 178
symptoms 269*t*
mast cell leukaemia (MCL) 170*b*, 172–3
serum tryptase level 174–5
treatment algorithm 181*f*
mast cell sarcoma 173
mastocytoma 169, 173
mastocytosis
disease burden assessment 277–9
MPN-SAF TSS mast cell 276
quality of life assessment 278
see also cutaneous mastocytosis; systemic mastocytosis
Mastocytosis Quality of Life Questionnaire (MQLQ) 178
Mastocytosis Society survey 278–9
Mastocytosis Symptom Assessment form (MSAF) 178
matrix metalloproteinases (MMPs), role in fibrosis 128*f*, 129–30
McCabe, W.R. 9
MCS Nes+ 129
mediator symptoms, systemic mastocytosis 179–80
megakaryocyte morphology 46–7, 48*f*
essential thrombocytosis 56–7
PMF 52
polycythaemia vera 59–60
prefibrotic PMF 47*b*, 55*f*
primary myelofibrosis 55–6
WHO diagnostic criteria for pre-PMF, PMF, ET, and PV 53*t*
melphalan
in myelofibrosis 143–4, 144*b*
prior to allo-SCT 257, 258*t*
midostaurin 184–5, 188
in MPN-eo 215*t*
Minot, G.R. 7
MIPSS70 261
molecular analysis, MPN-eo 212–13
molecular response assessment 239*t*, 240–1
molecular risk stratification 80, 91
phenotypic driver mutations 87*f*
CALR (calreticulin) mutations 83, 85–6
JAK2 mutations 80, 84–5
MPL mutations 83, 84
reduction of mutated allele burden 84–5
in PMF 90*f*
subclonal mutations 87–90, 88*t*
thrombosis risk 85–6
momelotinib 146
monitoring 235
BCR-ABL1 fusion gene 235–8
CSF3R mutations 244–5
in developing countries 246–7
emerging technologies 245–6
JAK2 mutations 244
in Ph-negative classic MPN 241–3
MPL and *CALR* mutations 244
mutation testing 241
post-transplantation
in CML 254–5
in myelofibrosis 257
treatment response assessment 238–41, 239*t*
monoclonal mast cell activation syndrome (MMAS) 173
diagnostic decision-making 178
monosomy 7 28, 195–7, 199
montelukast 180
MPL mutations 22–3, 29*t*, 36*f*, 37, 80, 152–3, 288
frequency 24*f*
monitoring 244
MPL Baltimore 24–5
MPL^{S505N} 24–5
murine models 40–1
myelodysplastic/ myeloproliferative overlap neoplasms 201
myelofibrosis 128
post-transplantation 257
prognostic significance 83, 84, 87*f*, 137
subclonal mutations 88*t*

MPN 10 see Myeloproliferative Neoplasm Symptom Assessment Form Total Symptom Score
MPN-eo see eosinophilia-associated MPN
MPN Quartile Study 276–7
MPN-Symptom Assessment Form (MPN-SAF) 114–15
mRNA splicing gene mutations 26
multipotent stromal cell expressing nestin (MSC Nes+) 129
murine models 38–9
  chronic myelomonocytic leukaemia 197
  effect of *JAK2*^{V617F} on HSCs 41–2
  evaluation of novel therapies 39
  influence of STATs on MPN phenotype 39–40, 40*t*
  of leukaemic transformation 228
  MPL mutations 83
  TET2 mutations 42–3
  thrombopoietin signalling pathway 40–1
mutation-augmented prognostic scoring system (MAPSS) 179
Mutation-Enhanced International Prognostic Scoring System (MIPSS) 137–9, 138*t*
mutation types 19–20
MYB 225
MYC
  overexpression 98–100
myelodysplastic/myeloproliferative overlap neoplasms (MDS/MPN) 192*f*, 192–5, 202
  atypical chronic myeloid leukaemia 200–1
  chronic myelomonocytic leukaemia 195–8
  clinical features 194–5
  genetics 194, 195*t*
  incidence and aetiology 192–4
  juvenile myelomonocytic leukaemia 199–200
  key points 202–3
  leukaemic transformation
    genetics 228
    incidence 225
  with ringed sideroblasts and thrombocytosis (MDS/MPN-RS-T) 158, 201–2
  unclassifiable MPN (MPN-U) 202
  WHO diagnostic criteria 193*t*
myelofibrosis 127, 287
  allogeneic stem cell transplantation 250, 255–63
    after leukaemic transformation 262–3
    bone marrow fibrosis regression 257–60, 260*t*
    clinical trials 258*t*
    conditioning regimens 256–7
    development in Europe 260*f*
    donor source 261
    molecular markers and residual disease 257
    relapse management 263
    results 256–7
    role of disease risk scores 261, 262*f*
    splenectomy and spleen size reduction 262
  bone marrow morphology 132
  clinical features 130–1, 269*t*
  clinical trials
    overall response rate 293–5
    overall response rate as an endpoint 293–6
    overall survival as an endpoint 290–2
    progression-free survival as an endpoint 292–3
    ReTHINK study 289
  complications 132
  diagnosis 133
    flowchart 136*f*
    screening tests 135*t*
  disease burden 268, 277
  leukaemic transformation 132–3, 223
    incidence 223–4
  management 139–49
    of anaemia 140–1
    future directions 149
    high-risk patients 144–6
    hydroxyurea (hydroxy carbamide) 143–4
    intermediate-1 patients 139–44
    intermediate-2 patients 144–6
    investigational therapies and strategies 146–8, 147*t*
    JAK2 inhibitors 141–3, 142*f*
    low-risk and asymptomatic patients 139
    low risk symptomatic patients 139–44
    monitoring 148
    personalized treatment approach 146
    response criteria 148*f*, 149
    ruxolitinib, PROs 280–1
    of splenomegaly and constitutional symptoms 141–4, 144*b*
    see also allogeneic stem cell transplantation
  peripheral blood 131*f*, 131–2
  prognostic scores 138*t*
  prognostic tools 272
  risk stratification and prognostic factors 137–9, 288–9
  treatment goals 288–9
  see also primary myelofibrosis
Myelofibrosis Symptom Assessment Form (MF-SAF) 273*t*, 276
  development of modified score 280–1, 281*f*
  use in COMFORT studies 297–8
myelofibrotic progression
  association with *MPL* mutation 84
  diagnosis 133, 134*t*
    flowchart 136*f*
  essential thrombocytosis 155
  epidemiology 127
  polycythaemia vera 116
    epidemiology 127
    haematopathology 60
  risk of 52
  WHO diagnostic criteria 57*t*
myeloid and lymphoid neoplasms with eosinophilia (MPN-eo)
  clinical features 210–12
    bone marrow morphology 211
    organ involvement 211–12
    peripheral blood 210

clonal eosinophilia as a consequence of point mutations 209
cytogenetics and molecular analyses 212–13
T-cell clonality analyses 213
diagnostic procedures 214*t*
treatment 214–18, 215*t*
FIP1L1-PDGFRA positive MLN-eo in chronic phase 214–17
other *PDGFR* fusion genes in chronic phase 217
other TK fusion genes 218
PDGFR fusion genes in blast phase 217, 218*f*
tyrosine kinase fusion genes 207, 208*f*
WHO classification 2016 206*t*
myeloproliferative disorders (MPDs), use of term 2
myeloproliferative neoplasms (MPN)
introduction of term 2
shared features 33
Myeloproliferative Neoplasm Symptom Assessment Form (MPN-SAF) 273*t*, 276
use in RESPONSE study 298
Myeloproliferative Neoplasm Symptom Assessment Form Total Symptom Score (MPN-SAF TSS/ MPN-10) 140*f*, 148, 273*t*, 276
MPN-SAF TSS mast cell 276, 279
relationship to PGIC 280–1, 282*t*
relationship to risk scores 270–1
MYSEC-PM (Myelofibrosis Secondary to PV and ET-Prognostic Model) 155, 261

N

Najean, Y. 9
natural history of MPN 223
chronic myeloid leukaemia 95
polycythaemia vera 116
Neumann, Ernst 4
next generation sequencing (NGS) 246
NF1 mutations 195*t*, 199
nilotinib 12, 105
adverse effects 107, 108*t*
clinical trials 105, 106*t*
discontinuing therapy 110
dose 74
in leukaemic transformation 230–1
molecular structure 102*f*
in MPN-eo 218
pharmacokinetics 71
post-transplantation 254–5
in systemic mastocytosis 183–4
treatment response 67*t*
see also tyrosine kinase inhibitors
'non-classic' MPN 46
Nowell, Peter 7, 20–1
NRAS mutations 27, 28, 29*t*, 88*t*
juvenile myelomonocytic leukaemia 199

O

objective response rate (ORR), as a trial endpoint 287–8
Ohno, Susumu 7–8
omalizumab 180
OPA score 277–8
OPTIC study 106
organic cation transporter 1 (OCT1) 71
Osler, W. 6
osteoporosis/ osteopenia, systemic mastocytosis 177–8
management 180
osteosclerotic PMF, bone marrow morphology 56
overall response rate (ORR)
clinical trials 293–6
as a trial endpoint 293, 299
overall survival (OS)
clinical trials 290–2, 291*t*
as a trial endpoint 287–8, 290, 299
oxymetholone, anaemia management 140
Ozer, F.L. 9

P

p190 *BCR-ABL1* transcript 236–7, 237*f*
P190 protein 69–70
p210 *BCR-ABL1* transcript 236–7, 237*f*
p230 *BCR-ABL1* transcript 236–7, 237*f*
P230 protein 69–70
PACE study 106
pacritinib 146
panobinostat 147*t*
paraesthesias, essential thrombocytosis 155
Parkes-Weber, F. 6
pathogenesis 33*f*, 33–4
atypical CML and CNL 35
CML 34–5
cooperating mutations 37
inflammatory cytokines 38
JAK2^{V617F}
murine models 38–9
phenotype determination 37–8, 38*f*
murine models 38–9
influence of STATs on MPN phenotype 39–40, 40*t*
TET2 mutations 42–3
thrombopoietin signalling pathway 40–1
Philadelphia chromosome and BCR-ABL1 34–5
Ph-negative MPN 35
CALR (calreticulin) mutations 36
JAK2 mutations 35–6
MPL mutations 37
mutational landscape 36*f*
systemic mastocytosis and hypereosinophilic syndrome 35
Patient Global Impression of Change (PGIC), relationship to MSA-TSS 280–1, 282*t*
patient-reported outcome (PRO) tools 273*t*, 276
patient-reported outcomes (PROs)
clinical trials 297–8
as a trial endpoint 281–3, 287–8, 297–8, 299
validation for FDA/EMA submission 280–1
PCR techniques 236–8
emerging technologies 245–6
JAK2 mutation assays 243
PDGFRA mutations 194
PDGFRB mutations 194
imatinib resistance 216*f*, 216
PDGFR translocations 35

pegylated interferons
in chronic myeloid leukaemia 108–9
effect on mutated allele burden 84–5
in essential thrombocytosis 161
in polycythaemia vera 120
see also interferons
peripheral blood
chronic myeloid leukaemia 96*f*, 96
chronic myelomonocytic leukaemia 197
MPN-eo 210, 214*t*
myelofibrosis 131*f*, 131, 135*t*
phenotypic driver mutations 80, 91
CALR (calreticulin) mutations 83, 85–6
frequencies 83*f*
impact on survival 87*f*
JAK2 mutations 80
JAK2^{V617F} levels 84
MPL mutations 83, 84
see also CALR (calreticulin) mutations; *JAK2* mutations; *MPL* mutations
Philadelphia chromosome 20*f*, 20–1, 34–5, 96–7, 97*f*, 235
detection of 235–6
discovery of 7–8, 16–17
origin 98*f*
phlebotomy, polycythaemia vera 118–19
Ph-negative MPN, pathogenesis 35
CALR (calreticulin) mutations 36
JAK2 mutations 35–6
MPL mutations 37
mutational landscape 36*f*
phototherapy, mastocytosis 181
pioglitazone, study in CML 108–9
pipobroman 119–20
and risk of leukaemic transformation 224
platelet derived growth factor (PDGF), role in fibrosis 128*f*, 129–30
platelets, first descriptions of 2, 4
point mutations 19–20
clonal eosinophilia 209
polycythaemia vera (PV) 287
aetiology 114
bone marrow morphology 48*f*
clinical features 269*t*
symptom-burden 114–15
thrombosis 59, 115
clinical trials
measuring time-to-vascular-event 296–7
of ruxolitinib 295
diagnosis 46, 116
differentiation
from ET 156
WHO diagnostic criteria 117*b*
disease burden 270–1
epidemiology 114
genomic landscape 22–3, 114
mutation frequencies 24*f*, 83*f*
somatic mutations 29*t*
haematopathology 58–60
initial-stage disease 59–60
historical background 6–7, 8–9, 10–11, 114
hydroxyurea resistance and intolerance criteria 121*t*
JAK2 mutations 59
allelic burden 242
management 117–23, 242, 277
flow chart 122*f*
high thrombotic risk patients 119–22
low thrombotic risk patients 118–19
during pregnancy 123*b*
risk stratification 118
summary 122–3
of thrombosis in unusual sites 117*b*
myelofibrotic progression
diagnosis 133, 134*t*
epidemiology 127
WHO diagnostic criteria 57*t*
natural history 116
pathogenesis 33*f*
JAK2 mutations 35–6, 37–8, 38*f*
post-ET transformation 156
prognostic tools 272
risk factors for survival 116, 119–20
thrombosis risk stratification 85–6
WHO diagnostic criteria 53*t*, 81*t*
Polycythaemia Vera Study Group (PVSG) 10–11
pomalidomide 141
ponatinib 12, 106, 250–2
adverse effects 107, 108*t*
molecular structure 102*f*
in MPN-eo 218
see also tyrosine kinase inhibitors
portal hypertension, myelofibrosis 130
post-ET myelofibrosis, WHO diagnostic criteria 57*t*
post-PV myelofibrosis
haematopathology 60
WHO diagnostic criteria 57*t*
PRC2 (polycomb repressor complex 2) 26
prefibrotic PMF
bone marrow morphology 48*f*
diagnosis 55*f*, 156–8
bone marrow morphology 55*f*, 132
diagnostic criteria 46–7, 47*b*, 53*t*
haematopathology 52
prognosis 52, 156–8
pregnancy
essential thrombocytosis 165
polycythaemia vera 123*b*
systemic mastocytosis 181
primary familial congenital polycythaemia (PFCP) 24–5
primary myelofibrosis (PMF) 127
allogeneic stem cell transplantation 255–63
after leukaemic transformation 262–3
bone marrow fibrosis regression 257–60, 260*t*
clinical trials 258*t*
conditioning regimens 256–7
development in Europe 260*f*
donor source 261
molecular markers and residual disease 257
relapse management 263
results 256–7

role of disease risk scores 261, 262*f*
splenectomy and spleen size reduction 262
bone marrow morphology 48*f*, 132
clinical features 55–6, 130–1
complications 132
diagnosis 133
flowchart 136*f*
screening tests 135*t*
WHO criteria 53*t*, 81*t*, 134*b*
disease burden 277
epidemiology 127
evolution to leukaemia 132–3
genomic landscape 22–3
CALR (calreticulin) mutations 244
JAK2 mutations 242–3
MPL mutations 244
mutation frequencies 24*f*, 83*f*
somatic mutations 29*t*
haematopathology 55–6
historical background 4, 9
leukaemic transformation 223
management 139–49
of anaemia 140–1
future directions 149
high-risk patients 144–6
hydroxyurea (hydroxy carbamide) 143–4
intermediate-1 patients 139–44
intermediate-2 patients 144–6
investigational therapies and strategies 146–8, 147*t*
JAK2 inhibitors 141–3, 142*f*
low-risk and asymptomatic patients 139
low risk symptomatic patients 139–44
monitoring 148
personalized treatment approach 146
response criteria 148*f*
of splenomegaly and constitutional symptoms 141–4, 144*b*
see also allogeneic stem cell transplant
molecular risk status 89–90
impact on survival 90*f*
occurrence of HMR mutations 90*t*
pathogenesis 33*f*
JAK2 mutations 35–6
MPL mutations 37
pathophysiology 127–30, 128*f*
cytokines 129–30
haematopoietic niche 129
JAK/STAT pathway activation 128–9
mutations 128–9
peripheral blood 131*f*, 131–2
prefibrotic
bone marrow morphology 48*f*
diagnosis 52, 55*f*
diagnostic criteria 46–7, 47*b*
prognosis 52
prognostic scores 138*t*
prognostic tools 272
risk stratification and prognostic factors 137–9
subclonal mutations 89–90
thrombocytosis 156–8
PRM-151 147*t*
prognostic factors
chronic myeloid leukaemia 70, 73–5, 74*b*, 100
age 64–7
age and comorbidities 71–2
cytogenetics 68–9
gene expression profile screening 70
pharmacological 71
on second-line treatment 72
transcript type and transcript level 69–70
myelofibrosis 137–9
polycythaemia vera, symptom-burden 114–15
systemic mastocytosis 179
prognostic scores and tools 73, 224, 272, 288–9
chronic myeloid leukaemia 64–8, 100, 100*t*
baseline prognostic factors 65*t*
response and outcome by risk 66*t*
EBMT risk score 252
myelofibrosis 137–9, 138*t*
outcome after allo-SCT 261, 262*f*
systemic mastocytosis 187–8
progression-free survival (PFS)
clinical trials 292–3
as a trial endpoint 287–8, 292, 299
PROUD-PV trial 120
PTPN11 mutations 195*t*, 199
PVSG 01 trial 118

Q

quality of life (QoL)
assessment in clinical trials 297–8
impact of disease burden 271
systemic mastocytosis 178, 278

R

radiation exposure, CML risk 95
radiophosphorus
introduction of 10
and risk of leukaemic transformation 224
radotinib 108–9
RAS mutations 96–7
and leukaemic transformation 225–7
myelodysplastic/ myeloproliferative overlap neoplasms 194
RB mutations 88*t*, 98–100
reactive oxygen species (ROS), and leukaemic transformation 225
red blood cells, first descriptions of 2
red cell mass (RCM) measurement 9, 116
reduced intensity conditioning (RIC), allo-SCT 256–7, 258*t*
refractory anaemia with ringed sideroblasts (RARS) 26
pathogenesis 33*f*
refractory anaemia with ringed sideroblasts and thrombocytosis (RARS-T, MDS/MPN-RS-T) 158, 201–2, 203
RELIEF trial 120–1
RESPONSE trial 120–1, 295
use of PROs 298

restriction enzyme digestion 243
ReTHINK study 289
reverse transcription (RT)-PCR 236–8
ring sideroblasts 51, 58, 158
RARS 26, 33*f*
RARS-T 158, 201–2, 203
risk stratification 288–9
essential thrombocytosis 160*t*
myelofibrosis 137–9
polycythaemia vera 118
see also molecular risk stratification
ristocetin cofactor activity 163
ropeginterferon alfa-2b 120
Rosenthal, 6–7
Rowley, Janet 7–8, 8*f*, 20–1, 235
RUNX1 mutations 26, 28, 29*t*, 37, 88*t*
myelodysplastic/ myeloproliferative overlap neoplasms 194, 195*t*
CMML 195–7
systemic mastocytosis 175, 179, 187
Russell, R.P. 8–9
ruxolitinib 35, 120–1, 122–3, 288
adverse effects 142–3
in atypical chronic myeloid leukaemia 201
clinical trials
overall response rate 293–5
overall survival as an endpoint 290–2, 291*t*
progression-free survival as an endpoint 292–3
COMFORT-2 study 79
discontinuing therapy 142–3, 143*f*
effect on mutated allele burden 84–5
historical background 11
in leukaemic transformation 230, 230*t*
in MPN-eo 218
in myelofibrosis 141–3, 142*f*, 144*b*, 242–3, 277
continuation with HSCT 146–8
prior to allo-SCT 262
patient-reported outcomes 280–1
in polycythaemia vera 118, 242
clinical trials 295
ReTHINK study 289

S

Sanger sequencing 246
sapacitabine 198
Schultze, Max 4
secondary polycythaemia, historical background 8–9
second-generation TKIs 105
study results 106*t*
second-line treatment, prognostic factors 72
selective KIT D816 inhibition 186
SETBP1 mutations 27, 29*t*, 35, 96–7
and leukaemic transformation 225
myelodysplastic/ myeloproliferative overlap neoplasms 194, 195*t*
aCML 200
juvenile myelomonocytic leukaemia 199
in systemic mastocytosis 175
SF3B1 mutations 26, 28, 29*t*, 88*t*
myelodysplastic/ myeloproliferative overlap neoplasms 194, 195*t*
MDS/MPN-RS-T 201
SH2B3 mutation 88*t*
Shakespeare, William 2
skeletal surveys, systemic mastocytosis 177–8
skin involvement
MPN-eo 211
see also cutaneous mastocytosis
SMD4 mutations 88*t*
smouldering systemic mastocytosis (SSM) 170*b*, 171
serum tryptase leve l 174–5
treatment algorithm 181*f*
SOCS mutations 88*t*
Sokal score 64–8, 73, 100
baseline prognostic factors 65*t*
prediction of probability of molecular response 67*t*
response and outcome by risk 66*t*
sonidegib 147*t*
sorafenib 218
spleen response, COMFORT studies 293–5, 294*f*
spleen size reduction, prior to allo-SCT 262
splenectomy 141, 144*b*
prior to allo-SCT 262
and risk of leukaemic transformation 224
splenic irradiation 143–4, 144*b*
splenomegaly
essential thrombocytosis 154
imaging studies 177–8
management 141, 143–4
JAK2 inhibitors 141–3, 142*f*
MPN-eo 211
myelofibrosis 130
prognostic significance in CML 67–8, 71–2
systemic mastocytosis 170*b*, 179
spliceosome inhibitors 201–2
splicing machinery gene mutations 26, 28
SRSF2 mutations 26, 27, 28, 29*t*, 88*t*
frequency in PMF 90*t*
and leukaemic transformation 225–7
myelodysplastic/ myeloproliferative overlap neoplasms 194, 195*t*
MDS/MPN-RS-T 201
prognostic significance 89–90, 116, 137
in systemic mastocytosis 175–7, 179, 187
Stat1, murine studies 40
Stat3, murine studies 40
Stat5, murine studies 39
STATs
knockout mouse models 39–40, 40*t*
STAT1/STAT5 balance 37–8, 38*f*
stem cell factor (SCF) 35
stem cell transplantation
historical background 11

see also allogeneic stem cell transplantation
STIM1 (Stop Imatinib) study 110
STOP (Stopping Second Generation TKIs) study 110
subclonal mutations 87–90, 88t
sunitinib 218
surgery
patients with essential thrombocytosis 165
patients with systemic mastocytosis 181
SUZ12 mutations 88t
myelodysplastic/ myeloproliferative overlap neoplasms 194
symptom assessment, MPN 10 140f
symptom assessment tools 273t, 276
symptoms 269t
systemic mastocytosis 268–70
see also disease burden
systemic mastocytosis (SM) 169, 176–7f, 268
classification 169, 170b
aggressive SM 172
indolent SM 169–71
mast cell leukaemia 172–3
smouldering SM 171
SM with associated haematological neoplasms, 172
well-differentiated SM 173
clinical features 268–70, 269t
mediator symptoms 179–80
diagnostic criteria 169, 170t
diagnostic decision-making 178–9
diagnostic evaluation 174
additional mutations 175–7
imaging studies 177–8
KIT mutation analysis 175–7
serum tryptase level 174–5
disease burden 268–70
assessment 277–9
future directions 187–8
gene mutations 28, 29t
KIT gene structure and mutations 176–7f
MPN-SAF TSS mast cell 276
pathogenesis 33f, 35
quality of life assessment 278
survival and prognostic factors 179
treatment 179–80
anaphylaxis management 180
avapritinib 186
of bone disease 180
cladribine 183
of cutaneous lesions 181
DCC-2618 186
haematopoietic stem cell transplantation 186–7
interferon alpha 182
mast cell activation management 180
perioperative management 181
during pregnancy 181
tyrosine kinase inhibitors 183–6
treatment algorithm 181f
systemic mastocytosis with associated haematologic neoplasm (SM-AHN) 170b, 172
future directions 188
treatment algorithm 181f

T

T3151 mutation 105, 250–2
T-cell clonality analyses, MPN-eo 213
TET (Ten-Eleven-Translocation) proteins 25–6
TET2 mutations 19–20, 25–6, 27, 28, 29t, 37, 88t
and leukaemic transformation 225–8, 227t
murine models, concomitant $JAK2^{V617F}$ 42–3
myelodysplastic/ myeloproliferative overlap neoplasms 194, 195t
CMML 195–7
prognostic significance 89–90
in systemic mastocytosis 175–7
thalidomide
in anaemia 141, 144b
clinical trials 290, 292
third-generation TKIs 106
Thomas, Donald 11
THPO (thrombopoietin) mutations 24–5
thrombocytosis
5q-syndrome 158
chronic myeloid leukaemia 158
diagnosis 157f, 158b
MDS/MPN-RS-T 201–2
in prefibrotic PMF 156–8
reactive 158
refractory anaemia with ringed sideroblasts and marked thrombocytosis 158
see also essential thrombocytosis,
thrombosis 268
abdominal vein 117b
cerebral vein 117b
clinical trials measuring time-to-vascular-event 296–7
in essential thrombocytosis 154–5
in myelofibrosis 132
in polycythaemia vera 115, 117
early-stage disease 59
risk stratification 118
risk stratification 85–6, 118, 154–159
IPSET score 86t
time-to-vascular-event (TTE), as an endpoint in clinical trials 296–7
total body irradiation (TBI), prior to allo-SCT 253–4, 256, 258t
TP53 mutations 27, 29t, 88t, 98–100
and leukaemic transformation 225–7, 227t
myelodysplastic/ myeloproliferative overlap neoplasms 195t
TPSAB1 mutations 173
transformation to AML see leukaemic transformation
transforming growth factor-beta (TGF-β), role in fibrosis 129–30
treatment goals 288–9
treatment response assessment 238–41, 239t
mutation testing 241

triple negativity 91
- essential thrombocytosis 153
- frequency 83*f*
- impact on survival 85–6, 87*f*
- primary myelofibrosis 128

trisomy 8 27, 28, 202
tryptase, serum level 174–5, 210
Turk, W. 6
tyrosine kinase activity, BCR-ABL1 34–5
tyrosine kinase fusion genes 207, 208*f*
- in CEL-NOS 209

tyrosine kinase inhibitors (TKIs) 9–10, 12, 34–5, 94, 238
- adverse effects 107, 108*t*
- discontinuing therapy 110
- dose 74
- first-generation 102–5
- molecular structures 102*f*
- monitoring TKI therapy 101*b*
- pharmacogenetics 71
- pharmacokinetics 71
- resistance to 102–5
  - associated mutations 104*f*
  - mutation testing 241
- second-generation 105
- second-line treatment, prognostic factors 72, 73*t*
- in systemic mastocytosis 183–6
  - dasatinib and nilotinib 183–4
  - imatinib 184
  - masitinib 184
  - midostaurin 184–5, 188
- third-generation 106
- treatment response
  - ELN guidelines 101*t*
  - prognostic significance 100
- trials in mice 39
- *see also* imatinib

U

U2AF1 mutations 28, 29*t*
- myelodysplastic/myeloproliferative overlap neoplasms 195*t*
  - MDS/MPN-RS-T 201
- in systemic mastocytosis 175

UK-PT1 study 159–60
unclassifiable MPN (MPN-U) 46, 51
uniparental disomy (UPD) 19*f*, 19–20, 27
urine studies, systemic mastocytosis 177–8
UTX mutations 28, 29*t*

vaccine therapies, chronic myeloid leukaemia 108–9
Vainchencker, William 22–3
Vaquez, Louis 6
variant translocations (VT) 68–69
vascular endothelial growth factor (VEGF), role in fibrosis 128*f*, 129–30
vascular toxicity, tyrosine kinase inhibitors 107
vasomotor symptoms, essential thrombocytosis 155
Vaughan, J.M. 7
Velpeau, Alfred 2
venesection, polycythaemia vera 118–19
venous thrombosis 154–5
Virchow, Rudolf 4, 5*f*
visual disturbance, essential thrombocytosis 155
vitamin D 180
von Willebrand disease 155
vorinostat 121–2

Ward, H.P. 9
Wasserman, L.R. 6–7, 10–11
well-differentiated systemic mastocytosis (WDSM) 173
white blood cell count, prognostic significance in pre-PMF 52
white blood cells, first descriptions of 2
work, impact of disease burden 271
World Health Organization classification (2016) 16*t*, 46, 81*t*
- diagnostic criteria
- for ET 156, 157*b*
- for PMF 134*b*
- for post-ET MF and post-PV MF 57*t*
- for pre-PMF, PMF, ET, and PV 53*t*
- for PV 117*b*
- impact in classic MPN 46–7
- myelodysplastic/myeloproliferative overlap neoplasms 193*t*
- myeloproliferative neoplasms with eosinophilia 206*t*
- reproducibility of morphological criteria 47–50
  - study details 49*t*, 50*t*

Y

Y chromosome loss 28
- prognostic significance 68–9

Z

ZRSR2 mutations 28, 29*t*
- myelodysplastic/myeloproliferative overlap neoplasms 195*t*
- in systemic mastocytosis 175